Medical Complications of Kidney Transplantation

Medical Complications of Kidney Transplantation

Editor: Rowen Griggs

AMERICAN
MEDICAL PUBLISHERS
www.americanmedicalpublishers.com

AMERICAN
MEDICAL PUBLISHERS
www.americanmedicalpublishers.com

Cataloging-in-publication Data

Medical complications of kidney transplantation / edited by Rowen Griggs.
p. cm.
Includes bibliographical references and index.
ISBN 979-8-88740-248-2
1. Kidneys--Transplantation. 2. Kidneys--Transplantation--Complications.
3. Kidneys--Disease--Complications. 4. Kidneys--Diseases--Treatment.
5. Nephrology. I. Griggs, Rowen.
RD575 .M43 2023
617.461 059 2--dc23

American Medical Publishers,
41 Flatbush Avenue,
1st Floor, New York,
NY 11217, USA

ISBN 979-8-88740-248-2 (Hardback)

Contents

Preface

The kidneys are two bean-shaped organs located below the rib cage. Each kidney is roughly the size of a fist. If the kidneys lose their function, waste products may accumulate and can potentially lead to life-threatening risks. The most frequent reason for requiring a kidney transplant is loss of kidney function, which causes kidney failure or end-stage chronic kidney disease. A kidney transplant is a type of surgery in which a diseased kidney is replaced with a healthy kidney. The kidney can be taken from either a living donor or deceased organ donor. There are some complications associated with kidney transplants, such as infection, temporary kidney failure, blockage of the blood vessels that supply the new kidney, and inappropriate functioning of the newly replaced kidney. After the transplant, medicines should be consumed to convince the immune system to not attack the transplant and accept it. This book contains some path-breaking studies on kidney transplantation. It provides significant information to help develop a good understanding of the medical complications associated with this medical procedure. Researchers and students in this field will be assisted by this book.

This book is the end result of constructive efforts and intensive research done by experts in this field. The aim of this book is to enlighten the readers with recent information in this area of research. The information provided in this profound book would serve as a valuable reference to students and researchers in this field.

At the end, I would like to thank all the authors for devoting their precious time and providing their valuable contribution to this book. I would also like to express my gratitude to my fellow colleagues who encouraged me throughout the process.

Editor

1

Post-Transplant Anaemia

Bhadran Bose and David Mudge
Princess Alexandra Hospital, Brisbane
Australia

1. Introduction

Anaemia, as a complication of end stage kidney disease (ESKD), is well studied (Eschbach and Adamson 1985). Reports indicate that anaemia in this patient population is associated with numerous morbidities, but predominantly cardiovascular complications such as left ventricular hypertrophy and heart failure (Wizemann, Schafer et al. 1993; Harnett, Foley et al. 1995). Contrary to the ample data available regarding anaemia in ESKD population, much less is known about the epidemiology of post-transplant anaemia (PTA), and only few studies have systematically investigated this issue (Saito, Fujiwara et al. 1998; Yorgin, Scandling et al. 2002; Mix, Kazmi et al. 2003; Vanrenterghem, Ponticelli et al. 2003).

A successful renal allograft will correct not only the excretory functions of the kidney but also the endocrine functions (through the restored synthesis of erythropoietin and vitamin D) including the correction of anaemia. However, in the majority of transplant recipients, the renal graft does not function optimally. It is well known that renal excretory functions are not restored completely, but the extent to which renal endocrine functions are restored is only recently becoming better understood. A recent European survey of ten transplant centres revealed a prevalence of PTA as high as 42% (Molnar et al, 2011).

PTA may occur at any time after renal transplantation. Early PTA (from the time of surgery until 3 months post-operatively) is most likely to be related to pre-transplant anaemia of ESKD, the surgery itself, iron deficiency, immunosuppression, inflammation or infection (Miles, Markell et al. 1997; Turkowski-Duhem, Kamar et al. 2005) or some combination of these. Later PTA is more likely to be related to consequences of long-term immunosuppression (particularly anti-metabolite medications) or a failing allograft. All the published large scale studies to date have focused mainly on late PTA (Miles, Markell et al. 1997; Vanrenterghem, Ponticelli et al. 2003; Turkowski-Duhem, Kamar et al. 2005), and there are a lack of studies looking at the management of early PTA, in particular, the optimal management of iron deficiency at the time of kidney transplantation.

The importance of PTA is that it is one of the commonest complications after kidney transplantation, that it is strongly associated with cardiovascular morbidity (the primary cause of death of kidney transplant recipients, accounting for approximately one half of such deaths), and that its optimal treatment, either with iron, erythropoietin, or other agents, has yet to be determined by large-scale randomised controlled trials.

2. Prevalence

PTA remains a common complication after kidney transplantation, with an incidence ranging from nearly 80% at day 0 to as low as 25% at 1 year (Saito, Fujiwara et al. 1998;

Yorgin, Scandling et al. 2002; Mix, Kazmi et al. 2003; Vanrenterghem, Ponticelli et al. 2003). To date, there are very few published studies of PTA, and very few presenting data on interventions for PTA.

One of the largest studies (Vanrenterghem, Ponticelli et al. 2003) was published in the *American Journal of Transplantation*, and included 4,263 kidney transplant patients from 72 centres in 16 European countries (**TR**ansplant **E**uropean **S**urvey on **A**naemia **M**anagement [TRESAM] survey). The patients were divided into four cohorts and assessed at 6 months (n=1003), 1 year (n=960), 3 years (n=1254) and 5 years (n=1046) after kidney transplantation. Recipients of multiple organs, pregnant women and children aged <10 years were excluded from the study.

Demographic data indicate that the patients included in the TRESAM survey were representative of the European transplant population. Approximately 60% of patients were male and 40% were female, and these proportions were similar in the four cohorts. The mean (SD) age of transplant recipients at transplantation was 45.5 (13.1) years, although patients who had received their transplant more recently were significantly (p=0.01) older at transplantation than patients who had received their transplant 5 years ago. The proportion of patients in this survey who had received their kidney from a living donor was relatively low (~10%). The most prevalent underlying kidney disease in the TRESAM survey was chronic glomerulonephritis (29.8-37.0% across the four cohorts). The prevalence of diabetic nephropathy was uncharacteristically low (6.5-7.5%) by contemporary standards. The most frequently occurring co-morbidities were coronary artery disease (13.0-16.1%), hepatitis B/C (9.3-10.8%) and type 2 diabetes mellitus (8.7-10.1%).

Pre-transplant haemoglobin (Hb) concentrations in one study were significantly higher in patients who had received their transplant more recently than in patients who had received their transplant 5 years earlier, suggesting progressive anaemia with time. In that study, the mean Hb concentrations were 11.9 g/dL in the 6 month cohort *vs* 10.8 g/dL in the 5 year cohort (p<0.01; Eschbach and Adamson, 1985)

Anaemia, defined as Hb concentration ≤ 13 g/dL for male patients and ≤ 12 g/dL for female patients, was present in 38.6% of patients overall in this survey, and was equally distributed between the sexes. Of these patients, 11.6% had moderate anaemia (Hb concentration >11 and ≤ 12 g/dL for male patients and >10 and ≤11g/dL for female patients), while 8.5% had severe anaemia (Hb concentrations ≤11g/dL for male patients and ≤10 g/dL for female patients). In patients with a serum creatinine levels >2 mg/dL, 60.1% were considered anaemic, whereas in patients with a serum creatinine level ≤ 2 mg/dL, only 29.0% of patients were considered anaemic (p<0.01). The findings of the TRESAM survey were in agreement with the results published by a contemporary American group (Yorgin, Scandling et al. 2002). The aforementioned 5-year follow up of the TRESAM survey (Molnar et al, 2011) reported similar rates of anaemia at 42% overall, suggesting that the problem is not improving over time despite awareness of the problem.

The group from Boston, MA undertook a retrospective longitudinal cohort study (Mix, Kazmi et al. 2003) to characterise changes in haematocrit (Hct) following kidney transplantation and to identify factors associated with those changes. The study included 240 patients who underwent kidney transplantation in Tufts-New England Medical Centre, Boston, MA. Hct levels were available for 94% of patients at 1-month follow-up and for 95-100% of patients at subsequent follow-up intervals. At the time of transplant surgery, 22% (95% CI 16%, 28%) of the cohort had Hct < 30%. The mean Hct rose from its nadir of 33% (95% CI 27%. 39%), both at the time of transplantation and at 1 month after transplantation, to a peak of 40% (95% CI 34%, 46%) 12 months after transplantation, and declined thereafter. During the first year after transplantation, the proportion of patients with Hct <36% steadily decreased from 76% (95% CI 70%, 82%) at transplantation to 21% (95% CI 15%, 27%) at 12 months after transplantation. The proportion of patients with Hct < 33% declined over a shorter time interval, from 48% (95% CI 42%, 54%) at transplantation to 7% (95% CI 3%, 11%) at 6 months after transplantation. These data closely reflect the European experience as previously described.

3. Risk factors for PTA

In the post-transplant setting anaemia may be contributed to by blood loss, iron deficiency, bone marrow suppression by anti-proliferative agents (mycophenolate, azathioprine), erythropoietin deficiency, and inflammation (Table 1). The relative contributions of these components may be difficult to ascertain in an individual patient and may often be due to a combination of these factors.

Early PTA	Late PTA
Immunosuppressive agents	↓ red cell survival
Surgical blood loss	Immunosuppressive agents
Frequent blood sampling	↓erythrocyte production
Drugs-ACEi/ARB	Low excretory +/- endocrine graft function
Iron deficiency	EPO resistance
Delayed graft function	
Persistent uraemic toxins	

ACEi=Angiotensin converting enzyme inhibitor, ARB=Angiotensin Receptor Blocker.
EPO resistance is defined as the need of ≥300IU/Kg/week.

Table 1. Common risk factors for PTA

3.1 Early PTA

A prospective study (Turkowski-Duhem, Kamar et al. 2005) published in *Transplantation* attempted to identify independent predictors of anaemia at 6 months and 12 months post-transplant. The authors studied 99 patients who had undergone kidney transplantation at Toulouse University Hospital between January 2001 and January 2002. Anaemia as defined by WHO criteria was observed in 38.6% of patients, which is a very similar rate to that found in other published studies from the same era.

Immunosuppressive treatment, particularly with antimetabolite drugs, is one of the most likely contributors to PTA. The purine synthesis inhibitors, azathioprine and mycophenolate mofetil (MMF), are known to cause anaemia (Gossmann, Kachel et al. 1993; de Sevaux, Hilbrands et al. 1998; Kuypers, Claes et al. 2004; Shipkova, Spielbauer et al. 2004). Macrocytosis was present in the majority of the patients in those studies treated with azathioprine. Mammalian target of rapamycin (mTOR) inhibitors (e.g., sirolimus) are also associated with PTA, and particularly with microcytosis even in the absence of iron deficiency (Thaunat, Beaumont et al. 2007). In that study nearly all patient received concomitant MMF and for the 42.3% who received induction therapy with rabbit antithymocyte globulin (ATG), the incidence of PTA was lower than previously reported values, at only 25% at 1 year post-transplantation. This could merely reflect selection bias.

Some recent report suggests that sirolimus-based therapy was an independent factor of PTA (Augustine, Knauss et al. 2004). For example, the prevalence of PTA was 31% with MMF-based immunosuppression and as high as 57% with sirolimus-based immunosuppression. Through mTOR inhibition, sirolimus blocks S6 kinase activity and consequently impairs cell replication in an erythroid cell line (Jaster, Bittorf et al. 1996) leading to anaemia.

One other obvious contributor to post-transplant anaemia is iron deficiency. Iron deficiency, defined by low ferritin and a low transferrin saturation, was present in 17% (Mahmud, Aziz et al. 2002) and 34.6%(Kim, Park et al. 2003) of anaemic patients in the post-transplant setting. Patients coming to kidney transplantation are known to be frequently iron deficient both in absolute and functional terms (Lorenz, Kletzmayr et al. 2002).

Many studies have demonstrated that the occurrence of PTA is related to renal allograft function, with declining function related to worsening anaemia as is seen in the chronic kidney disease (CKD) population. The results of the TRESAM survey showed a strong correlation between Hb levels and graft function expressed as serum creatinine and creatinine clearance: the majority of anaemic patients had creatinine levels > 2 mg/dL (Vanrenterghem, Ponticelli et al. 2003). Turkowski-Duhem found an effect of post-transplant renal function on haemoglobin levels at 6 months. Both delayed graft function (DGF) and renal allograft function, defined by creatinine clearance, were independent factors associated with the occurrence of anaemia at 12 months post transplantation(Turkowski-Duhem, Kamar et al. 2005). In another study it was reported that at both 6 and 12 months post transplantation higher serum creatinine values (defined as each 1 mg/dL increase in serum creatinine level) were significant independent risk factors for anaemia (Shibagaki and Shetty 2004). Similarly, in a further study (Yorgin, Scandling et al. 2002) serum CO_2, blood urea nitrogen (BUN) and creatinine correlated with anaemia at 1 year post transplantation (Yorgin, Scandling et al. 2002). These findings were explained by the decreased production of erythropoietin (Kuypers, Claes et al.) and also the increase in erythropoietin (EPO) resistance relative to the decline in renal excretory function in the early 1990's. (van Dullemen, Luykx-de Bakker et al. 1992).

In the TRESAM survey, transplant recipients who had experienced one or more rejection episodes, or who had received a second or third graft, had lower haemoglobin levels than recipients without rejection episodes or recipients with a first transplant. An analysis using DNA microarrays identified a cluster of genes related to haemoglobin synthesis and/or erythropoiesis that was altered in kidneys with renal allograft rejection compared with normal allograft kidneys (Chua, Barry et al. 2003).

Another factor relevant to early PTA is cytomegalovirus (CMV) infection. Turkowski-Durhem showed on univariate analysis that at 12 months post transplantation, the prevalence of CMV seropositivity was significantly higher in those presenting with anaemia (78%) than in those without anaemia (51%), suggesting CMV infection might be a predisposing factor to PTA. However, on multivariate analysis, CMV status was no longer a significant predictor. . Mix et al. found that positive CMV donor status and negative recipient status (CMV D+/R-) was a factor independently associated with a greater likelihood of PTA, in this case defined as a haematocrit (Hct) <36% at 6 months post transplantation (Mix, Kazmi et al. 2003). These two observations suggest that CMV infection itself, and/or the use of drugs to prevent or treat CMV infection/disease, might result in a degree of bone-marrow suppression leading to PTA.

Angiotensin converting enzyme (ACE) inhibitor therapy is known to induce anaemia (Gossmann, Kachel et al. 1993), and has been used to treat post-transplant erythrocytosis

(Rostaing, Boisseau et al. 1995). The TRESAM survey reported that the use of ACE inhibitors or angiotensin II receptor blockers (ARB's) was associated with a higher odds ratio for anaemia (OR=1.55); they also found that it increased the risk of severe anaemia. Winckelmayer et al. observed that patients taking ACE inhibitors had significantly lower Hct levels compared with patients not taking them. In addition, a significant curvilinear dose-response relationship was found between ACE inhibitor dose and Hct level.
Turkowski-Durhem also observed that the platelet count at day-7 post transplantation was an independent predictive factor for anaemia at both 6 months (OR 0.12 (0.03-0.48); P=0.002) and 12 months (OR 0.096 (0.01 -1.04); P=0.05), i.e. more anaemic patients had a significantly lower platelet count (<200X10^9/L) than non-anaemic patients (72% vs. 38% at 6 months, and 65% vs. 45% at 12 months). The significance of the association with platelet counts at day-7 post transplant, and the occurrence of PTA at 6 and 12 months, persists even after excluding patients that received induction therapy with ATG because the latter can result in thrombocytopenia. There was no explanation given for this observation, although it could just represent a different measure of overall bone marrow suppression
The other causes of early PTA have been attributed to blood loss at the time of surgery, frequent blood sampling and the persistent effect of uraemic toxins.

3.2 Late PTA

PTA that occurs late after transplantation has been attributed to decreased red blood cell survival (Najean, Rain et al. 1997), erythrocyte hypoproduction due to iron deficiency (Teruel, Lamas et al. 1989; Beshara, Birgegard et al. 1997; Miles, Markell et al. 1997), low excretory graft function (Miles, Markell et al. 1997), and immunosuppressive agents (Solheim, Albrechtsen et al. 1987; Yoshimura, Oka et al. 1989; Creemers, van Boven et al. 1993; Zazgornik 1997).
A retrospective longitudinal analysis (Yorgin, Scandling et al. 2002) of adult renal transplant recipients was published in *American Journal of Transplantation* looking at the prevalence, severity and predictors of late PTA. The study population of adults (>18 years) transplanted during 1995 at Stanford University (n=88) and University of North Carolina (n=40) were selected. Post-transplant anaemia was a common problem which affected 30% of the study population at least once during the first 5 years after transplant. Recurrence of PTA was common (50%) and the prevalence and severity of anaemia increased with time after transplantation.
Renal excretory function is strongly correlated with anaemia in adult renal transplant recipients. Yet the effect of renal excretory function on anaemia is not absolute, as a small proportion of anaemic patients have creatinine clearance values > 75 mL/min/1.73 m^2 (i.e. normal), whereas conversely, some non-anaemic patients have creatinine clearance < 50 mL/min 1.73 m^2.(Yorgin, Scandling et al. 2002). A study by van Dullemen et al. demonstrated that EPO production decreases and EPO resistance increases proportionally to the decline in renal excretory function (van Dullemen, Luykx-de Bakker et al. 1992). Other factors not related to declining renal excretory function include DGF, acute tubulointerstitial rejection (Besarab, Caro et al. 1987; Heidenreich, Tepel et al. 1995), chronic rejection (Heidenreich, Tepel et al. 1995) and possibly long-term calcineurin inhibitor toxicity (Jensen, Hansen et al. 1994) may contribute to PTA by leading to diminished EPO production.
Since renal tubular injury may be attributable to DGF, allograft rejection and calcineurin inhibitor toxicity in renal transplant recipients, and that all of these complications are

frequent, another factor which has been evaluated as an important indicator of renal tubular function is serum total CO_2. In one study, Anaemic patients had lower serum total CO_2 values (p=0.019 at 1 year post transplant and p<0.0001 at 5 years post transplant) (Yorgin, Scandling et al. 2002). The authors speculate that the presence of metabolic acidosis is a surrogate indicator of renal tubular injury, diminished renal excretory function and diminished EPO production, however this hypothesis has not been tested.
Yorgin et al also found that few anaemic patients were ever treated with EPO or even iron therapy. This finding may demonstrate a need for increased awareness of anaemia and increased concern about subnormal Hct by the patient's primary nephrologists and transplant physicians.

4. Treatment of PTA

There is a paucity of good quality and large scale intervention trials for PTA in the transplant literature, although some registry studies and multi-centre surveys do shed some light on practice patterns. For example, in the TRESAM survey rates of ESA use were reported. Surprisingly, of the 3969 patients overall for whom the use of erythropoietic therapy was documented, only 207 (5.2%) had received an erythropoietin-stimulating agent (ESA) for the treatment of anaemia. Even more striking was the fact that among the group of anaemic patients (n=1539), only 10% had received an ESA or other specific therapy. Of the 343 patients with severe anaemia, 17.8% were treated with erythropoietic therapy (Fig 1).

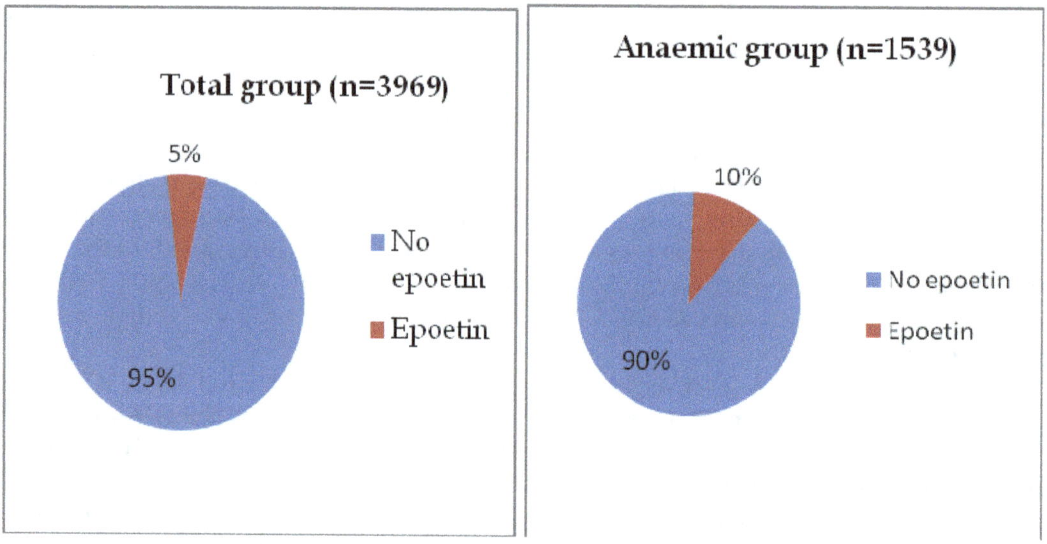

Fig. 1. Epoetin treatment in the TRESAM survey.

Possible reasons for the reluctance of nephrologists to correct anaemia in transplant patients include a relative paucity of published studies on intervention strategies for PTA, an under-recognition of the importance of the problem in terms of contribution to overall cardiovascular risk (also due to lack of specific studies demonstrating this) and finally the "psychological factor" of concerns regarding the efficacy and safety of therapy. In terms of safety of therapy, there have been concerns regarding the normalisation of Hb concentrations with ESA in the CKD population and. A few studies, involving small number of patients, have suggested that transplant recipients treated with epoetin develop hypertension, which requires treatment with anti-hypertensive drugs (Muirhead 1999; Kim, Park et al. 2003). However, to date, there have been no indications that patients treated with erythropoietic therapy after transplantation show a more rapid deterioration of their allograft function(Muirhead 1999).

4.1 Erythropoietin-stimulating agent use

Several small-scale studies suggest that ESA may be an effective treatment for post-transplant anaemia (Traindl, Barnas et al. 1994; Muirhead 1999; Kim, Park et al. 2003). The study done by *Lezaic* (Lezaic, Djukanovic et al. 1995) suggested that the response to erythropoietic therapy of patients with anaemia post-transplant is comparable with that of anaemia due to other forms of renal failure. As EPO resistance is common in these patients, they should be evaluated for secondary or tertiary hyperparathyroidism, hypothyroidism, haemolysis, and GI blood loss if a reticulocyte spike is not detected 7 days post transplantation.

Several recent studies in the CKD literature (Pfeffer et al. 2009, Drueke et al 2006) regarding haemoglobin targets have resulted in concern over the potential for increasing the risk of stroke and possibly malignancy-related death when haemoglobin targets of >13 mg/dL are aimed for. The optimum Hb target for kidney transplant recipients remains unknown. Future trials will need to assess these endpoints in the post-transplant situation in order to establish the safety of ESA in this setting.

4.2 Iron therapy

Replacement of depleted iron stores are necessary for the correction of PTA. Functional iron deficiency is a common problem in CKD populations and may also be a problem in kidney transplant recipients. The best form of iron replacement in this setting is yet to be established. Oral iron is poorly absorbed, often not tolerated, and may interfere with the absorption of immunosuppressants. Intravenous iron has been used to replenish iron stores (Macdougall 1999) in transplant recipients as it has been in CKD patients in order to get around the problems of oral iron supplements. But a study currently in press but whose protocol was recently published (Mudge, Tan et al. 2009) showed that intravenous versus oral iron was not associated with a reduction in PTA, but did lead to a non-significant reduction in gastro-intestinal side-effects, numerically fewer blood transfusions and was equally efficacious in the treatment of post-transplant anaemia.

The measurement of iron status in post-kidney transplant patients, as in CKD patients, remains problematic. Existing measurements include serum iron, ferritin, and transferrin saturation. Ferritin is elevated in the setting of inflammation and therefore may not be indicative. New measures of iron status such as hepcidin show promise for more accurate estimation of iron status in this setting, but as yet a reference range has not been elucidated.

4.3 Other treatments

Other nutritional parameters such as B vitamins (B12, folate etc) are important in the pathogenesis of anaemia, and patients who have been treated with haemodialysis prior to transplantation are at risk of B-group vitamin deficiencies due to the removal of these water soluble vitamins with long-term dialysis, and especially with extended-hours dialysis

(Coveney, 2010). Most such patients would be supplemented with B-group vitamins during their dialysis treatment however.

5. Conclusions

PTA is a common problem in kidney transplant recipients and further studies are needed to better determine the relative contributions of iron deficiency, EPO deficiency, and bone marrow suppression, with a view to better determining the optimum strategy for its correction in individual patients. Anaemia is a risk factor for cardiovascular events and may be a contributor to the high cardiovascular event rate seen in kidney transplant recipients.

6. References

Augustine, J. J., T. C. Knauss, et al. (2004). "Comparative effects of sirolimus and mycophenolate mofetil on erythropoiesis in kidney transplant patients." American journal of transplantation : official journal of the American Society of Transplantation and the American Society of Transplant Surgeons 4(12): 2001-2006.

Besarab, A., J. Caro, et al. (1987). "Dynamics of erythropoiesis following renal transplantation." Kidney international 32(4): 526-536.

Beshara, S., G. Birgegard, et al. (1997). "Assessment of erythropoiesis following renal transplantation." European journal of haematology 58(3): 167-173.

Chua, M. S., C. Barry, et al. (2003). "Molecular profiling of anemia in acute renal allograft rejection using DNA microarrays." American journal of transplantation : official journal of the American Society of Transplantation and the American Society of Transplant Surgeons 3(1): 17-22.

Coveney, N., Polkinghorne, K.R., Linehan, L. et al. (2010). "Water-soluble vitamin levels in extended hors hemodialysis." Hemodialysis International Nov 24. doi: 10.1111/j.1542-4758.2010.00505.x. [Epub ahead of print]

Creemers, G. J., W. P. van Boven, et al. (1993). "Azathioprine-associated pure red cell aplasia." Journal of internal medicine 233(1): 85-87.

de Sevaux, R. G., L. B. Hilbrands, et al. (1998). "A randomised, prospective study on the conversion from cyclosporine-prednisone to cyclosporine-azathioprine at 6 months after renal transplantation." Transplant international : official journal of the European Society for Organ Transplantation 11 Suppl 1: S322-324.

Drueke, T.B. et al (2006). "Normalization of hemoglobin level in patients with chronic kidney disease and anemia." New England Journal of Medicine 355(20): 2071-2084.

Eschbach, J. W. and J. W. Adamson (1985). "Anemia of end-stage renal disease (ESRD)." Kidney international 28(1): 1-5.

Gossmann, J., H. G. Kachel, et al. (1993). "Anemia in renal transplant recipients caused by concomitant therapy with azathioprine and angiotensin-converting enzyme inhibitors." Transplantation 56(3): 585-589.

Harnett, J. D., R. N. Foley, et al. (1995). "Congestive heart failure in dialysis patients: prevalence, incidence, prognosis and risk factors." Kidney international 47(3): 884-890.

Heidenreich, S., M. Tepel, et al. (1995). "Prognostic value of serum erythropoietin levels in late acute rejection of renal transplants." American journal of kidney diseases : the official journal of the National Kidney Foundation 25(5): 775-780.

Jaster, R., T. Bittorf, et al. (1996). "Inhibition of proliferation but not erythroid differentiation of J2E cells by rapamycin." Biochemical pharmacology 51(9): 1181-1185.

Jensen, J. D., H. E. Hansen, et al. (1994). "Increased serum erythropoietin level during azathioprine treatment in renal transplant recipients." Nephron 67(3): 297-301.

Kim, H. C., S. B. Park, et al. (2003). "Anemia following renal transplantation." Transplantation proceedings 35(1): 302-303.

Kuypers, D. R., K. Claes, et al. (2004). "Clinical efficacy and toxicity profile of tacrolimus and mycophenolic acid in relation to combined long-term pharmacokinetics in de novo renal allograft recipients." Clinical pharmacology and therapeutics 75(5): 434-447.

Lezaic, V., L. Djukanovic, et al. (1995). "Recombinant human erythropoietin treatment of anemia in renal transplant patients." Renal failure 17(6): 705-714.

Lorenz, M., J. Kletzmayr, et al. (2002). "Anemia and iron deficiencies among long-term renal transplant recipients." Journal of the American Society of Nephrology : JASN 13(3): 794-797.

Macdougall, I. C. (1999). "Strategies for iron supplementation: oral versus intravenous." Kidney international. Supplement 69: S61-66.

Mahmud, S. N., R. Aziz, et al. (2002). "Anemia characteristics after renal transplantation." Transplantation proceedings 34(6): 2428.

Miles, A. M., M. S. Markell, et al. (1997). "Anemia following renal transplantation: erythropoietin response and iron deficiency." Clinical transplantation 11(4): 313-315.

Mix, T. C., W. Kazmi, et al. (2003). "Anemia: a continuing problem following kidney transplantation." American journal of transplantation : official journal of the American Society of Transplantation and the American Society of Transplant Surgeons 3(11): 1426-1433.

Mudge, D. W., K. S. Tan, et al. (2009). "Intravenous versus oral iron supplementation for correction of post-transplant anaemia in renal transplant patients." BMC nephrology 10: 14.

Muirhead, N. (1999). "Erythropoietin and renal transplantation." Kidney international. Supplement 69: S86-92.

Najean, Y., J. D. Rain, et al. (1997). "Red cell and platelet kinetics in chronic cytopenias following transplantation." Hematology and cell therapy 39(5): 233-236.

Pfeffer, M.A., Burdmann, M.D., Chen, C.Y., et al. (2009). "A trial of darbepoetin alfa in type 2 diabetes and chronic kidney disease" New England Journal of Medicine 361(21): 2019-32

Rostaing, L., M. Boisseau, et al. (1995). "Correction of post-renal transplant erythrocytosis by enalapril." Scandinavian journal of urology and nephrology 29(4): 399-406.

Saito, S., T. Fujiwara, et al. (1998). "Anemia following renal transplantation." Transplantation proceedings 30(7): 3025-3026.

Shibagaki, Y. and A. Shetty (2004). "Anaemia is common after kidney transplantation, especially among African Americans." Nephrology, dialysis, transplantation : official publication of the European Dialysis and Transplant Association - European Renal Association 19(9): 2368-2373.

Shipkova, M., B. Spielbauer, et al. (2004). "cDNA microarray analysis reveals new candidate genes possibly linked to side effects under mycophenolate mofetil therapy." Transplantation 78(8): 1145-1152.

Solheim, B. G., D. A. Albrechtsen, et al. (1987). "Hemolytic anemia in cyclosporine-treated recipients of kidney or heart grafts from donors with minor incompatibility for ABO antigens." Transplantation proceedings 19(5): 4236-4238.

Teruel, J. L., S. Lamas, et al. (1989). "Serum ferritin levels after renal transplantation: a prospective study." Nephron 51(4): 462-465.

Thaunat, O., C. Beaumont, et al. (2007). "Late introduction of sirolimus induces anemia in renal transplant recipients." Transplantation 83(9): 1283; author reply 1284.

Traindl, O., U. Barnas, et al. (1994). "Recombinant human erythropoietin in renal transplant recipients with renal anemia." Clinical transplantation 8(1): 45-48.

Turkowski-Duhem, A., N. Kamar, et al. (2005). "Predictive factors of anemia within the first year post renal transplant." Transplantation 80(7): 903-909.

van Dullemen, H. M., S. Luykx-de Bakker, et al. (1992). "Inhibitors of recombinant human erythropoietin in chronic renal failure." The Netherlands journal of medicine 41(1-2): 56-63.

Vanrenterghem, Y., C. Ponticelli, et al. (2003). "Prevalence and management of anemia in renal transplant recipients: a European survey." American journal of transplantation : official journal of the American Society of Transplantation and the American Society of Transplant Surgeons 3(7): 835-845.

Wizemann, V., R. Schafer, et al. (1993). "Follow-up of cardiac changes induced by anemia compensation in normotensive hemodialysis patients with left-ventricular hypertrophy." Nephron 64(2): 202-206.

Yorgin, P. D., J. D. Scandling, et al. (2002). "Late post-transplant anemia in adult renal transplant recipients. An under-recognized problem?" American journal of transplantation : official journal of the American Society of Transplantation and the American Society of Transplant Surgeons 2(5): 429-435.

Yoshimura, N., T. Oka, et al. (1989). "Cyclosporine-associated microangiopathic hemolytic anemia in a renal transplant recipient." The Japanese journal of surgery 19(2): 223-228.

Zazgornik, J. (1997). "Azathioprine induced macrocytosis and red cell aplasia in renal transplant patients." Nephrology, dialysis, transplantation : official publication of the European Dialysis and Transplant Association - European Renal Association 12(3): 628.

2

Antibody-Mediated Kidney Allograft Rejection

Xu Haiyan and He Xiaozhou
Third Affiliated Hospital of Soochow University, Changzhou, China

1. Introduction

Successful kidney transplantation improves the quality of life and increases survival when compared with long-term dialysis. Renal transplantation is now a well established and the preferred treatment for most patients with end-stage renal disease (ESRD). In recent years, the short-term effects of kidney transplantation have been greatly achieved due to the improvement in immunosuppression medicines, better genotyping technology and monitoring methods. However, the long-term outcome of kidney transplantation has not been improved for long period. Among the various influencing factors, antibody-mediated kidney allograft rejection is now widely recognized as a major problem which decreases the long-term outcome. How many kinds of antibodies involved in the antibody-mediated rejection (AMR)? How do these antibodies produce? How do these antibodies injure the transplantated kidney function? How to eliminate these antibodies? How about the clinical effects when the new agents were applied? All these questions are being gradually and deeply studied.

2. Anti-HLA and MHC-class I related chain A antibody

At present, anti-HLA antibody (Lefaucheur et al., 2010) and anti-MHC-class I related chain Antibody (Zou et al., 2009) are the main cytotoxic antibodies, resulting in kidney allograft rejection and long-term kidney allograft survival.

2.1 Anti-HLA antibody

HLA (the human leukocyte antigen system) is the name of the major histocompatibilty complex (MHC) in humans. MHC molecules are divided into 2 main classes: HLA class I antigens (HLA-A, -B, and –C), presented on the surface of all nucleated cells and platelets; and HLA class II antigens (HLA-DR, -DQ, -DP, -DM and –DO), expressed on professional antigen-presenting cells, but also on the surface of vascular endothelial cells and renal tubular epithelial cells. There lie high polymorphism degree of the HLA system (more than 1600 alleles), so the individuals do not present identical sets of HLA antigens. After solid organ transplantation, HLA polymorphism confers immunological identity to the recipients, thus, the immune system can distinguish between self and non-self, and non-self may represent targets for the immune system. T cellular-mediated rejection (TCMR) and/or AMR will be initiated. As for AMR, donor specific anti-HLA antigens -I and -II alloantibodies would be produced.

The presence of alloantibodies against donor HLA-I and HLA-II antigens has been associated with hyperacute and accelarated graft rejection. Since HLA typing is strictly requested before renal transplantation (RTx), whatever cadaveric RTx, or living related or non-related RTx, the incidence of hyperacute and accelarated graft rejection have been greatly decreased.
However, some evidences suggest that donor specific antibody (DSA) is common in RTx recipients after 1 year of operation, which may be explained by the HLA polymorphism.

2.2 Anti-MHC-class I related chain A antibody (MICA)

MHC-class I related chain (MIC) has been reported to be an important polymorphic alloantigen system, consisting of MICA and MICB, and distributing on the peripheral blood lymphocytes, tissue endotheliocytes, and umbilical endotheliocytes, which also play a role in renal allograft rejection. Specific anti-MICA antibody can be found in sera of transplanted patients with allograft rejection (Zou et al, 2007). And the statistical analysis indicated that, anti-MICA antibodies were associated with the failure of a renal graft, regardless of good HLA typying (0 or 1 HLA mis matched) and PRA =0.
One report showed that, despite negative pretransplantation T- and B- lymphocyte flow cytometric crossmatches and blood group identity, two cases of hyperacute humoral rejection of living related kidney grafts happened (Grandtnerova et al, 2008). Retrospectively, antiendothelial IgG antibodies were detected on a panel of umbilical cord cells in the first case, and IgM antibodies against donor endothelial precursor cells were detected using a new endotheilal cell crossmatch kit in the second case. Standard crossmatch methods using donor lymphocytes failed to detect these pathogenic antibodies and did not predict the danger of hyperacute rejection.
Now, MIC typying is still not carried out in clinic. Were the antiendothelial IgG and IgM antibody all belonging to anti-MICA antibody? This question may be worth investigating.

2.3 Subtypes of alloantibodies

IgM-alloantibody and IgG-alloantibody are all common in the peripheral blood and intragraft of recipients, and they are all involved in kidney allograft rejection.
IgM antibodies against donor HLA antigens can be found before transplantation and also produced both early and late in the post-transplant course. IgM antibodies against donor HLA appear to be associated with decreased survival of kidney and heart allografts.
IgG1/IgG3 and IgM can specially bind to alloantigens, activate complement system, and play their immunological action. While IgG2 only weakly activate complement system, and IgG4 does not activate complement system. IgG1/IgG3 and IgM probably participate in AMR by this pathway.
This viewpoint is concordant to the observed evidence. For example, three cases of successful living donor kidney transplantation, showed strongly positive B lymphocyte flow cytometry owing to highly reactive DSA directed to HLA II antigens. IgG solid-phase subtypes analysis suggested that, more than 50% of these antibodies were represented by non-complement binding IgG2/IgG4 subtypes (Lobashevsky et al., 2010).
Now, new technologies are quickly developed. Some new methods based on solid phase multiplex platforms, such as ELISA, flow cytometry and luminex, have been applied in clinic. These methods can detect binding of serum antibodies to specific antigens independently of complement activation. And, using additional anti-IgM/IgG antibodies,

these new technologies can distinguish between IgM and IgG anti-HLA antibodies. Additionally, it can discriminate between HLA class I and class II antibodies, and more, single antigen methods allow identification of a unique HLA specificity.
With the help of development in detection technology, clinician can obtain more precise information and make rational decision.

2.4 Potential mechanism

After these antibodies are produced, they will attack their targets represented by the graft endothelial cells, complement system would be activated, coagulation cascade happened and other inflammation factors would be produced. This procedure may be the most classical procedure of AMR.
The microcirculation characteristic of microcirculation changes of AMR include of:
(1) Microcirculation inflammation (glomerulitis (g), peritubular capillaritis (ptc))(Einecke et al., 2009); (2) Microcirculation deterioration (transplant glomerulopathy (cg), medangial matrix increase (mm)); (3) Peritubular capillary basement membrane multilayering (ptcm-score) ; (4) Diffuse C4d positivity.
A key element in the pathology of AMR is capillaritis, which is associated with glomerulitis and anti-HLA antibodies. Over time it seems likely that capillaritis will induce peritubular capillary basement membrane multilayering as a time dependent feature of late AMR.

3. Antibody-producing cells

3.1 Characterization of intra-graft B cells

During renal allograft rejection, cluster-forming $CD20^+$ B cells in the rejected graft are likely derived from the recipient and composed of mature B cells. These cells are activated ($CD79a^+$), some of them contain memory B cells ($CD27^+$) and do not correlate with intra-graft C4d deposition or with donor-specific antibody detection.
Furthermore, several non-cluster forming $CD20^-$ B-lineage $CD38^+$ plasmablasts and plasma cells infiltrate in the rejected grafts and these cells strongly correlated with circulating donor-specific antibody, and to a lesser extent with intra-graft C4d.
Both $CD20^+$ B cells and $CD38^+$ cells correlated with poor response of the rejection to steroids. Reduced graft survival is associated with the presence of CD20 cells in the graft.
And, a specific subset of early lineage B cells appears to be antigen-presenting cells and which may support a steroid-resistant T-cell-mediated cellular rejection when these cells present in the rejected graft. Late lineage interstitial plasmablasts and plasma cells may also support AMR. These studies suggest that detailed analysis of interstitial cellular infiltrates may allow better use of B-cell lineage specific treatments to improve graft outcomes.

3.2 Plasma cells and memory B cells

Now the exact cellular mechanisms responsible for AMR are still not known. It seems likely that both pre-existing plasma cells and the conversion of memory B cells to new plasma cells play a role in the increased DSA production (Stegall et al., 2010).
There indeed normally exists very little amount of long-lived plasma cells, but they may not be able to produce enough pathological alloantibodies to injury the kidney allograft. Plasma cells, DSA and C4d are associated with each other in renal transplants developing chronic rejection by sequential graft biopsies detection. Bone-marrow-derived long-lived plasma

cells appear to be a major source of donor-specific alloantibody in sensitized renal transplant recipients. Memory B cells appear to be important in early acute AMR, but few basic have been performed.

3.3 Potential survival factor: BAFF

Some factors may survive the plasma cells or enhance the production of pathological alloantibodies. B cell activating factor belonging to TNF superfamily (BAFF) may be one of the most potential survival factors. BAFF is also termed Blys, TALL-1, zTNF4, THANK and TNFSF13b, is a nomotrimer, member of the TNF superfamilies, expressed on the cell surface or cleaved and secreted. BAFF specifically binds to BAFF receptor (BAFF-R, also known as BR3 (Thompson, et al., 2001)), and BAFF can also bind to other two receptors, transmembrane activator and calcium-modulator and cyclophilin ligand interactor (TACI) and B-cell maturation antigen (BCMA), shared with another TNF ligand, a proliferation-inducing ligand (APRIL) (Day, et al., 2005).

BAFF is expressed by monocyte-derived cells, such as monocytes, macrophages, dendritic cells, and activated T lymphocytes, which plays an important role in immune response (Mackay, F. and Schneider, P. 2009). The discovery of BAFF has shed new light on the importance of finely tuned B cell survival for B cell tolerance during B cell maturation and activation. Excessive production of BAFF is associated with the development of autoimmune diseases, because transgenic (Tg) mice that overproduce BAFF develop severe autoimmune disorders resemble systemic lupus erythematosus (SLE) and Sjogren's syndrome (SS) in humans, possibly as a result of improper B cell survival, predominantly affecting the maturing splenic transitional type 2 (T2) and the marginal zone (MZ) B cell populations. BAFF-induced autoimmunity in BAFF Tg mice appears to be highly dependent on B cells and possibly the production of autoantibodies. High levels of BAFF have been found in the blood of patients with autoimmune diseases, particularly SLE and SS. And BAFF is also found on T lymphocytes infiltrating labial salivary glands from patients with SS.

3.3.1 BAFF and rituximab

Rituximab can specially delete $CD20^+$ B lymphocytes, gradually applied to induce immunosuppression state at present. The impact of rituximab therapy on tertiary lymphoid organs associate with chronic active antibody-mediated rejection, a prototypic humoral chronic inflammatory condition. In certain patients, inflammatory microenvironment provides BAFF-dependent paracrine survival signal to B-cells in tertiary lymphoid organs, allowing them to escape rituximab-induced apoptosis, thereby thwarting therapeutic efficiency (Thaunat et al. 2008).

3.3.2 BAFF and alemtuzumab

BAFF is increased in renal transplant patients following treatment with alemtuzumab (Bloom et al. 2009). Alemtuzumab is an anti-CD52 monoclonal antibody that can deplete T and B cells and is used as induction therapy for renal transplant recipients. However without long-term calcineurin inhibitor (CNI) therapy, alemtuzumab-treated patients have a prospensity to develop alloantibody and may undergo AMR.

These data suggest associations between BAFF signal and AMR in alemtuzumab-treated patients.

3.3.3 BAFF and renal transplantation

In view of special bioactivity of BAFF, experiments have been carried through to explore the expression characteristic of BAFF and its potential bioactivity in renal allograft rejection, and some significant results were obtained.

3.3.3.1 BAFF expression and serum PRA

The FACS (Fluorescence Activated Cell Sorter) results indicated that, cell surface BAFF was abnormally highly expressed on peripheral T lymphocytes of some kidney transplant recipients, especially in those recipients for more than 5 years (Fig.1).

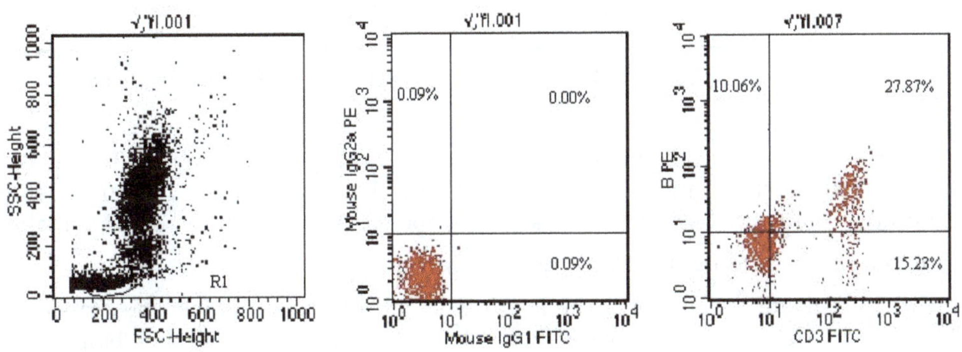

Fig. 1. BAFF expression on CD3+ T lymphocytes in RTx recipients after 5 yrs' operation

The real-time PCR (Polymerase Chain Reaction) results showed that BAFF mRNA levels gradually increased along with the prolonged transplantation time, and BAFF mRNA levels were consistent with BAFF protein levels in different groups (Fig.2).

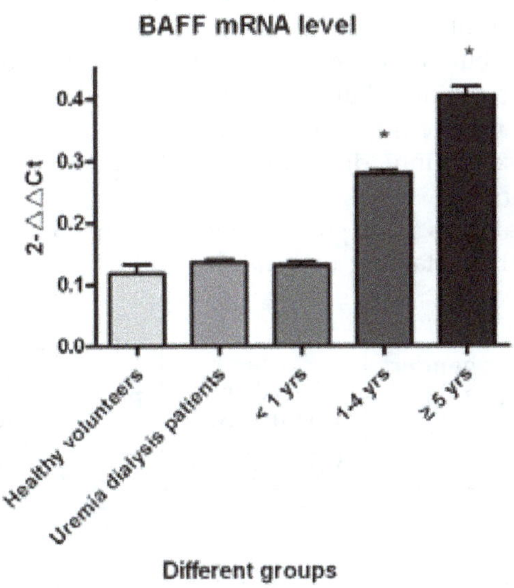

Fig. 2. BAFF mRNA levels in peripheral blood monocytes of RTx recipients after operation with different periods (<1 yr, 1-4 yr and ≥5 yr)

Healthy volunteers and uremia dialysis patients as controls
To investigate the correlation of transplanted renal function and BAFF expression, transplanted renal function was stratified and these data were statistically analyzed. In abnormal renal function group, BAFF was abnormally highly expressed on peripheral T lymphocytes, and the expression level was about as high as that in ≥ 5 years group. And there was statistically significant association between anti-HLA I & II antibodies level and BAFF expression level (Tab.1).

	anti-HLA I & II antibodies	
CD257	Person Correlation	.587**
	Sig (2-tailed)	.008

Table 1. The correlation analysis of BAFF expression and serum PRA (panel reactive antibody)

The results indicated that BAFF expression was correlated with gradually decreasing transplant renal function, and BAFF may be involved in immune regulating network of kidney transplantation, which was the first report about BAFF and kidney transplantation.

3.3.3.2 BAFF and its receptors in the allograft rejection tissues

To further investigate the role of BAFF in AMR in renal transplantation, the correlation of BAFF and C4d deposition in excised transplanted kidney and protocol biopsies were investigated. The results showed that, BAFF could not only be found in renal allograft tissues, including AR and IF/TA (Interstitial Fibrosis/Tubular Atrophy) tissues, but also was highly expressed in these allograft sections, compared to protocol biopsy sections. BAFF can regulate the development of transitional B lymphocytes and survival of plasmacytoid lymphocytes, which implies that the BAFF signal may participate in AMR. To test this presumption, C4d and IgG were also detected in these allograft sections by immunohistochemistry. The results showed that BAFF expression significantly correlated with C4d deposition. The intensity and percentage score of BAFF were similar to those of C4d. BAFF mainly distributed in the perinephric tubular epithelial cell cytoplasm and cytomembrane, similar to the distribution of C4d. There was IgG deposition in BAFF high-expression sections, but its intensity and percentage score were much weaker than BAFF. IgG deposition was also mainly distributed in the perinephric tubular epithelial cell cytoplasm and cytomembrane.
The patients' clinical materials were shown in Tab.2. And the representative examples of immunohistochemical (IHC) staining of BAFF and C4d in renal allograft rejection tissues were listed in Fig. 3.

groups		**gender** Male/ female	**Age (year) (means±SD)**	**PRA(%)**	**HLA-DR non-matched level**	**POD(day, means±SD)**
Graft failure	AR(n=10)	6/4	39±10 (19~58)	17±4.1	0.8±0.6 (0~2)	9±8
	UAC(n=9)	4/5	42±8 (32~56)	5±4.2	0.7±0.7 (0~2)	1875±784
Graft normal	Protocol renal biopies (n=10)	7/3	37±5 (26~48)	7.4±3.5	0.7±0.7 (0~2)	17±4

Table 2. All the accepted patients' clinical materials

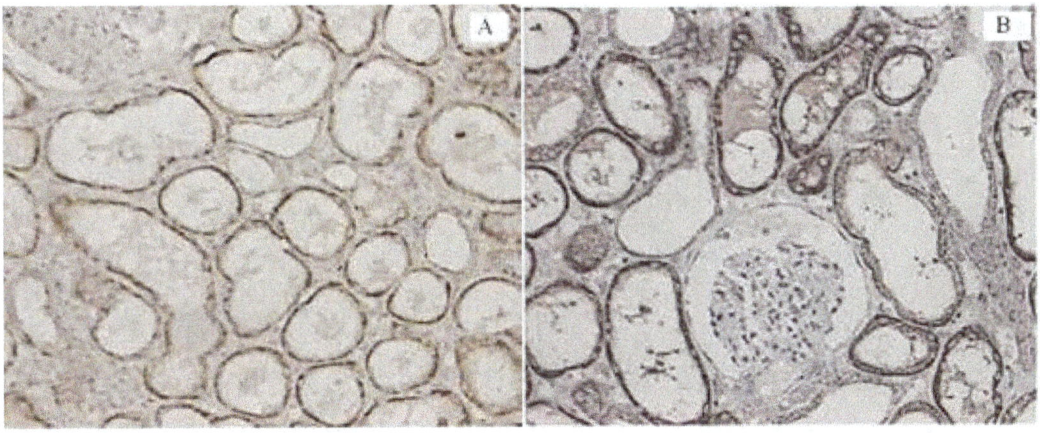

Fig. 3. Representative examples of immunohistochemical staining of BAFF and C4d in renal allograft rejection (original mannification 200X).Positive staining was observed as a dark brown color. Renal allograft rejection tissues showed strong expression of C4d (A) and BAFF (B).

We performed further study by IHC to investigate the receptors of BAFF involved in the renal allograft rejection. The TACI, BCMA and BAFF-R (BAFF receptor, BR3) were all detected. And the APRIL, much high homogenicity with BAFF, was also done. Meanwhile, the plasma cell marker CD138 was also investigated.

The obtained data showed that, high immunogenicity of BAFF, APRIL and their receptors, TACI, BCMA and BAFF-R, and CD138 can be found in renal allograft rejection tissues (including of acute and chronic rejection) (Fig.4), while these molecules all have low immunogenicity in other etiological tissue (excluding of acute and chronic rejection).

All data were analyzed according to C4d expression. In C4d negative group, BAFF, BAFF-R, BCMA and CD138 were all low immunogenicity, while APRIL and TACI have high immunogenicity. In C4d positive group, BAFF, BAFF-R, BCMA, APRIL, TACI and CD138 were all high immunogenicity. The statistical analysis suggested that, the expression of BAFF, BAFF-R, BCMA and CD138 significantly correlated with C4d deposition (Fig.5). These results suggest that BAFF signal may participate in AMR, and APRIL signal may simultaneously participate in cell-mediated and antibody-mediated rejection.

4. Diagnosis of AMR

4.1 Diagnosis of acute AMR

AMR may occur early or late, may be acute or chronic and is associated with poor renal allograft function and survival. According to the speed of rejection, three AMR conditions are now recognized: hyperacute, subacute and chronic AMR.

The following items are required in diagnosis of acute AMR:

1. Histopathological evidence of either acute tubular injury (with no other identifiable cause for it), glomerulitis, endothelitis or capillaritis with neutrophil or mononuclear cell infiltratem capillary thrombosis;
2. Serologica evidence of circulating antibodies;
3. Diffuse C4d positivity in peritubular capillaries (PTC).

These diagnosis criteria are based on Banff 2005 guidelines, in which, C4d deposition in the peritubular capilary (PTC) is considered as the mark of AMR.

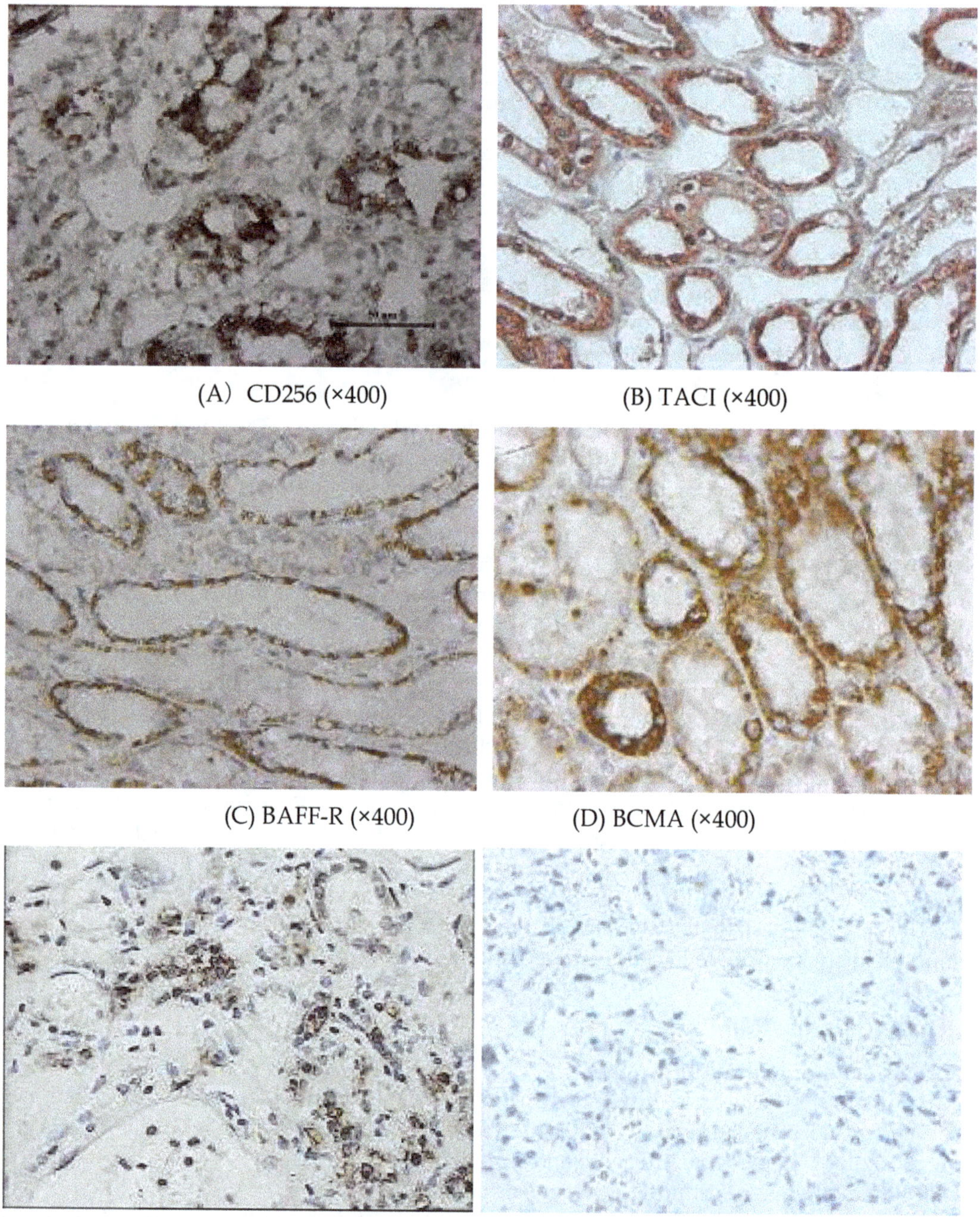

(A) CD256 (×400)

(B) TACI (×400)

(C) BAFF-R (×400)

(D) BCMA (×400)

(E) CD138 (×400)

(F) IgG isotype (×400)

Fig. 4. The representative IHC staining results of APRIL, TACI, BAFF-R, BCMA and CD138 were listed (×400). The APRIL, BAFF-R,BCMA and CD138 signal were developed with 3,3'-diaminobenzidine tetrahydrochloride (DAB), the dark brown particles were the positive signal. And TACI signal was developed with 3-amino-9-ethycarbozole (AEC), the red particle was the positive signal. (F): the IgG isotype of the used antibodies.

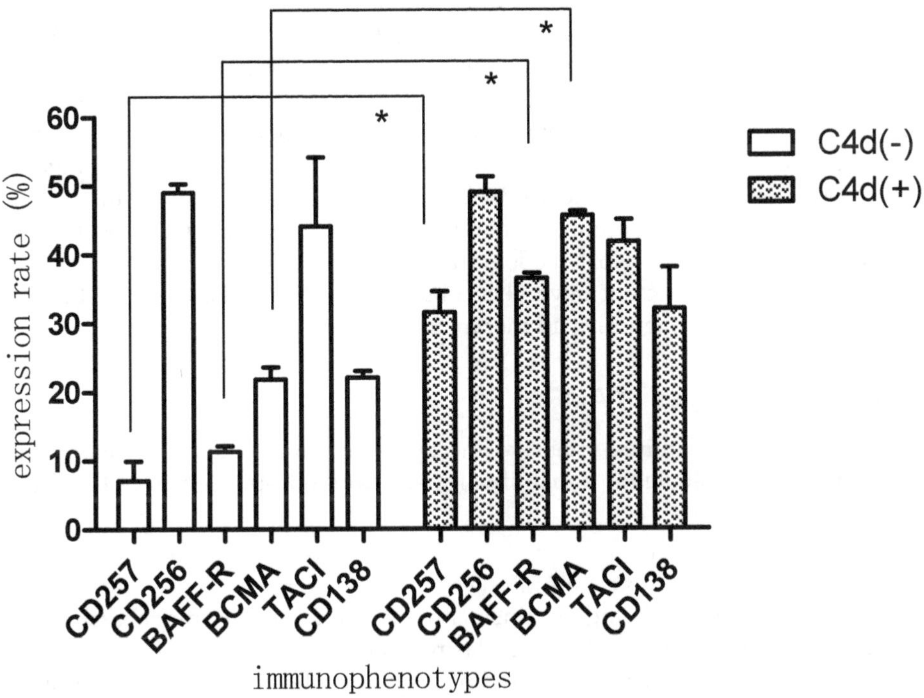

Fig. 5. All data was analyzed according to C4d immunoreactivity, C4d(-) represented C4d negative group and C4d(+) represented C4d positive group. There were significant difference of the expression rate of BAFF, BAFF-R and BCMA between C4d(-) group and C4d(+) group. $P<0.05$ was considered as statistical significance. * $P<0.05$.

4.2 Suspicious for AMR

However, C4d staining is found to be not completely useful in diagnosis of AMR with the advancement of knowledge about AMR. For example, C4d staining in post-reperfusion renal biopsy is not useful for the early detection of AMR when CDC crossmatching is negative (David-Neto et al., 2010). In ABO-incompatible transplant cases, AMR is difficult to be diagnosed by C4d analysis.

Banff 09 meeting discussed several aspects of solid organ transplants with a special focus on antibody mediated graft injury, and revised the diagnosis indexes.

Because C4d may not be sensitive in the diagnosis of AMR: many cases of transplant glomerulopathy with anti-HLA are C4d negative (Sis et al., 2009). Therefore, the recent update of the Banff classification introduced the diagnostic category "**suspicious for AMR**" if C4d (in the presence of antibody) or alloantibody (in the presence of C4d) cannot be demonstrated but morphologic evidence of antibody-mediated tissue injury is present. Moreover, in microarray studies, expression of endothelial transcripts was increased in biopsies with DSA and associated with graft loss even in C4d negative biopsies.

4.3 Remained questions

The risk for graft loss is not captured well by the current Banff diagnoses because many cases with AMR features (anti-HLA and microcirculation changes) were C4d negative and thus given other diagnosis. However, when AMR is redefined as the presence of HLA antibody and microcirculation changes, regardless of C4d status, it is the most frequent phenotype associated with subsequent graft loss. In contrast, nonspecific scarring (IFTA), calcineurin inhibitor toxicity and TCMR are rare diagnosis in grafts that subsequently failured. Thus, antibody-mediated microcirculation injury accounts for the majority of kidneys presenting with indications for biopsy and subsequently failing, but many cases are C4d negative.

Subclinical AMR seems to be complicated by a substantial proportion of positive-crossmatch transplantations even in the absence of allograft dysfunction, and may result in chronic histological abnormalities and shorten allograft function (Loupy et al., 2009).

So, although much advancement have been obtained in diagnosis, there is still absent of specific marker to aid the diagnosis and therapeutic of AMR.

5. Therapeutic strategies of AMR

Once AMR happen, it requires intensive therapy, but no standard treatment has been established now. To eliminate the alloantibodies and antibody-producing cells are the main strategy of AMR treatment.

5.1 Therapeutic strategies of acute AMR

Now, several strategies are being routinely applied, such as plasmapheresis, high-dose intravenous immunoglobulin (IVIG) and plasmapheresis (PP) with low-dose IVIG. Some new interventions have been applied in clinic, such as the use of rituximab (anti-CD20 chimeric antibody)(Rodriguez et al. 2010; Takagi et al., 2010), bortezomib (a proteasome inhibitor-mediated plasma cell depletion)(Raghavan et al. 2010; Walsh et al., 2010), and eculizumab (recombinant human C5-inhibitor)(Lonze et al., 2010; Tillou et al.,2010), for preventing acute AMR. These methods are promising therapeutic avenues currently under investigation.

IVIG has many ideal advantages as a therapy for AMR.

1. It can down regulate B-cell activation and antibody production.
2. It can induce anti-inflammatory cytokines and contain blocking antiidiotyic antibodies to anti-HLA antibodies;
3. IVIG has the unique ability to block complement-mediated injury through inhibition of C3 activation.

Rituximab (anti-CD20 chimeric antibody) can deplete B cells and interfere with antigen-presenting cell (APC) activity of B cells subsequently decreasing T-cell activation,

Bortezomib is one kind of proteasome inhibitors. The preliminary results indicate that bortezomib therapy provides effective reduction in DSA levels with long-term suppression in transplant recipients.

Bortezomib therapy's advantages:

1. It provides effective treatment of AMR and TCR with minimal toxicity.
2. It provides sustained reduction in iDSA and non-iDSA levels.

While, other center reported that, Bortezomib treatment did not significantly decrease DSA within the 150-day posttreatment period in any patient; lack of efficacy on long-lived plasma cells. So, one cycle of bortezomib alone does not decrease DSA levels in sensitized kidney transplant recipients in the time period studied. These results underscore the need to evaluate this new desensitization agent properly in prospective, randomized and well-controlled studies (Sberro-Soussan et al., 2010).

5.2 Therapeutic strategies of subacute and chronic AMR

Now, there seems to have not any good methods to treatment the subacute and chronic AMR. Although subacute and chronic AMR are not immediately result in the graft loss, they cause chronic histological injury and shorten allograft function. Many evidences have suggested that AMR is the important factor influencing the long-term of kidney allograft. Thus, great efforts are still needed to resolve this problem.

6. Conclusion

In summary, recent advances in the diagnosis and treatment of AMR has allowed for significant improvements in the outcome of a condition usually associated with rapid graft failure. However, much work needs to be done to better understand the immunologic processes leading to AMR and how current therapies can be best used to effectively prevent and treat it.

7. References

Bloom, D.; Chang, Z.; Pauly, K.; et al. (2009) BAFF is increased in renal transplant patients following treatment with alemtuzumab. *Am J Transplant*. Vol. 9(8):1835-45.

David-Neto, E.; David, DS.; Ginani, GF.; et al. (2010) C4d staining in post-reperfusion renal biopsy is not useful for the early detection of antibody-mediated rejection when CDC crossmatching is negative. *Nephrol Dial Transplant*. 2010, Vol 26(4):1388-92.

Day, ES.; Cachero, TG.; Qian, F.; et al. (2005) Selectivity of BAFF/Blys and APRIL for binding to the TNF family receptors BAFFR/BR3 and BCMA. *Biochemistry*. Vol.44(6):1919-31.

Einecke, G.; Sis, B.; Reeve, J.; et al. (2009) Antibody-mediated microcirculation injury is the major cause of late kidney transplant failure. *Am J Transplant*. Vol.9(11):2520-31.

Lefaucheur, C.; Loupy, A.; Hill, GS.; et al. (2010) Preexisting donor-specific HLA antibodies predict outcome in kidney transplantation. *J Am Soc Nephrol*. Vol.21(8):1398-406.

Lonze, BE.; Dagher, NN.; Simpkins, CE.; et al. (2010) Eculizumab, bortezomib and kidney paired donation facilitate transplantation of a highly sensitized patient without vascular access. *Am J Transplant*. Vol.10(9): 2154-60.

Lobashevsky, A.; Rosner, K.; Goggins, W.; et al. (2010) Subtypes of immunoglobulins (Ig)-G antibodies against donor class II HLA and cross-match results in three kidney transplant candidates. *Transpl Immunol*. Vol.23(1-2):81-5.

Loupy, A.; Suberbielle-Boissel, C.; Hill, GS.; et al. (2009) Outcome of subclinical antibody-mediated rejection in kidney transplant recipients with preformed donor-specific antibodies. *Am J Transplant*. Vol.9(11): 2561-70.

Mackay, F. and Schneider, P. (2009) Cracking the BAFF code. *Nature Reviews / Immunology*. Vol 9:491-502.

Rodriguez, F.; Rincon, A.; Bucalo, L.; et al. (2010) Treatment of acute antibody-mediated rejection: a single-center experience. *Transplant Proc*. Vol.42: 2848-50.

Raghavan, R.; Jeroudi, A.; Achkar, K.; et al. (2010) Bortizomib in kidney transplantation. *J Transplant*. 2010.pii:698594.

Sherro-Soussan, R.; Zuber, J.; Suberbielle-Boissel, C.; et al. (2010) Bortezomib as the sole post-renal transplantation desensitization agent does not decrease donor-specific anti-HLA antibodies. *Am J Transplant*. Vol.10(3):681-6.

Sis, B.; Jhangri, GS.; Bunnag, S.; et al. (2009) Endothelial gene expression in kidney transplants with alloantibody indicates antibody-mediated damage despite lack of C4d staining. *Am J Transplant.* Vol.9(10):2312-23.

Stegall, MD.; Gloor, JM. ((2010) Decipering antibody-mediated rejection: new insights into mechanisms and treatment. *Curr Opin Organ Transplant.* Vol.15(1):8-10.

Takagi, T.; Ishida, H.; Shirakawa, H.; et al. (2010) Evaluation of low-dose rituximab induction therapy in living related kidney transplantation. *Transplantation.* Vol.89(12):1466-70.

Thaunat, O.; Patey, N.; Gautreau, C. et al. (2008) B cell survival in intragraft tertiary lymphoid organs after rituximab therapy. *Transplantation.* Vol. 85(11): 1648-53.

Thompson, JS.; Biller, SA.; Qian, F.; et al. (2001) BAFF-R, a newly identified TNF receptor that specially interacts with BAFF. *Science.* Vol.293(5537):2108-11.

Tillou, X.; Poirier, N.; Le Bas-Bernardet, S.; et al. (2010) Recombinant human C1-inhibitor prevents acute antibody-mediated rejection in alloimmunized baboons. *Kidney Int.* Vol.78(2):152-9.

Walsh, RC.; Everly, JJ.; Brailey, P.; et al. (2010) Proteasome inhibitor-based primary therapy for antibody-mediated renal allograft rejection. *Transplantation.* Vol.89(3):277-84.

Zou, Y.; Stastny, P.; Susal, C.; et al. (2007) Antibodies against MICA antigens and kidney-transplant rejection. *N Engl J Med.* Vol. 357(13):1293-300.

Zou Y and Stastny P. (2009) The role of major histocompatibility complex class I chain-related gene A antibodies in organ transplantation. *Curr Opin Organ Transplant.* Vol.14(4):414-8.

3

Perioperative and Long-Term Safety of Living Kidney Donors

Masahiko Okamoto
Department of Organ Interaction Research Medicine
Kyoto Prefectural University of Medicine
Japan

1. Introduction

Because securing the safety of living kidney donor is essential to the continued success of this procedure, in this chapter we will review articles which focused not only on recipient outcome but also on living kidney donor to clarify what is known and what should be known in this field.

2. Indication for living kidney donor

For the perioperative and long-term safety, medical indication for living kidney donor is substantial issue. However, criteria for living kidney donor has been often derived empirically on a temporary basis and might vary by country, region and institute. Here, we summarize newly-developed guideline for the indication of living kidney donation which is internationally accepted such as the consensus of Amsterdam forum guideline (Delmonico F. 2005) and OPTN/UNOS guideline (Table 1). Then they were compared with the results of survey of US transplant center concerning evaluating living kidney donors (Mandelbrot DA, et al. 2007).

2.1 Age

There is no description of age limitation of living kidney donor in Amsterdam forum guideline. However age younger than 18 years old is attributed to contraindication in OPTN/UNOS guideline. Half of the institute did not set the upper limit of age, although widely accepted upper limit is 65 years old and some other institute set the cutoffs of 55, 60,70 and 75 years old (Mandelbrot DA, et al. 2007).

2.2 Obesity

Obesity was defined by a body mass index (BMI) of >30 kg/m^2. All potential donors should have BMI determined at initial evaluation because of data suggesting an association between obesity and kidney disease. In most guideline, BMI above 35 kg/m^2 is thought to be contraindication especially when other comorbid conditions are present. And obese patients should be encouraged to lose weight before kidney donation and should not to donate if they have other associated comorbid conditions. According to the survey of US transplant centers, about one-half of programs use a BMI cutoff of 35 kg/m^2, while 10%

exclude donors with BMI over 30 kg/m^2 and 20% exclude donors with BMI over 40 kg/m^2 (Mandelbrot DA, et al. 2007).

	Amsterudam Forum (2005)	OPTN/UNOS (2007)
Age	no description	<18 years old
Obesity	BMI>35kg/m^2	BMI>35kg/m^2
Renal function	GFR<80ml/min or 2SD below normal	CCr<80ml/min
Urinalysis abnormality	u-pro>300mg/day	u-pro>300mg/day
	persistant microhematuria	
Hypertension	BP>140/90 by ABPM	BP>130/90(50yo), anti-HT medication≥3
Diabetes	FBS≥126 or 2hr BS≥200	2hr BS≥140
Dyslipidemia	no excluison	no description
History of malignancy	depend on kind of malignancy	recent malignancy

BMI: Body mass index, GFR: Glomerular filtration rate, SD: Standard deviation, CCr: Creatinine clearance, BP: Blood pressure, ABPM: Ambulatory blood pressure monitoring, FBS: Fasting blood sugar, BS: Blood sugar

Table 1. Contraindication for living kidney donor

2.3 Renal function

The first substantial issue is which measurement should be adapted to estimate renal function of potential living donors. Creatinine clearance calculated by 24-hour urine collections has been used most frequently, however, may under- or overestimate glomerular filtration rate (GFR) in patients with normal or near normal renal function. Estimated GFR values are easy way but not standardized in this population. These methods may be replaced or supplemented by inulin clearance in cases of borderline GFR determination although it is a complicated method. In most program, a GFR<80 ml/minute or 2 standard deviations below normal (based on age, gender, and BSA corrected to 1.73/m^2) generally preclude donation (Delmonico F. 2005). According to the survey of US transplant center, few programs now have no specific cutoff, and no programs use 40 or 60 mL/min/1.73 m^2 as cutoffs (Mandelbrot DA, et al. 2007).

2.4 Proteinuria

Proteinuria should be assessed as a standard part of the donor work up. Dipstick measurements of proteinuria are not enough in the assessment of a prospective living donor. According to the survey of US transplant center, most programs use a 24-hour urine collection for protein. Some programs rely on a spot urine protein to creatinine ratio, and almost one-half of programs now use urinary albumin as a screen. As for cutoff level of proteinuria, more than 300 mg/24-hour of urineprotein is widely accepted as a contraindication to donation. Microalbuminuria determination is also reccomended, although its value as an international standard of evaluation for kidney donors has not been determined (Delmonico F. 2005).

2.5 Hematuria

Isolated microscopic hematuria may not be a contraindication to donation. Red blood cells (RBCs) with glomerular origin have a dysmorphic appearance observed by phase-contrast microscopy and automated RBC analysis. Patients with persistent microscopic hematuria should not be considered for kidney donation unless urine cytology and a complete urologic work up are performed. If urological malignancy and stone disease are excluded, a kidney biopsy may be indicated to rule out glomerular pathology such as IgA nephropathy.

2.6 Hypertension

Hypertension has been considered to be a contraindication in potential renal transplant donors. Some patients with easily controlled hypertension who meet other defined criteria may represent a low-risk group for development of kidney disease and may be acceptable as kidney donors. Hypertension exclusion criteria have become more flexible compared with previous survey (Bia MJ, et al. 1995). In recent survey, while 47% of programs exclude donors on any antihypertensive medication, 41% exclude donors if they are taking more than one medication, and 8% exclude donors taking more than two medications (Mandelbrot DA, et al. 2007). Blood pressure criteria tend to be looser if the donor is older, or if end organ damage is ruled out.

2.7 Diabetes

Diabetes is associated with an increased risk of postsurgical complications and future development of renal failure compared to the general population. Therefore, individuals with a history of diabetes or fasting blood glucose ≥126 mg/dl on at least two occasions or 2-hour glucose with OGTT ≥200 mg/dl are thought to be contraindication for living kidney donation in Amsterdam forum guideline. OPTN/UNOS guideline adapts more strict cutoff level where 2hr BS≥140 are considered to be contraindication for living kidney donation.

According to the survey of US transplant center, almost one-half of programs exclude donors based on elevated fasting blood glucose (FBG), but various cutoffs are used to define 'elevated' (from >100 mg/dl to >120mg/dl). Most programs exclude based on abnormal oral glucose tolerance test or Type II diabetes.

2.8 Dyslipidemia

Dyslipidemia should be included along with other risk factors in donor risk assessment, but dyslipidemia alone does not generally exclude kidney donation.

2.9 History of malignancy

Living kidney donors should be screened by standard medical guidelines to exclude malignancy. A prior history of malignancy may only be acceptable for donation if prior treatment of the malignancy does not decrease renal reserve or place the donor at increased risk for end stage renal disease (ESRD) and if prior treatment of malignancy does not increase the operative risk of nephrectomy. The history of melanoma, renal or urological malignancy, choriocarcinoma, hematologic malignancy, lung cancer, breast cancer and monoclonal gammopathy generally precludes living donation (Pham, PC, et al 2007).

3. Being donor with medical abnormality

Due to the extreme shortage of organ donors worldwide, the indications for live kidney donation have been expanding in terms of medical status, and now include patients with mild hypertension, older age, and mild decline of renal function. Individuals with isolated medical abnormalities (IMAs) are undergoing living donor nephrectomy more frequently. Knowledge of health risks for these living donors is important for donor selection, informed consent and follow-up. One systematical review with living kidney donors with preexisting IMA showed perioperative outcomes for donors with and without IMAs were similar (Young A, et al 2008). However, few studies reported longer term rates of hypertension, proteinuria or renal function. Studies were frequently retrospective and without a comparison group. Centers may accept some IMA donors considering the small risk of ESRD developing as result of the IMA (Bia MJ, et al. 1995). Some long-term follow-up study of IMA donors will be described below.

3.1 Being donor having hypertension

When seeing the relatively short-term outcomes of hypertensive donors, white subjects with moderate, essential hypertension and normal kidney function have no adverse effects regarding blood pressure, GFR, or urinary protein excretion during the first year after living kidney donation. Although further studies are essential to confirm long-term safety, these data suggest that selected hypertensive patients may be accepted for living kidney donation (Textor SC, et al. 2004).

One more study confirmed the long-term safety of hypertensive donors. When 674 live kidney donors were divided into two groups, survival rates in hypertension (HT)-group (N=54) by 20 years were equivalent as compared with non- HT group (N=620). Prevalence of renal dysfunction and ESRD were not increased in HT-group, while prevalence of HT and HT with medication was increased (Okamoto M. unpublished data). Those results demonstrated that those who have HT were able to donate their kidney safely with little major long-term morbidity by strict evaluation and careful postoperative follow-up.

3.2 Being donor having proteinuria

There were one long-term follow-up study of 70 renal outcome 25 years after donor nephrectomy in US single center (at the Cleveland Clinic). By this analysis patients with mild or borderline proteinuria before donation (0.160 g /24 hour) may represent a subgroup at particular risk for the development of significant proteinuria (>0.8 g /24 hour) 20 years or greater after donation (Goldfarb DA, et al. 2001).

3.3 Being donor having glucose intolerance

There were one report concerning long-term coutome of living kidney donors who donated kidneys having glucose intolerance (GI). In this study, 444 donor nephrectomies were divided into GI group and non-GI group according to the results of 75g-oral glucose tolerance test (75g-OGTT). Survival rates in the GI group up to 20 years were equivalent to those in the non-GI group. None of the patients with diabetes mellitus (75g-OGTT: DM pattern, n=27) had developed severe diabetic complications or ESRD at a mean follow-up point of 88±71 (range, 14-225) months. These results suggested that individuals who have GI without diabetic complication may be able to donate their kidney safely with little major morbidity if strict evaluation is performed before transplant (Okamoto M, et al. 2010).

3.4 Transplant outcomes from isolated medical abnormality (IMA) donors

According to the meta-analysis of 12 studies, recipients of kidneys from older donors had poorer 5-year patient and graft survival than recipients of kidneys from younger donors. However, few transplant outcomes were described for other IMA, namely, obesity, hypertension, reduced GFR, proteinuria and hematuria. This disconnect between donor selection and a lack of knowledge of recipient outcomes should give transplant decision-makers pause and sets an agenda for future research (Iordanous Y, et al. 2009).

4. Perioperative issue in living kidney donation

The first major concern regarding living kidney donation is the incidence of perioperative deaths and serious surgical complications. Although it is considered to be a relatively safe procedure, risk of death for the donor is generally estimated as being around 0.02-0.03%. Perioperative mortality and complications of donor nephrectomy including pulmonary embolism, pneumothorax, and less seriously, wound infection, unexplained fever and urinary tract infection will be described below.

4.1 Perioperative mortality

Donor safety is of paramount importance in living donor transplantation. Yet, living donor deaths actually occur (Ratner LE, et al. 2010). According to the survey of 171 United States kidney transplant centers, two donors (0.02%) out of 10,828 living donors died from surgical complications between 1999 and 2001 (Matas AJ, et al. 2003). However, in separate report from the various transplant center, there are little report of a donor death (Siebels M,et al. 2003, Jones KW, et al. 1997, Johnson EM, et al. 1997, Blohme I, et al. 1992).

4.2 Possible surgical complication

There are some surgical complication specific to living donor nephrectomy. Special care must be taken to prevent them.

4.2.1 Deep vein thrombosis/pulmonary embolism

Deep vein thrombosis/pulmonary embolism are most serious complication following living donor nephrectomy. Actually one specified death was caused by pulmonary embolism (Matas AJ, et al. 2003). We reported one case of pulmonary embolism which was diagnosed in relatively early period and successfully recovered with anti-coagulant therapy and transient mechanical ventilation (Ushigome H, et al. 2003). It is very important for surgeons to realize that this can develop in any case of living donor nephrectomy. Every effort should be made to prevent it by enough hydration, intermittent pneumatic compression (IPC) and, if necessary, prophylactic anti-coagulant therapy.

4.2.2 Pneumothorax

Pneumothorax also occurs because of anatomical reason, which sometime needs pleural drainage. The report from US single center (University of Minnesota) described 13 (1.5%) pneumothoraces (6 required intervention, 7 resolved spontaneously) among 871 living donor nephrectomies (Johnson EM, et al. 1997).

4.2.3 Bleeding

Bleeding is the most common cause of reoperation especially laparoscopic nephrectomy. According to the survey of United States kidney transplant centers, 26 donors (0.24%) out of 10,828 living donors needed reoperation because of bleeding (Matas AJ, et al. 2003). By a report of Swedish single center through a retroperitoneal approach, there were 5 cases (1.02%) of postoperative haemorrhage requiring reoperation out of 490 living donor nephrectomies (Blohme I, et al. 1992).

4.2.4 Incisional hernia

Incisional hernia can occur as in other laparotomic surgery and needs reoperation. According to the survey of United States kidney transplant centers, 22 donors (0.20%) out of 10,828 living donors needed reoperation because of hernia (Matas AJ, et al. 2003).

4.2.5 Femoral nerve compression

Femoral nerve compression may occur because it exists on the psoas muscle and it can be compressed by would retractor.

4.2.6 Wound infections, hematomas or seromas

Wound infections, hematomas or seromas happen most frequently after living donor nephrectomy as a minor complication. They usually resolve without major operation.

4.2.7 Pneumonias, atelectasis and urinary tract infections

Pneumonias and atelectasis also happens as a complication of general anesthesia. They tend to occur at an opposite site of nephrectomy because of lateral recumbent position. Urinary tract infections also happen as in other surgical procedure due to insertion of urethral catheter.

4.3 Risk factors for perioperative complications

Transplant professionals should avoid possible risk for living kidney donors. A couple of report analyzed the risk factor for them. According to analysis of live donors drawn from a mandated national registry of 80 347 live kidney donors in the United States between 1994 and 2009, surgical mortality was higher in men than in women (RR=3.0), in black vs. white and Hispanic individuals (RR=3.1), and in donors with hypertension vs. without hypertension (RR=27.4) (Segev DL, et al. 2010). The report from US single center (University of Minnesota) described that the analysis, by logistic regression, among 871 living donor nephrectomies identified significant risk factors for perioperative complications were male gender (vs. female), pleural entry (vs. no pleural entry), and weight > or = 100 kg (vs. < 100 kg) (Johnson EM, et al. 1997).

5. Long-term follow-up of living kidney donor -Survival, renal function, complication

The long-term consequences after kidney donation are not fully understood. However, most long-term follow-up studies of living kidney donors find no decrease in long-term survival. And most of the data suggested that the donors had normal renal function, with an incidence of hypertension comparable to that expected in the age-matched general population, while other demonstrated that donor nephrectomy is associated with mild proteinuria and hypertension. The Long-term follow-up study of living kidney donor concerning survival rate, renal function and various complications will be described including our Japanese experiences (Table 2).

Author	year	Subject	Tx done	No.	retrieval rate	HT	ESRD	die	Survival rate
Najarian JS	1992	single center	1963-1970	135	NA	32%	not stated	15	NA
Fehrman-Ekholm I	1997	single center	1964-1994	459	93%	35%	not stated	41	29% better
Fehrman-Ekholm I	2001	single center	1964-1995	451	77%	38%	1	49	NA
Goldfarb DA	2001	single center	1963-1975	180	38%	48%	2	24	NA
Ramcharan T	2002	single center	1963-1979	773	60%	similar	5	84	NA
Ellison MD	2002	UNOS registry		NA	NA	NA	56	NA	NA
Thiel GT	2005	naitonal registry	1993-2005	737	85%	35%	0	9	NA
Gossmann J	2005	single center	1973-2001	152	93%	30%	0	7	NA
Ibrahim HN	2009	single center	1963-2007	3698	NA	32%	11	268	Similar to NP
Okamoto M	2009	single center	1972-2006	601	80%	30.1%	4	55	better than NP

No.: total number of donor, HT: hypertension, ESRD: end-stage renal disease, UNOS: United Network for Organ Sharing, NA: not accessed, NP: Normal population

Table 2. Report of long-term outcome after living kidney donation

5.1 Long-term survival following living kidney donation

Most long-term follow up studies of living kidney donors find no decrease in long-term survival. By analysis of 430 previous living kidney donors in Swedish single center, the survival rate of 20 years was 29% better than the expected survival rate calculated by using national registers. They concluded that the better survival among donors is probably due to the fact that only healthy persons are accepted for living kidney donation (Fehrman-Ekholm I, et al. 1997). Moreover, the analysis of 481 previous Japanese living kidney donors also showed that the survival rate of kidney donors was better than the age- and gender-matched cohort from the general population, and the patterns and causes of death were similar with the general population (Okamoto M, et al. 2009). The study of larger numbers of donors as many as 3698 who donated kidneys during the period from 1963 through 2007 for a longer follow-up period in US single institute (University of Minnesota) also ascertained that the survival of kidney donors was similar to that of controls who were matched for age, sex, and race or ethnic group (Ibrahim, HN, et al. 2009). The overall evidence suggests that living kidney donors have survival similar to that of non-donors.

5.2 Hypertension following living kidney donation

Hypertension is thought to be one of major concerns following living kidney donation. However, a couple of study demonstrated no increase of hypertension after living donor nephrectomy. By a 15-year experience on 162 living donors in Italy, Long-term incidence of hypertension in living donors was similar to the general population (Sansalone CV, et al. 2006). Furthermore, the analysis of 402 donor nephrectomy in Sweden showed that, although hypertension was present in 38% of the donors, the age-adjusted prevalence of hypertension among donors was not higher than in the general population (Fehrman-Ekholm I, et al. 2001).

On the other hands, some study demonstrated increase of hypertension after living donor nephrectomy. Another analysis of 75 donors, in US single center (University of Missouri), showed that the prevalence of hypertension was significantly increased compared with age/sex matched data from epidemiological studies of the general population, especially in those over the age of 55 years (Saran R, et al. 1997). Also, in a live kidney donor cohort with a 93% retrieval rate of the 152 donors, mean blood pressure had increased from 125 ± 15/79 ± 11 to 134 ± 19/81 ± 9 mmHg ($p < 0.01$) which remained significantly below normal. (Gossmann J, et al. 2005). One Meta-analysis showed kidney donors may have a 5 mmHg increase in blood pressure within 5 to 10 years after donation over that anticipated with normal aging (Boudville N, et al. 2006). Future controlled, prospective studies with long periods of follow-up will better delineate the risk of hypertension following living kidney donation.

5.3 Proteinuria following living kidney donation

Most reported data suggested that proteinuria increased in living kidney donor population, although follow-up period and measurement of proteinuria and/or microalbuminuria differed by report.

German experience at a single center of 102 living kidney donors for 35 years showed microalbuminuria was found in 22.6% of the donors (Schostak M, et al. 2004). Another study showed, in a live kidney donor cohort with a 93% retrieval rate of the 152 donors, fifty six percent of donors developed proteinuria (>150 mg/day), but only 10% had albuminuria (Gossmann J, et al. 2005). By analysis of 402 outcome after donor nephrectomy in Sweden, significant proteinuria (> or =1.0 g/L) was found in 3% and slight proteinuria (<1.0 g/L) in 9% of the donors and proteinuria was associated with hypertension and a lower GFR (Fehrman-Ekholm I, et al. 2001).

One Meta-analysis, which analyzed a total of 5048 donors from forty-eight studies with an average follow-up of 7 years after donation (range 1-25 years), demonstrated that the average 24-h urine protein was 154 mg/day and concluded that kidney donation results in small increases in urinary protein. (Garg AX, et al. 2006).

5.4 Renal function following living kidney donation

Renal function is the greatest concerns at a long time after living kidney donation. In a report from Saudi Arabia of 25 living kidney donors, total kidney function measured as creatinine clearance showed significant drop by 36% of the pre donated value. However, remaining kidney clearance increased by an average of 34% of the pre donated level as measured by Tc 99m DTPA renography. Compensatory hypertrophy of the remaining kidney measured by ultrasound attributed to an increase in the renal volume of 15% (Shehab AB, et al. 1994). Other investigator shows 25% decrease of GFR with mean time after uninephrectomy of 11 years. (Gossmann J, et al. 2005), and 27% decrease of with mean patient follow-up of 25 years (Goldfarb DA, et al. 2001).

In a Swedish study, the average estimated GFR (12 years after donation) was 72±18% of the age-predicted value. The ratio of the estimated to the predicted GFR showed no correlation to the time since donation, indicating that there is no accelerated loss of renal function after donation (Fehrman-Ekholm I, et al. 2001). These results demonstrated that although living kidney donor lose GFR by 15-25%, they usually do not show the accelerated loss of renal function if they do not have risk factor for chronic renal disease (CKD). One unique study examined renal function >20 years after donation by comparing that with siblings. They showed no significant difference in serum creatinine (1.1±0.01 vs 1.1±0.03 mg/dl), blood urea nitrogen (17±0.5 vs 17±1.2 mg/dl) and creatinine clearance (82±2 vs 89±3.3 ml/min) between 57 donors (mean age 61±1) and 65 siblings (mean age 58±1.3) (Najarian JS, et al. 1992).

5.5 ESRD in previous donor

Although the Swiss Organ Living Donor Health Registry showed no ESRD in 737 living kidney donors between 1993 and January 2005 (Thiel GT, et al. 2005), there were considerable reports of ESRD of previous kidney donor as below.

In a survey which used the Organ Procurement and Transplantation Network (OPTN) database, a total of 56 previous living donors were identified as having been subsequently listed for cadaveric kidney transplantation. They concluded that living renal donation has long-term risks that may not be apparent in the short term and that the numbers reported underestimate the actual number of living donors with renal failure, because they include only patients listed for a kidney transplant. (Ellison MD, et al. 2002). In analysis of 402 donor nephrectomy in Sweden, no donor died in uremia or had dialysis treatment before death. However, three donors developed renal disease, and one was in dialysis treatment. In two of these cases, hereditary factors were possibly involved (Fehrman-Ekholm I, et al. 2001). In Mexican experience, they present four kidney donors who developed ESRD thereafter, three becoming kidney recipients (Gracida C, et al. 2001). Other two case reports described kidney donors who developed ESRD (Ladefoged J, et al. 1992, al Shohaib S, et al. 1995). By analysis of 464 outcomes after donor nephrectomy at University of Minnesota, 84 had died and 380 were alive. Of the 84 donors who had died, three were known to have had kidney failure. Of the 380 still alive, three had abnormal kidney function and two had undergone transplantation (Ramcharan T, et al. 2002).

One study carefully investigated the association between postoperative clinical courses and changes in renal function in eight donors who developed chronic kidney disease (CKD) stage 5 or ESRD. According to their findings, except for one donor who developed ESRD caused by a traffic accident, none of the donors developed progressive renal dysfunction immediately after donation. Their renal functions remained stable for a long period, but started to decline after developing new comorbidities, especially risk factors known as progression factors (proteinuria or hypertension) or accelerating factors (cardiovascular event or infection) of CKD (Kido R, et al. 2009). However, the overall evidence suggests that their risk of ESRD is not increased.

6. Ethical issue and quality of life (Q.O.L.) in living kidney donation

Most published reports have indicated healthy psychological status and improved quality of life (Q.O.L.) in living kidney donors. However, there have been some reports of depression and disrupted family relationships after kidney donation. The reasons of negative results were mainly related to poor outcome of the kidney recipient, or long-lasting major pain or disappointment about medical handling before and after organ donation. Ethical issue and Q.O.L. in living kidney donation will be described.

6.1 Ethical issue in living kidney donation

Not only medical aspect but also ethical aspect is very important part to continue living kidney transplantation. The general public's concerns of living kidney donation is the length of a hospital stay, out-of-pocket expenses, size and appearance of a scar, and the donor risk of developing kidney failure (Boulware LE, et al. 2002). In this respect, it is quite important process to inform prospective donor of these issues. Especially, a long-term medical risk with potential living donors is a vital aspect of informed consent. According to a survey of 203 practitioners in 35 countries, risks of hypertension, proteinuria or kidney failure requiring dialysis were frequently discussed (usually over 80% of practitioners discussed each medical condition). However, many practitioners do not believe these risks are increased after donation, with surgeons being less convinced of long-term sequelae compared with nephrologists. Thus, transplant professionals vary in the long-term risks they communicate to potential donors. (Housawi AA, et al. 2007).

Moreover, the expansion of living donor kidney transplantation to include significant numbers of donors with little to no preexisting relationship to the candidate has caused concern in the medical community regarding as donor psychological status, motivation, knowledge about donation and the potential for undue pressure to donate under some circumstances. (Dew MA, et al. 2007). Another rare but delicate issue in living-related kidney donation is discovering misattributed paternity. In a survey, the prevalence of misattributed paternity ranges between approximately 0.25% and 0.5% of all living kidney donations. Opinions about revealing this information were quite variable by practitioners (Young A, et al. 2009).

6.2 Quality of life (Q.O.L.) in living kidney donation

Same as medical risk, Q.O.L. in living kidney donors is substantial issue to continue this procedure. According to the experience in German single institute of 102 living kidney donors, everyday life was managed as well as before surgery after 2-4 wk by the highest percentage (42%) of patients, but working capacity was only regained after 1-3 months by a comparable percentage (44%). Forty-six percent had a very good and 33% a good feeling after the kidney donation. The relationship to the recipient had intensified in most cases. Ninety-one percent would again decide in favor of a donation (Schostak M, et al. 2004). By another survey, majority of living kidney donors had an excellent Q.O.L. As a group, they scored higher than the national norm on the SF-36, a standardized Q.O.L health questionnaire. However, 4% were dissatisfied and regretted the decision to donate. Further, 4% found the experience extremely stressful and 8% very stressful. Multivariate analysis found that relatives other than first degree and donors whose recipient died within 1 year of transplant were more likely to say they would not donate again if it were possible. Further, donors who had perioperative complications and female donors were more likely to find the overall experience more stressful (Johnson EM, et al. 1999).

Women considering kidney donation frequently ask whether a nephrectomy will impact their ability to have children (Nevis IF, et al. 2009). There is a single-center survey which described 490 pregnancies in 239 donors after donation. Compared to pregnancies before donation, pregnancies after donation had increased rates of gestational diabetes (0.7% vs. 2.7%), gestational hypertension (0.6% vs. 5.7%), preeclampsia (0.8% vs. 5.5%), prematurity (4.0% vs. 7.1%) and fetal loss (11.3% vs.19.2%). The authors reported that these incidences of adverse events observed in donors were similar or better than expected levels for the general population (Ibrahim H et al. 2009). Therefore, pregnancy after kidney donation is not necessarily contraindication although it is better to avoid.

7. Financial Issue in living kidney donation

Many nations have programs that help living donors with their financial costs while donors in other regions of the world are without support. Moreover some living kidney donors encounter difficulties obtaining life insurance, despite the surveys of insurance companies reporting otherwise.

7.1 Reimbursement for living kidney donation

The financial risk of living donation is theoretically well covered by different insurances. However, some of the donors had to cover some expenses by themselves (Wolters HH, et al. 2003). It is proposed to reimburse donor risk by a package of specific benefits (life insurance, health insurance and a small amount of cash) to minimize hazard and ensure donor interests. It will fund medical follow-up and enable data collection so that long-term risk can be accurately assessed (Gaston RS, et al. 2006).

One international research network examined legislation and programs that facilitate reimbursement, focusing on policy mechanisms, eligibility criteria, program duration and types of expenses reimbursed. According to their results, among 40 countries, reimbursement is expressly legal in 16, unclear in 18, unspecified in 6 and expressly prohibited in 1. Donor reimbursement programs exist in 21 countries; 6 have been enacted in the last 5 years. Lost income is reimbursed in 17 countries, while travel, accommodation, meal and childcare costs are reimbursed in 12 to 19 countries. Ten countries have comprehensive programs, where all major cost categories are reimbursed to some extent. These programs differ in operation and scope. Donors in other regions of the world are without support (Sickand M, et al. 2009). Effort should be taken to establish reimbursement system to facilitate living kidney donation where this procedure is performed.

7.2 Life insurance after living kidney donation

Being an organ donor may affect one's ability to obtain life, disability and health insurance. According to a systematic review, almost all companies would provide life and health insurance to living organ donors, usually with no higher premiums. However, concern about insurability was still expressed by 2%–14% of living organ donors in follow-up studies, and 3%–11% of donors actually encountered difficulties with their insurance (Yang RC, et al. 2007).

In another study, researchers contacted offices of life insurance companies in five major cities in Canada to obtain life insurance for fictitious living kidney donors and paired controls. As a result, all donor and control profiles received a quote, with no significant difference in the premium quoted. More time was spent on the phone for donor compared to control profiles, although difference was small. Age, gender, family history of kidney disease and new-onset hypertension had no further effect on donor insurability in regression analysis. They found no evidence that kidney donors were disadvantaged in the first step of applying for life insurance (Yang RC, et al. 2009).

8. Conclusion

Because securing the safety of donor is essential to the continued success of living kidney transplantation, we have reviewed important issues, namely, indication, donation with medical abnormality, perioperative problem, long-term follow-up, ethical issue, Q.O.L. and financial issue in living kidney donation. The background quite differ by region, therefore, it seems to be difficult to build a international standard. Regular follow-up of kidney donors is recommended in order to manage their complications effectively and to detect health problem early in those who may develop it. National registry is necessary to enable data collection so that long-term risk can be accurately assessed.

9. Reference

al Shohaib, S. (1992). Chronic renal failure following living-related kidney donation. *Nephron.* Vol. 71, No. 4, pp. 468, ISSN 0028-2766

Bia, MJ., Ramos, EL., Danovitch, GM., Gaston, RS., Harmon, WE., Leichtman, AB., Lundin, PA., Neylan, J. & Kasiske, BL. (1995). Evaluation of living renal donors. The current practice of US transplant centers. *Transplantation.* Vol. 60, No. 4, pp. 322-327, ISSN 0041-1337

Blohme, I., Fehrman, I. & Norden, G. (1992). Living donor nephrectomy. Complication rates in 490 consecutive cases. *Scand J Urol Nephrol.* Vol. 26, No. 2, pp. 149-53, ISSN 0036-5599

Boudville, N., Prasad, GV., Knoll, G., Muirhead, N., Thiessen-Philbrook, H., Yang, RC., Rosas-Arellano, MP., Housawi, A., Garg, AX. & Donor Nephrectomy Outcomes Research (DONOR) Network. (2006). Meta-analysis: risk for hypertension in living kidney donors. *Ann Intern Med.* Vol. 145, No. 3, pp. 185-196, ISSN 0003-4819

Boulware, LE., Ratner, LE., Sosa, JA., Tu, AH., Nagula, S., Simpkins, CE., Durant, RW. & Powe, NR. (2002). The general public's concerns about clinical risk in live kidney donation. *Am J Transplant.* Vol. 2, No. 2, pp. 186-193, ISSN 1600-6135

Delmonico, F. & Council of the Transplantation Society. (2005). A Report of the Amsterdam Forum On the Care of the Live Kidney Donor: Data and Medical Guidelines. *Transplantation.* Vol. 79, (6 Suppl), S53-66, ISSN 0041-1337

Dew, MA., Jacobs, CL., jowsey, SG., Hanto, R., Miller, C. & Delmonico, FL. (2007). Guidelines for the Psychosocial Evaluation of Living Unrelated Kidney Donors in the United States *Am J Transplant.* Vol. 7, No. 5, pp. 1047-1054, ISSN 1600-6135

Ellison, MD., McBride, MA., Taranto, SE., Delmonico, FL. & Kauffman, HM. (2002). Living kidney donors in need of kidney transplants: a report from the organ procurement and transplantation network. *Transplantation*. Vol. 74, No. 9, pp. 1349-1351, ISSN 0041-1337

Fehrman-Ekholm, I, Elinder, CG, Stenbeck, M, Tyden, G. & Groth, CG. (1997). Kidney donors live longer. *Transplantation*. Vol. 64, No. 7, pp. 976-978, ISSN 0041-1337

Fehrman-Ekholm, I., Duner, F., Brink, B., Tyden, G. & Elinder, CG. (2001). No evidence of accelerated loss of kidney function in living kidney donors: results from a cross-sectional follow-up. *Transplantation*. Vol. 72, No. 3, pp. 444-449, ISSN 0041-1337

Garg, AX., Muirhead, N., Knol,l G., Yang, RC., Prasad, GV., Thiessen-Philbrook., H, Rosas-Arellano, MP., Housawi ,A., Boudville, N. & Donor Nephrectomy Outcomes Research (DONOR) Network. (2006). Proteinuria and reduced kidney function in living kidney donors: A systematic review, meta-analysis, and meta-regression. *Kidney Int*. Vol. 70, No. 10, pp. 1801-1810, ISSN 0085-2538

Gaston, RS., Danovitch, GM., Epstein, RA., Kahn, JP., Matas, AJ. & Schnitzler, MA. (2006). Limiting financial disincentives in live organ donation: a rational solution to the kidney shortage. *Am J Transplant*. Vol. 6, No. 11, pp. 2548-2555, ISSN 1600-6135

Goldfarb, DA., Matin, SF., Braun, WE., Schreiber, MJ., Mastroianni, B., Papajcik, D., Rolin, HA., Flechner, S., Goormastic, M. & Novick, AC. (2001). Renal outcome 25 years after donor nephrectomy. *J Urol*. Vol. 166, No. 6 pp. 2043-2047, ISSN 0022-5347

Gossmann, J., Wilhelm, A., Kachel, HG., Jordan, J., Sann, U., Geiger, H., Kramer, W. & Scheuermann, EH. (2005). Long-term consequences of live kidney donation follow-up in 93% of living kidney donors in a single transplant center. *Am J Transplant*. Vol. 5, No. 10, pp. 2417-2424, ISSN 1600-6135

Gracida, C., Espinoza, R. & Cancino, J. (2004). Can a living kidney donor become a kidney recipient? *Transplant Proc*. Vol. 36, No. 6, pp. 1630-1631, ISSN 0041-1345

Housawi, AA., Young, A., Boudville, N., Thiessen-Philbrook., H, Muirhead, N., Rehman, F., Parikh, CR., Al-Obaidli, A., El-Triki, A. & Garg, AX. Donor Nephrectomy Outcomes Research (DONOR) Network. (2007). Transplant professionals vary in the long-term medical risks they communicate to potential living kidney donors: an international survey. *Nephrol Dial Transplant*. Vol. 22, No. 10, pp. 3040-3045, ISSN 0931-0509

Ibrahim, H., Akkina, S., Leister, E., Gillingham, K., Cordner, G., Guo, H., Bailey, R., Rogers, T. & Matas, AJ. (2009). Pregnancy outcomes after kidney donation. *Am J Transplant*. Vol. 9, No. 4, pp. 825–834, ISSN 1600-6135

Ibrahim, HN., Foley, R., Tan, L., Rogers, T., Bailey, RF., Guo, H., Gross, CR & Matas, AJ.(2009). Long-term consequences of kidney donation. *N Engl J Med*. Vol. 360, No. 5, pp. 459-469, ISSN 0028-4793

Iordanous, Y., Seymour, N., Young, A., Johnson, J., Iansavichus, AV., Cuerden, MS., Gill, JS., Poggio, E., Garg, AX. & Donor Nephrectomy Outcomes Research (DONOR) Network. (2009). Recipient outcomes for expanded criteria living kidney donors: the disconnect between current evidence and practice. *Am J Transplant*. Vol. 9, No. 7, pp. 1558-1573, ISSN 1600-6135

Johnson, EM., Remucal, MJ., Gillingham, KJ., Dahms, RA., Najarian, JS. & Matas, AJ. (1997). Complications and risks of living donor nephrectomy. *Transplantation*. Vol. 64, No. 8, pp. 1124-1128, ISSN 0041-1337

Johnson, EM., Anderson, JK., Jacobs, C., Suh, G., Humar, A., Suhr, BD., Kerr, SR., Matas, AJ. & Nevis, IF. (1999). Long-term follow-up of living kidney donors: quality of life after donation. *Transplantation*. Vol. 67, No. 5, pp. 717-721, ISSN 0041-1337

Jones, KW., Peters, TG., Charlton, RK., Lenz, BJ., Walker, GW., Repper, S., Crews, MJ., Antonucci, LE. & Peters, EJ. (1997).Current issues in living donor nephrectomy. *Clin Transplant*. Vol. 11, No. 5 Pt 2, pp. 505-510, ISSN 0902-0063

Kido, R., Shibagaki, Y., Iwadoh, K., Nakajima, I., Fuchinoue, S., Fujita, T. & Teraoka, S. (2009). How do living kidney donors develop end-stage renal disease? *Am J Transplant*. Vol. 9, No. 11, pp. 2514-2519, ISSN 1600-6135

Ladefoged, J. (1992). Renal failure 22 years after kidney donation. *Lancet*. Vol. 339, No. 8785, pp. 124-125, ISSN 0140-6736

Mandelbrot, DA., Pavlakis, M., Danovitch, GM., Johnson, SR., Karp, SJ., Khwaja, K., Hanto, DW. & Rodrigue, JR. (2007). The medical evaluation of living kidney donors: a survey of US transplant centers. *Am J Transplant*. Vol. 7, No. 10, pp. 2333-2343, ISSN 1600-6135

Matas, AJ., Bartlet,t ST., Leichtman, AB. & Delmonico, FL. (2003). Morbidity and mortality after living kidney donation, 1999-2001: survey of United States transplant centers. *Am J Transplant*. Vol. 3, No. 7, pp. 830-834, ISSN 1600-6135

Najarian, JS., Chavers, BM., McHugh, LE. & Matas, AJ. (1992). 20 years or more of follow-up of living kidney donors. *Lancet*. Vol. 340, No. 8823, pp. 807-810, ISSN 0140-6736

Nevis, IF. & Garg, AX. (2009). Donor Nephrectomy Outcomes Research (DONOR) Network. Maternal and fetal outcomes after living kidney donation. *Am J Transplant*. Vol. 9, No. 4, pp. 661-668, ISSN 1600-6135

Okamoto, M., Akioka, K., Nobori, S., Ushigome, H., Kozaki, K., Kaihara, S. & Yoshimura, N. (2009). Short- and long-term donor outcomes after kidney donation: analysis of 601 cases over a 35-year period at Japanese single center. *Transplantation*. Vol. 87, No. 3, pp. 419-423, ISSN 0041-1337

Okamoto, M., Suzuki, T., Fujiki, M., Nobori, S., Ushigome, H., Sakamoto, S. & Yoshimura, N. (2010). The consequences for live kidney donors with preexisting glucose intolerance without diabetic complication: analysis at a single Japanese center. *Transplantation* Vol. 89, No. 11, pp. 1391-1395, ISSN 0041-1337

Pham, PC., Wilkinson, AH. & Pham, PT. (2007). Evaluation of the potential living kidney donor.Am J Kidney Dis. Vol. 50, No. 6, pp. 1043-1051, ISSN 0272-6386

Ramcharan, T. & Matas, AJ. (2002). Long-term (20-37 years) follow-up of living kidney donors. *Am J Transplant*. Vol. 2, No. 10, pp. 959-964, ISSN 1600-6135

Ratner, LE. & Sandoval, PR. (2010). When Disaster Strikes: Death of a Living Organ Donor. *Am J Transplant*. Vol. 10, No. 12, pp. 2577-2581, ISSN 1600-6135

Sansalone, CV., Maione, G., Aseni, P., Rossetti, O., Mangoni, I., Soldano, S., De Roberto, A., Minetti, ME., Perrino, ML. & Civati, G. (2006). Early and late residual renal function and surgical complications in living donors: a 15-year experience at a single institution.*Transplant Proc*. Vol. 38, No. 4, pp. 994-995, ISSN 0041-1345

Schostak, M., Wloch, H., Muller, M., Schrader, M., Offermann, G. & Miller, K. (2004). Optimizing open live-donor nephrectomy - long-term donor outcome. *Clin Transplant.* Vol. 18, No. 3, pp. 301-305, ISSN 0902-0063

Segev, DL., Muzaale, AD., Caffo, BS., Mehta, SH., Singer, AL., Taranto, SE., McBride, MA. & Montgomery, RA. (2010). Perioperative mortality and long-term survival following live kidney donation. *JAMA.* Vol. 303, No. 10, pp. 959-966, ISSN 0098-7484

Shehab, AB., Shaheen, FA., Fallatah, A., Sheikh, IA., Gabal, MS. & Al-Koussi, M. (1994). Residual renal function after living related kidney donation. Is it enough? An early report. *J Egypt Public Health Assoc.* Vol. 69, No. 5-6, pp. 379-395, ISSN 0013-2446

Sickand, M., Cuerden, MS., Klarenbach, SW., Ojo, AO., Parikh, CR., Boudville, N., Garg, AX. & Donor Nephrectomy Outcomes Research Network. (2009). Reimbursing live organ donors for incurred non-medical expenses: a global perspective on policies and programs. *Am J Transplant.* Vol. 9, No. 12, pp. 2825-2836, ISSN 1600-6135

Siebels, M., Theodorakis, J., Schmeller, N., Corvin, S., Mistry-Burchardi, N., Hillebrand, G., Frimberger, D., Reich, O., Land, W. & Hofstetter, A. (2003). Risks and complications in 160 living kidney donors who underwent nephroureterectomy. *Nephrol Dial Transplant.* Vol. 18, No. 127, pp. 2648-2654, ISSN 0931-0509

Textor, SC., Taler, SJ., Driscoll, N., Larson, TS., Gloor, J., Griffin, M., Cosio, F., Schwab, T., Prieto, M., Nyberg, S., Ishitani, M. & Stegall, M. (2004). Blood pressure and renal function after kidney donation from hypertensive living donors. *Transplantation.* Vol. 78, No. 2, pp. 276-282, ISSN 0041-1337

Thiel, GT., Nolte, C. & Tsinalis, D. (2005). The Swiss Organ Living Donor Health Registry (SOL-DHR). *Ther Umsch.* Vol. 62, No. 7, pp. 449-457, ISSN 0040-5930

Ushigome, H., Yasui, H., Okamoto, M., Akioka, K., Nakamura, K., Kadotani, Y., Ohmori, Y., Oka, T. & Yoshimura, N. (2003). Pulmonary embolism in a living-related kidney transplantation donor. *Surg Today.* Vol. 33, No. 5, pp. 399-402, ISSN 0941-1291

Wolters, HH., Heidenreich, S. & Senninger, N. (2003). Living donor kidney transplantation: chance for the recipient--financial risk for the donor? *Transplant Proc.* Vol. 35, No. 6, pp. 2091-2092, ISSN 0041-1345

Young, A., Storsley, L., Garg, AX., Treleaven, D., Nguan, CY., Cuerden, MS. & Karpinski, M. (2008). Health outcomes for living kidney donors with isolated medical abnormalities: a systematic review. *Am J Transplant.* Vol. 8, No. 9, pp. 1878-1897, ISSN 1600-6135

Young, A., Kim, SJ., Gibney, EM., Parikh, CR., Cuerden, MS., Horvat, LD., Hizo-Abes, P., Garg, AX. & Donor Nephrectomy Outcomes Research (DONOR) Network. (2009). Discovering misattributed paternity in living kidney donation: prevalence, preference, and practice. *Transplantation.* Vol. 87, No. 10, pp. 1429-1435, ISSN 0041-1337

Yang, RC., Thiessen-Philbrook, H., Klarenbach, S., Vlaicu, S., Garg, AX. & Donor Nephrectomy Outcomes Research (DONOR) Network. (2007). Insurability of living organ donors: a systematic review. *Am J Transplant.* Vol. 7, No. 6, pp. 1542-1551, ISSN 1600-6135

Yang, RC., Young, A., Nevis, IF., Lee, D., Jain, AK., Dominic, A., Pullenayegum, E., Klarenbach, S., Garg, AX. & Donor Nephrectomy Outcomes Research (DONOR) Network. (2009). Life insurance for living kidney donors: a Canadian undercover investigation. *Am J Transplant*. Vol. 9, No. 7, pp. 1585-1590, ISSN 1600-6135

4

Transplantation in Diabetics with End-Stage Renal Disease

Elijah Ablorsu
Department of Nephrology and Transplant Services
University Hospital of Wales, Cardiff,
United Kindgdom

1. Introduction

Pancreas transplantation is well recognised and established treatment for selected patients with type-1 diabetes. Furthermore, this treatment remains the only therapeutic modality to offer excellent and reliable glycemia control, without the administration of insulin in type-1 diabetics.
It is well documented that combination of pancreas and kidney transplant (i.e. Simultaneous Pancreas and Kidney Transplantation or Pancreas After Kidney Transplantation) gives to patients who suffer from type-1 diabetes and End-Stage Renal Failure superior outcomes, improved patients' survival and better quality of life compared to other therapeutic modalities.
In this chapter will be reviewed current status of pancreas transplantation with focus on recipient selection, management and outcomes.

2. Diabetic Nephropathy

2.1 Definition

Diabetic nephropathy (DN) has been acknowledged as the most common disorder leading to End-Stage Renal Failure (ESRF) in adults (Fig. 1). Renal disease is associated with higher morbidity and mortality in diabetics compared to patients who do not suffer from diabetes. Approximately 0.5% of the population in developed countries (United States and Europe, i.e. Western societies) is thought to have diabetes (ADA, 1999). It is well known that DN is the most common diabetic complication. Patients with type-1 diabetes have the highest risk of developing nephropathy, but those with type-2 have significant risk, too. This condition develops in 50% of type-1 diabetics progressively over a period of 10 to 15 years. In contrast, people suffering from type-2 diabetes can undergo a more variable course and approximately 30% of them will develop DN at some point.

2.2 Etiology

The patho-physiologic mechanisms of diabetic nephropathy are not completely understood yet, but they include hyperglycemia (causing hyperfiltration and renal injury), glycosylation of circulating and intrarenal proteins, hypertension, and abnormal intrarenal hemodynamics.

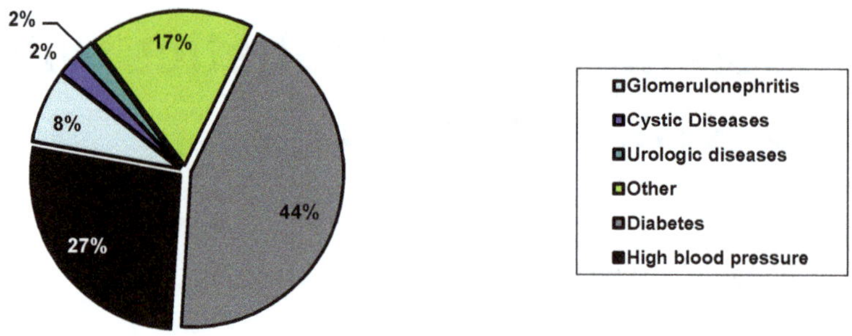

Fig. 1. Primary Causes of Kidney failure (Collins et al., 2008).

For DN are typically three major histological changes that seem to have a similar prognostic impact. Mesangial expansion is induced by hyperglycaemia, causing matrix production or glycosylation of matrix proteins. Another common feature is glomerular sclerosis caused by intraglomerular hypertension; induced by renal vasodilatation or from ischemic injury induced by the hyaline narrowing of the vessels supplying glomeruli. Glomerular basement membran thickening is another common feature, too.

2.3 Secondary complication of diabetes

Among patients with DN we see an increased prevalence of other secondary diabetic complications. Hypertension significantly increases diabetes-related morbidity and is the second most common cause of morbidity in diabetics. It has been documented that hypertension increases mortality in diabetics with renal failure by 37 folders (MacLeod & McLay, 1998). Hypertension also contributes to the developing of DN, microvascular and macrovascular complications.

Diabetic micro and macroangiopatic complications develop simultaneously and have a widespread effect on many organs as well as participating on the development of various diseases (diabetic nephropathy, retinopathy, coronary artery disease, peripheral vascular disease, cerebrovascular disease, etc).

Diabetic retinopathy is the leading cause of visual loss in diabetics due to retinal damage. This condition affects up to 80% of patients who have suffered from diabetes for more than 10 years (Kertes & Johnson, 2007). The main mechanism of diabetes induced retinal damage is a combination of cytotoxic effect of high blood glucose levels and hypertension. Characteristic retinal lesions include the formation of retinal capillary microaneurysms, extensive vascular permeability, vascular occlusion, angio proliferation and basement membrane thickening (Matthew et al., 1997). Some studies have demonstrated (Wong et al., 2008) that the prevalence of retinopathy rises with the increasing duration and severity of the diabetes. However, good glycaemia control reduces retinopathy development by more than 40% (TDCCTG, 1993).

In some diabetics, mainly in patients with long standing or poorly controlled diabetes, symptoms of hypoglycaemia (e.g. palpitation, sweating, tremor, headache, etc.) do not occur. The absence of these symptoms during hypoglycaemia is called hypoglycaemic unawareness. Patients suffering from this condition have a lack of warning signals and cannot actively correct their hypoglycaemia before plasma glucose falls to extremely low levels. The main factor responsible for the development of hypoglycaemic unawareness is autonomic diabetic neuropathy and brain desensitization to hypoglycaemia.

Absence of glucose homeostasis in diabetes also causes pathological damage and functional disturbance of the peripheral (motor and sensor) and autonomic nerves. Frequently, patients suffer from motor neuropathy: pain, paresthesia and anesthesia. Autonomic neuropathy (arrhythmia, postural hypotension, diabetic diarrhoea, gastroparesis, neurogenic bladder, impotence, etc) is less common than peripheral neuropathy, but is a more symptomatic and has limited therapeutic effect (Watkins & Edmonds, 1997).

The development of complications is related to the severity and length of diabetes, and its management involves glucose control and symptomatic treatment which seems to have a positive effect (Ward, 1997).

2.4 Management

In recent years, there has been significant progress in the management and treatment of diabetics. We have seen not only a reduced morbidity but also increased patients' survival and improved patients' quality of life. Median patient survival in recent years amongst this population has increased from 6 to 15 years (Wiesbauer et al., 2010).

It is well known that poor diabetic control is responsible for developing various diabetic complications; mainly DN. The risk of developing nephropathy is significantly reduced if HbA1c stays below 7.5-8.0% (Deferrari et al., 1998; Di Landro et al, 1998). For that reason the American Diabetes Association highlights in their "Guidelines for Glycemic Control" to target HBA1c level below 7% to achieve a normal or near normal glycemia (ADA, 2005).

It was documented in two large studies on a cohort of 1349 patients, the DCCT (Diabetes Controlled and Complication Trial) and EDIC (Epidemiology of Diabetes Intervention and Complications) that tight glycemic control decreases the risk of development of microvascular disease (retinopathy, nephropathy, and neuropathy) and even slows down established DN (TDCCTRG, 1993), (DCCT, 2003).

In brittle type-1 diabetes serum glucose levels can rapidly swing between extremely low and high levels. This can lead to the development of acute and life threatening conditions: keto-acidosis, coma or even death. Often patients have absent warning symptoms. In some diabetics it is difficult, and even impossible, to achieve a good glycemic control with conventional management.

Nowadays, varieties of insulin preparations are available. The type, the dose and the frequency of insulin doses depends on patient's individual factors. For type-1 diabetics "Basal-bolus insulin regiment" (a combination of high frequency boluses of short-acting insulin with long-acting insulin) is often used. Some people benefit from "Mixed insulin regiment". This includes a mixture of short and long-acting insulin delivered two to three times a day. Regardless of meticulous blood glucose monitoring and accurate insulin dosage, some patients may still have problems achieving an appropriate blood glucose level. These patients may be considered for an insulin pump. The disadvantage of this method is increased frequency of hypo/hyper glycemia episodes and also the fact that it requires a cannula implantation (Collins et al., 2007).

The innovations in insulin formulation and delivery have had a significant impact on the management of type-1 diabetes and they have improved glycaemic control. Despite this

progress, many patients cannot achieve a good degree of serum glucose control and keep suffering from frequent sudden hypoglycaemia episodes. These circumstances have a negative impact on patients' quality of life and can even be life threatening.
In addition, sufficient management of DN also includes rigorous treatment of hypertension in combination with conventional management of renal failure, hyperlipidemia, anaemia, etc.

3. Pancreas transplantation

The first pancreas transplant was performed at the University of Minnesota, in Minneapolis, on 17 December 1966 by the team led by Dr William Kelly and Dr Richard Lillehei (Kelly et all., 1967). A pancreas, together with a kidney, was implanted to a 28-year old woman. Immediately after the transplantation the patient became euglycemic, but unfortunately she died three months later from a pulmonary embolism with functioning grafts. The same team in Minneapolis, on 3 June 1969, performed the first successful pancreas transplant and the pancreas graft functioned for more than one year (Lillehei & et al., 1970). Early experiences with pancreas transplantation were disappointing, as they were associated with a high incidence of rejection, infectious complications and early graft failure. Progressively in the late 70's and early 80's the results of pancreas transplantation improved. First of all, the original Lillehei surgical technique was modified and refined. In 1988 Starz published a technique of anastomozing graft duodenum to the recipient jejunum for draining a pancreas graft exocrine secretion (Fig 2) (Starzl et al., 1988). Subsequently, his technique was adopted by other big pancreas transplant institutions; by Dr Hans Sollinger at the University of

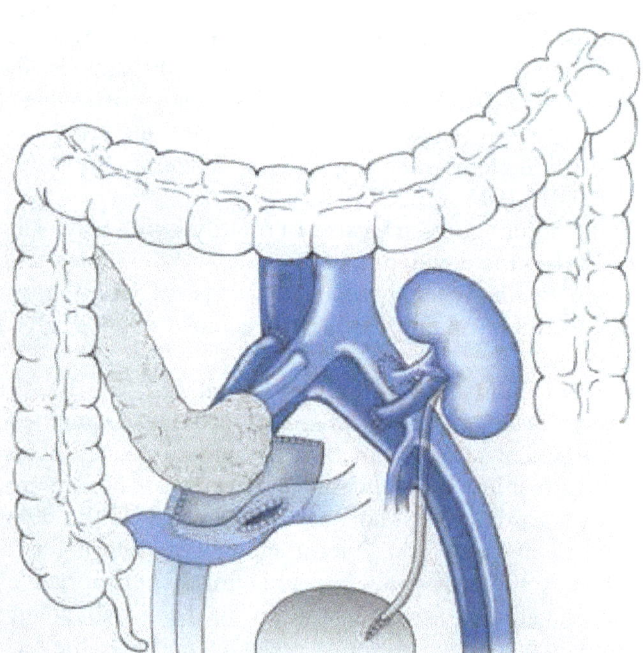

Fig. 2. The Enteric drainage technique in simultaneous pancreas and kidney transplantation. Pancreas graft duodenum is anastomosed side-to-side to the jejunum of a recipient.

Wisconsin and Dr Robert Corry at the University of Iowa. Later, all three centres employed to their routine practice the technique of draining graft duodenum to the bladder (Fig 3) (Sutherland et al., 1988; Sollinger & Belzer, 1988; Corry, 1988). Both techniques, with minimal modifications are still used these days. A number of studies compared the outcomes between bladder and enteric drained pancreas transplants. Most of them showed similar complication rates (Lo et al., 2001; Stratta et al., 2000), graft and patient survival (Sugitani et al., 1998).

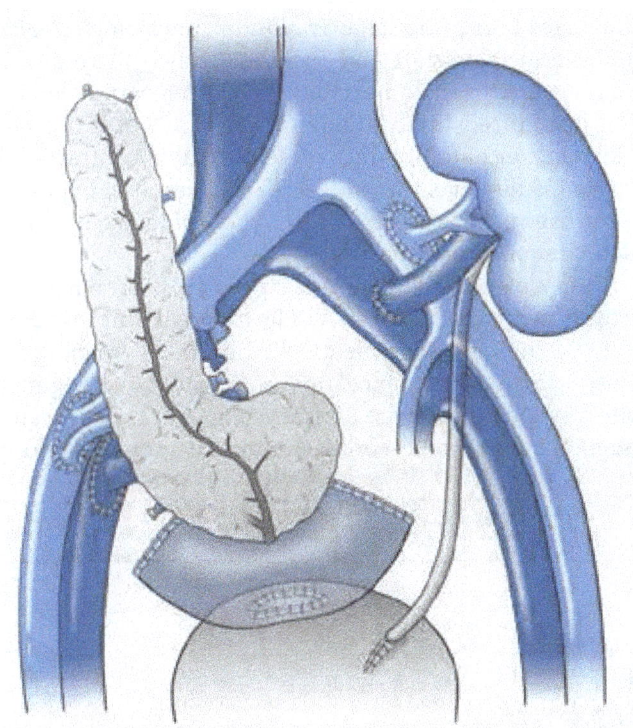

Fig. 3. The Bladder drainage technique in simultaneous pancreas and kidney transplantation. Pancreas graft duodenum is anastomosed side-to-side to the bladder of a recipient.

The Enteric Drainage pancreas technique compared (ED) to the Bladder Drainage pancreas technique (BD) is a more physiological option because it drains pancreatic enzymes into intestinal track. However, this technique is associated with a higher rate of surgical complications (anastomotic leak, chemical and infectious peritonitis, ileus, intra-abdominal abscess formation, etc.). A typical complication of bladder drainage technique is the recurrence of urinary track infections, haematuria, urethral strictures, prostatitis, pyeloneophritis, reflux pancreatitis, etc. Additionally to these complications, the urinary diversion of exocrine pancreas graft secretion potentiates excessive loss of bicarbonates, sodium and fluid. This results in acid-base and electrolytes disturbance (metabolic acidosis) and fluid depletion. Metabolic acidosis is even more exacerbated by renal dysfunction. For those reasons, serum electrolytes must be closely monitored in patients with bladder drained pancreas, patients must be well hydrated and receive bicarbonate supplements.

Enteric conversion is a surgical alternative to manage sever complications related to the bladder drainage of pancreas graft (Stephanian et al., 1992). The United Network for Organ Sharing (UNOS) and the International Pancreas Transplant Registry (IPTR) data from 2005 reports the overall conversion rate from BD to ED of 9% at 1 year and 17% at 3 years after transplant (Gruessner & Sutherland, 2005). The major indications for conversion were recurrent episodes of haematuria, graft pancreatitis, chronic urinary track infections, dehydration and bladder calculi (Jimenez-Romero, et al., 2009).

In terms of pancreas venous drainage there are two available variations: portal venous and systemic venous drainage. Portal drainage is a more physiological alternative, but with regards to the complication rate; graft and patient survival there are not any significant differences. Some data suggests that portal venous drainage is an important factor to determine peripheral insulin sensitivity (Radziuk et al., 1993). In portal venous drainage, serum glucose and insulin concentration recover to normal in contrast with systemic venous drainage, where plasma insulin levels are increased, as a result of bypassing liver circulation (Gu et al., 2002). Hyperinsulinemia contributes to hyperlipidemia, hypercholesterolemia and accelerate the development of atherosclerosis.

A milestone in the history of transplantation occurred in 1976, when Calne published the first clinical experiences with Cyclosporin-A. He reported improved graft and patients' survival in a cohort of 34 transplant recipients (32 kidneys, 2 pancreases and 2 livers) who received only Cyclosporin-A maintenance immunosuppressive regiment (Lillehei et al., 1979). A Cyclosporin-A helped to achieve a better control of rejection and minimise steroid dependence. Although, the introduction of new immunosuppressive drugs (tacrolimus,

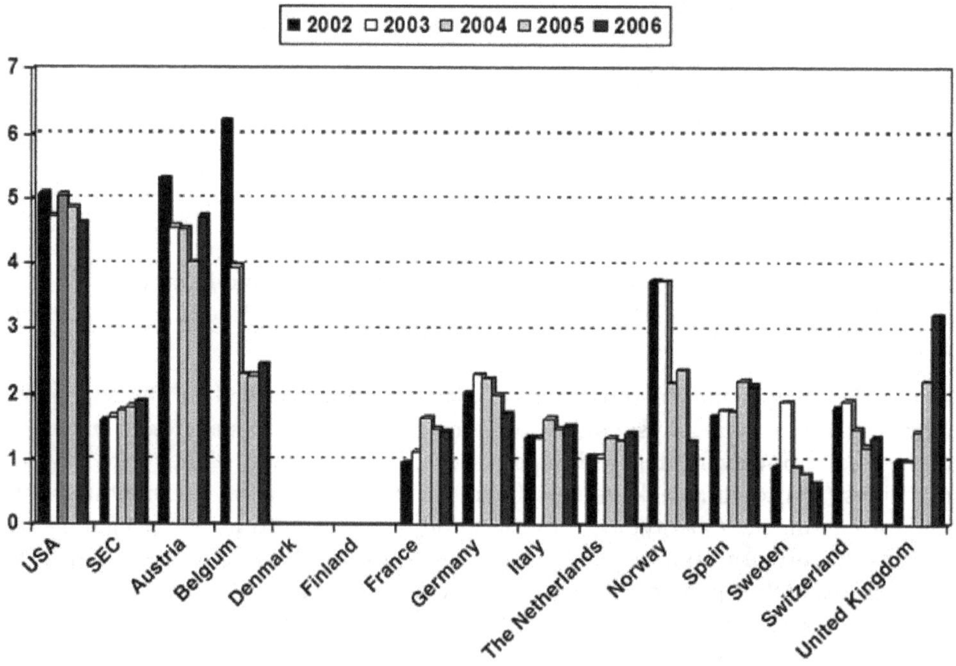

Fig. 4. Pancreas transplant activity rate (incidence per million population) in USA and 13 European countries considered together (SEC) and individually during the period 2002–06 (Gonzales-Posada et al. 2010).

	USA	Europe[a]	Austria	Belgium	Denmark	Finland	France	Germany	Italy	Netherlands	Norway	Spain	Sweden	Switzerland	UK
Population[b]															
2002	287.67	366.73	8.07	10.31	5.37	5.19	61.40	82.44	56.99	16.10	4.52	40.96	8.91	7.25	59.22
2003	290.34	368.82	8.10	10.36	5.38	5.21	61.83	82.54	57.32	16.19	4.55	41.66	8.94	7.31	59.44
2004	293.03	371.05	8.14	10.40	5.40	5.22	62.25	82.53	57.89	16.26	4.58	42.34	8.98	7.36	59.70
2005	295.73	373.34	8.21	10.45	5.41	5.24	62.64	82.50	58.46	16.30	4.61	43.04	9.01	7.41	60.06
2006	298.44	375.29	8.27	10.51	5.43	5.26	63.00	82.44	58.75	16.33	4.64	43.76	9.05	7.46	60.39
Pancreas Tx[c]															
2002	1460	591	43	64	0	0	59	161	77	17	17	69	8	13	59
2003	1373	614	37	41	0	0	70	191	77	17	17	74	17	14	59
2004	1483	657	37	24	0	0	103	187	95	22	10	74	8	11	86
2005	1444	678	33	24	0	0	92	165	87	21	11	96	7	9	133
2006	1386	718	39	26	0	0	90	141	90	23	6	94	6	10	193
Pancreas WL[d]															
2002	2835	897	38	56	0	0	189	180	245	15	11	47	20	6	90
2003	2747	877	42	56	0	0	199	145	213	14	11	75	19	5	98
2004	2388	918	36	53	0	0	178	158	216	34	13	79	14	8	132
2005	2071	920	38	34	0	0	169	169	197	40	10	87	15	16	145
2006	1984	1009	32	30	0	0	169	190	222	40	10	73	15	21	207
DD[e]															
2002	6190	6422	195	223	73	89	1198	1001	1020	202	62	1409	98	75	777
2003	6457	6598	187	248	75	85	1119	1110	1042	223	87	1443	114	95	770
2004	7150	6898	181	220	64	109	1291	1052	1203	228	90	1495	123	91	751
2005	7593	7159	200	237	63	85	1371	1185	1197	217	76	1546	128	90	764
2006	8024	7340	201	273	62	109	1442	1227	1231	200	76	1509	137	80	793

[a] All 13 countries.
[b] Million inhabitants.
[c] Tx = transplants.
[d] WL = waiting list.
[e] DD = deceased donors.

Table 1. Population, total number of pancreas transplants, pancreas waiting list and DD in USA and 13 European countries (Gonzales-Posada et al. 2010).

MMF, sirolimus, antibody based agents) contributed to further improved graft survival, reduction of rejection rate and the overall expansion of transplantation.

These days, pancreas transplantation has become a worldwide popular therapeutic alternative for type-1 diabetics. According to data from the United Network for Organ Sharing (UNOS) and the International Pancreas Transplant Registry (IPTR), more than 30,000 pancreas transplants have been performed worldwide (>22,000 reported from the United States and >8,000 from rest of the world) between December 1966 and 31 December 2008 (UNOS & IPTR, 2008). The majority pancreas transplants have been performed in North America and Western Europe (Fig 4), (Tab. 1) (Gonzales-Posada et al. 2010).

4. Indication of pancreas transplantation

At the present, Pancreas Transplantation is the only therapeutic modality that can achieve full insulin independence and euglycemic state in type-1 diabetic patients. It is well known that normoglycemia has a positive impact on preventing secondary diabetic complications. Therefore, this modality does not only improve patients' quality of life but also it has a positive impact on patients' medical conditions. Nevertheless, this therapeutic alternative is recommended only to a selected group of diabetics.

For a pancreas transplantation should be considered patients with brittle type-1 diabetes who suffer from secondary diabetic complications (diabetic nephropathy, diabetic retinopathy, diabetic neuropathy, diabetic gastro-enetopathy, etc); frequent hypoglycaemic episodes or hypoglycaemic unawareness and failure to achieve eu-glycemia even on intensive insulin treatment (insulin pump, etc.).

A detailed assessment of potential candidates for pancreas transplantation is mandatory because many of these patients have pre-existing cardiac diseases or other medical problems related to diabetes, and these may significantly increase per-operative morbidity, mortality and early graft failure.

4.1 Diabetes assessment

The first part of the evaluation is to determine the type of diabetes. It is generally accepted that pancreas transplantation should be reserved for type-1 diabetics. However, there are published data repording successes of pancreas transplantation also in type-2 diabetic patients. Nevertheless, a more strict patients' selection is required (Orlando et al., 2010). For diagnosis type-1 diabetes it is satisfactory to detect an absence or very low levels of C-peptide together with raised HbA1c (>7.5%). However, the patient's considered for pancreas transplantation cannot exceed insulin requirements beyond 1.5mg/kg/day; as this is the marker of peripheral insulin resistance. These patients do not achieve full insulin independence even with successful pancreas transplantation. Patients who are failing to achieve a reasonable serum-glucose control with conventional insulin treatment should be also considered for pancreas transplantation. Usually, they suffer from frequent hypo and hyper-glycemic episodes. Sever hypoglycaemia is the most common casualty in diabetics on insulin treatment. These complications are potentially life-threatening, associated with high morbidity and mortality rate.

4.2 Cardiac evaluation

Diabetes doubles the risk of developing cardio-vascular disease; coronary-artery disease, cerebro-vascular disease and peripheral vascular disease (Grundy et al., 1999). Over 50% of diabetics have some degree of coronary artery disease. Also, it is well known that diabetics suffer from accelerated atherosclerosis and a high incident of silent ischemia and cardio-myopathy compared to the non-diabetic population. Furthermore, cardio-vascular disease is the leading cause of death in the general population (35%) but diabetic patients are two times (67%) more likely to die due to this cause (Watkins, 2003).

The key purpose of the pre-transplant cardiac assessment is to identify risk factors (reversible ischemia, impaired left ventricular function, coronary artery disease, etc.) that may increase per-operative morbidity and mortality; and minimize them with the appropriate management and treatment. For cardiac evaluation standard echocardiography, Dobutamine stress echocardiography (DSE), exercise tolerance testing, nuclear (thalium) myocardial perfusion scan and formal coronary angiogram are routinely used. Because each of these tests has some limitations, there is not a consensus yet regarding which method has the highest predicting value.

Dobutamine stress echocardiography (DSE) is a non-invasive imaging modality which combines two-dimensional echocardiography with cardiovascular stress induced by dobutamine infusion. This test is sensitive to detect coronary artery disease in asymptomatic, high risk (diabetic, patients with peripheral vascular disease, etc.) patients.

The nuclear myocardial perfusion study (MPI) is a sensitive, non-invasive test for the assessment of myocardial perfusion, ejection fraction, wall motion and wall thickness. Stress radionuclide myocardial perfusion imaging, on the other hand, displays the downstream functional consequences of epicardial coronary artery disease in the myocardium. It also may visualize the regional effects of micro vascular endothelial dysfunction and impairment of regional coronary flow reserve.

DSE and MPI methods are generally accepted as standard and non-invasive screening studies useful to identify patients (diabetics with ESRF) with significantly increased risk of myocardial infarction or cardiac death (Rabbat et al., 2003; Cai et al., 2010). Nevertheless, they have low sensitivity and specificity to define coronary artery disease in patients with ESRD (Letine et al., 2010).

On the other hand, the coronary-angiogram (CA) offers high sensitivity to detect coronary-artery disease but it is limited in regards to predicting survival. This is mainly because myocardial infarction is more likely to be caused by plague instability rather than angiographic stenosis. Additionally, the contrast used for this test is nephro-toxic and it can have a catastrophic impact on impaired kidney function (Letine et al., 2010).

There is only one published study which directly compares doputamine stress echocardiography to coronary angiogram in renal transplant candidates (Herzog et al., 1999). Fifty potential transplant candidates underwent DSE followed by CA. Twenty of fifty DSE were positive for inducible ischemia. Sensitivity and specificity of DSE were 52% and 74%, respectively, for stenosis ≥50%; 75% and 71% for stenosis greater than 70%; 75% and 57% for stenosis greater than 75%. At the end the authors concluded that DSE is a good screening method, in spite of low sensitivity to detect coronary artery disease. For that reason, CA is reserved for high risk groups of patient with a previous history of cardiac problems (cardiac event, ishemic heart desease etc) or for patients with positive stress echocardiography or MPI scan.

4.3 Dietitian management

4.3.1 Pre-transplant assessment

A well balanced nutrition in transplant recipients plays a vital role in a pre and pos-transplant period to ensure the best possible outcomes. The role of a dietician is to evaluate the patient's nutrition status and design a nutrition plan for a pos-transplant period. For that reason it is important we ensure pre-operatively the following parameters:

a. *Good glucose control:* It is well documented (Kuo et al., 2010) that diabetes mellitus is a major predictor of cardiovascular morbidity and mortality in kidney transplant recipients. A recent study (Sato et al., 2010) analysed the outcomes of patients undergoing cardiac surgery and revealed that increased of HbA1c levels (>6.5%) predicts insulin sensitivity and increases the incidence of major complications. In addition, a well controlled diabetes improves gastroparesis and delays gastric empting (Reddy, 2010) as well as preventing other gastro intestinal symptoms including nausea, vomiting, bloating, early satiety and abdominal pain (Kashyap & Farrugia, 2010).
b. *Weight maintenance:* A Body Mass Index (BMI) ≥25kgs/m^2 is a strong predictive factor with significantly negative impact on long term renal graft outcomes (Cheung et al., 2010). So, in these patients weight loss is strongly recommended.

c. *Balanced nutrition status*: Prior to transplantation it is also crucial to optimize good nutrition status in patients with low BMI. According to some data (Meier-Kriesche et al, 2002) poor nutrition is associated with significantly worse patient and graft survival.
d. *Adequate electrolyte balance:* Patients with chronic renal failure may be on a low potassium, phosphate and low salt diets and fluid restrictions. Raised levels of potassium and phosphate are associated with increased mortality in these patients (Noori et al 2010; Ganesh et al., 2001).

4.3.2 Immediate pos-transplant management

The transplant recipient must receive adequate nutrition support (25-30 kcal/kg ideal body weight per day) during the first seven pos-operative days to avoid starvation and to enhance postoperative recovery (Braga et al., 2009). We should aim to identify the patient's post-transplant nutrition requirements prior to a surgery and in advance to design an individual sufficient nutrition plan.

The European Society for Clinical Nutrition and Metabolism (ESPEN) developed guidelines on enteral nutrition management after surgery (Weiman et al., 2006). These guidelines suggest that oral diet and supplements should be initiated early after surgery, where possible. Furthermore, enteral nutrition should be considered in patients with obvious under-nutrition and those whose oral intake will be inadequate (<60% of requirements) for 10 days after surgery. These patients should ideally have a naso-jejunal tube placed during surgery and feeding commenced on the first pos-operative day. According to these guidelines, parenteral nutrition is reserved for those patients who are unable to tolerate enteral feeding; due to complication including interstinal obstruction, ileus and sever shock (Braga et al., 2009).

4.3.3 Pos-transplant surveillance

In the long term, it is important to maintain a healthy weight and maintain good nutrition status. A team from the Netherlands (Hoogeveen et al., 2011) reports that 1-year post-transplant BMI is more strongly related to death and graft failure than pre-transplant BMI. According these data, patients who reached pos-transplant BMI>30 kg/m^2 have a 20-40% higher risk of death and graft failure compared to patients with lower BMI.

4.4 Other tests

A routine part of the pre-transplant assessment includes blood tests:

a. *Haematology Blood Tests:* Blood group identifying, antibody screen, full blood count, Thrombophilia screen, APTT, PT, and INR.
b. *Biochemistry Test:* Urea & electrolytes, creatinine, uric acid, calcium, phosphate, 24-hour urine collection (tested for protein/micro albuminuria and creatinine clearance), eGFR (radioisotope glomerular filtration rate if needed), liver function tests, amylase, thyroid function, fasting blood glucose, fasting and stimulated C-peptide levels if needed, fasting blood lipids.
   Additional studies may include oral or intravenous glucose challenge, anti-insulin and islet cell antibodies, proinsulin level and lipoprotein.
c. *Viral screen:* Hepatitis B and C, HIV, HTLV, BK virus, Polioma virus, Syphilis, Rubella, Epstein Barr Virus, Toxoplasma, Varicella-Zoster, Herpes , simplex, Cytomegalovirus.
d. *Immunology Blood Tests:* HLA typing and antibody screening.

5. Contraindications

Overall, contraindications to pancreas transplantation are the same as for kidney transplantation, and they are often determined by patient co-morbidity.

5.1 Absolute contraindications

a. Insufficient cardiovascular reserve:
   - Ejection fraction below 50%
   - Myocardial infarction within 6 months
   - Non-correctable coronary artery disease or refractory congestive heart failure

b. Non curable malignancy (excluding localised skin malignancy)
c. Active sepsis
d. Active peptic ulcer
e. Major psychiatric history likely to result in non-compliance
f. Inability to withstand surgery and immunosuppression

(UKT, 2003)

Some contraindications are relative and must be individually assessed and discussed with the responsible specialist on multidisciplinary bases and with the patient, too.

5.2 Relative contraindications

a. Cerebrovascular accident with long term impairment.
b. HIV (subject to discussion).
c. Chronic liver disease: Candidates with Hepatitis B/C need recent viral screen, LFT and assessment by hepatologist prior activating on a WL. The aim is to exclude active viral disease as well as advanced irreversible liver disease.
d. Body Mass Index greater than 30.
e. Malignancy: In patients with a history of cancer a cancer free interval from three to five years according the type of cancer, stage and cancer therapy are required. This issue must be discussed in detail with an oncologist. A valuable source of information is "Israel Penn International Transplant Tumor Registry" (www.ipittr.org).
f. Type-2 diabetes was originally an absolute contraindication to pancreas transplantation. However, a recently published review reports that selected group type-2 diabetics benefit from whole organ pancreas transplantation, too. Transplant outcomes (after SPK) are comparable between type 1 and 2 diabetics. But a strict patient selection is required; BMI less than 30 kg/m^2, insulin requirements <1.0 units/kg/day, C-peptide level less than 10 ng/ml, etc. (Orlando et al., 2010).
g. Extensive aorta/iliac and/or peripheral vascular disease.
h. Continued abuse of alcohol, smoking or other drugs.

(UKT, 2003)

6. Transplant alternatives for diabetic patients

For diabetic patients with ESRF three transplant alternatives are currently available: kidney transplantation (including cadaver and living donor kidney transplantation); Simultaneous Pancreas-Kidney Transplantation (SPK) and Pancreas After Kidney Transplantation (PAK). Each of them has some recognised advantages and disadvantages (Tab. 2).

	Advantages	Disadvantages
CKT	Provides better survival than dialysis options	Inferior to other transplant options with respect to kidney graft survival and patient survival
LRD	Minimizes waiting time, time spent on dialysis Very low early morbidity and mortality	Absence to normalize of blood glucose Inferior patient survival over time when compared with SPK recipients with functioning grafts
SPK	Glycemic control, with recent median pancreas graft survival of >10 years High-quality, deceased donor kidney graft	Higher morbidity and mortality due to larger operation If pancreas fails within the first year, outcomes are worse than LRD
PAK	Glycemic control If living donor kidney transplant, comparable/better patient and kidney graft survival than LRD	Two separate surgical procedures, increased mortality early postoperatively following pancreas transplant Historically inferior pancreas graft survival (35% at 10 years) than SPK

Table 2. Summary of advantages and disadvantages of transplant options for diabetic kidney disease (Wiseman, 2010).

6.1 Kidney transplantation

Kidney transplantation is a widely used and well accepted transplant option for patient with ESRF secondary to DN. It is indisputable that this alternative gives survival advantages to these patients over chronic dialysis. The estimated survival of a diabetic on dialysis is only 30-40% at five years, while kidney transplantation increases their 5 year survival to up to 70% for Cadaver Kidney Transplantation (CKT), and to up to 80% for Living Donor Kidney Transplantation (LRD) (Reddy et al., 2003; USRDS 1998; Cecka et al. 1997). As we know, LRD is associated with better outcomes due to a superior quality of kidney graft and reduced cold ischemia time. This type of transplantation has relatively low risk of post-transplant complications (10-12%) and compared to pancreas transplantation it is less traumatic, too. For that reason, a greater population of diabetic patients with ESRF is eligible for renal transplantation rather pancreas transplantation. A successfully treated ESRF with renal transplantation does not only improve overall patients' medical conditions (anaemia, hypertension, etc) but in many cases it also stabilises brittle diabetes.

6.2 Simultaneous pancreas and kidney transplantation

During recent years, Simultaneous Pancreas and Kidney Transplantation (SPK) has become the most popular transplant alternative and golden standard for type-1 diabetic with ESRF. Additionally to renal transplantation in these patients pancreas transplantation helps to achieve euglycemia, insulin independence and enhances patients' quality of life (Sureshkumar et al., 2006). Also, the tight glycaemic control prevents the recurrence of diabetic nephropathy and improves secondary diabetic complications; mainly diabetic retinopathy, cardiovascular disease, diabetic neuropathy, etc.

Overall, it has been proven that SPK gives some survival benefits to these patients. In one of the largest studies (Ojo et al., 2001) SPK was associated with a 10-year patient survival of 67% compared to 46% in a CKT recipient group. However, in comparison with the LRD benefit of SPK, in terms of patient and graft survival, it does diminish. Wisconsin experiences (Tab. 3) (Rayhill et al., 2000) have shown that patient and renal graft survival was not different between the LRD and the SPK groups, but it was significantly lower in the CKT group (Fig 5,6) (Young et al., 2009).
The main advantage of LRD is the low immunological risk and good quality kidney graft that participates on excellent kidney function and prolongs graft survival. However, only an additional pancreas transplant gives a protective role to prevent the recurrence of DN, maintain a good kidney function, improve the quality of life and eliminate secondary diabetic complications. On the other hand, we cannot forget that SPK is associated with a double level of morbidity (20-40%) and mortality (2-5%) compared to kidney transplantion. For that reason, younger patients with better medical conditions (Rayhill et al., 2000) should be considered for SPK.

	1y patient survival	5-y patient survival
LRDi	100%	94%
LRDh	99%	85%
SPK	96%	88%
CKT	94%	72%

	1y graft survival	5-y graft survival
LRDi	96%	85%
LRDh	94%	72%
SPK	87%	78%
CKT	86%	64%

LRDi - HLA-identical living related donor, LRDh - haplotype-identical living related donor

Table 3. The 1-year and 5-year pos-transplant outcomes (Rayhill et al., 2000).

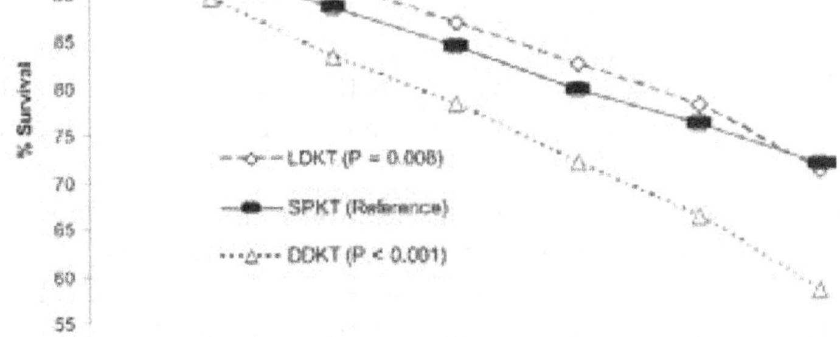

(LDKT - living donor kidney transplant; SPKT - simultaneous pancreas kidney transplant; DDKT - deceased donor kidney transplant).

Fig. 5. Unadjusted kidney graft survival by transplant type (Young et al., 2009).

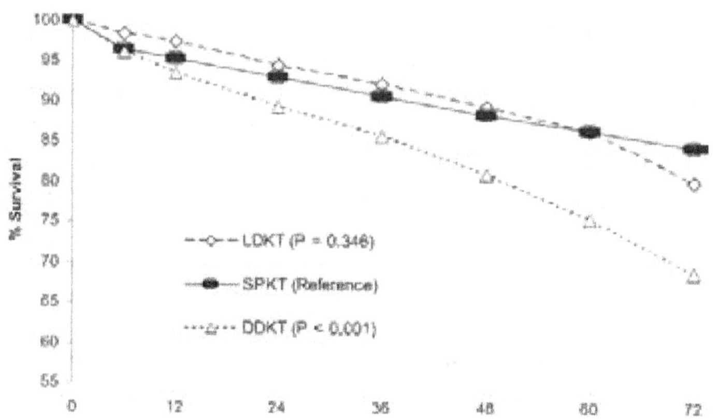

(LDKT - living donor kidney transplant; SPKT - simultaneous pancreas kidney transplant; DDKT - deceased donor kidney transplant).

Fig. 6. Unadjusted patient survival by transplant type (Young et al., 2009).

6.3 Pancreas after kidney transplantation

Historically, Pancreas After Kidney Transplantation (PAK) was not a very popular pancreas transplant alternative due to the inferior pancreas graft survival compared to SPK. The impact of pancreas graft on patients with kidney graft from two different donors was associated with high immunological graft failure. However, the development of new immunosuppressive regiments based on depleting antibody induction and Tacrolimus and MMF maintenance reduced the risk of immunological graft loss and improved graft survival outcomes. For those reasons, this alternative has become more popular (Larson et al., 2004).

Diabetic patients who have undergone kidney transplant or who underwent SPK and have lost pancreas graft might be today considered for PAK. With increased frequency, this two-stage procedure involves a living donor kidney transplantation followed by a cadaver pancreas transplant (PALK). This alternative has the advantage of a short waiting time and of a superior quality kidney graft (Kleinclauss et al., 2009). The second great advantage of PAK is performing major pancreas transplant surgery on a non-uremic patient. This minimizes the risk of per-operative morbidity and mortality related to renal failure.

Pominipanin analysed data of the Organ Procurement Transplant Network/United Network of Organ Sharing (OPTN/UNOS) database and compared outcomes of SPK with CKT and PALK. He reports that renal graft outcomes were superior in PALK compared to SPK. The 1-year pancreas graft survival was marginally higher for the SPK cohort (86%) vs. 80% for PALK. The overall patient survival was better in PALK compared to SPK (Fig 7 a,b). Even this study showed that PAK is an alternative with competitive results to SPK.

6.4 Simultaneous cadaver pancreas and living donor kidney transplantation

At present, SPK and PAK are the most common options for uremic type-1 diabetics. SPK is a one-stage procedure and this is its main advantage over PAK. On the other hand, PAK has the advantage of involving living donor with superior quality of kidney graft function and subsequently of performing pancreas transplantation on a non-uremic patient. Simultaneous Cadaver Pancreas and Living Donor Kidney Transplantation (SPLK) is an innovative approach that merges some benefits of both alternatives; superior quality of living donor kidney and s single procedure with shorter waiting time for cadaver pancreas graft.

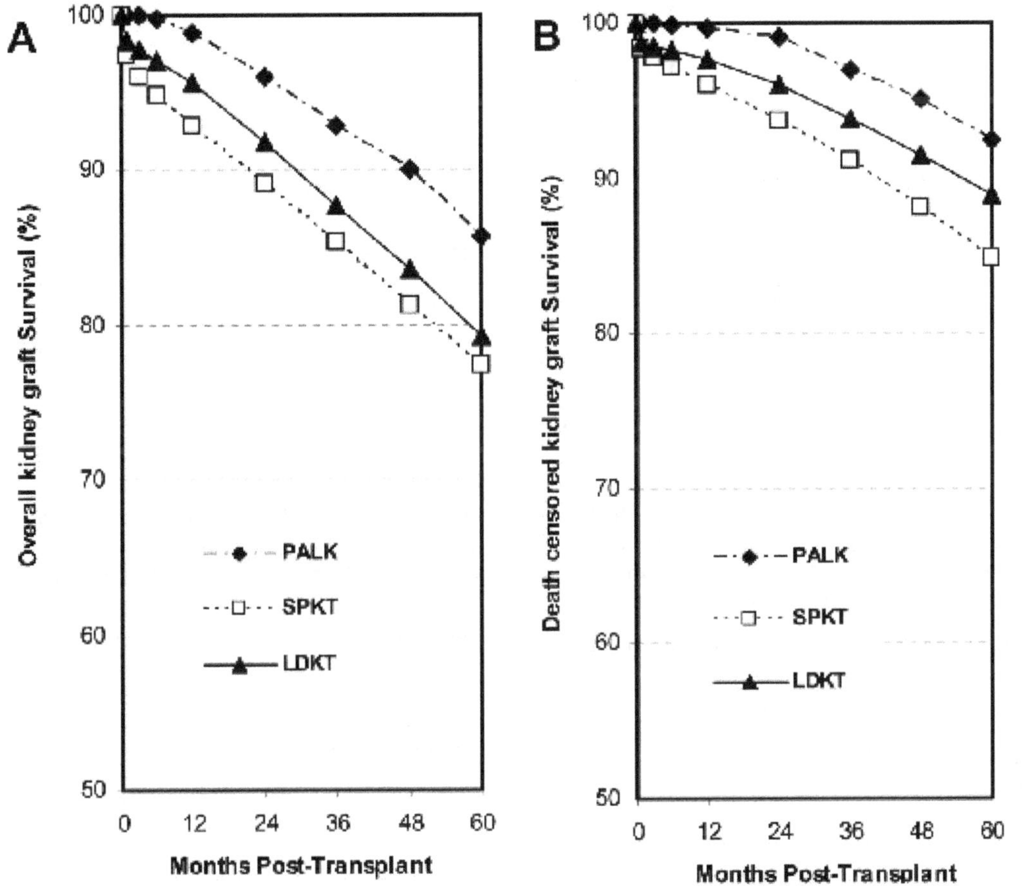

No at risk						
PALK	807	755	669	547	403	283
SPKT	5580	4457	3527	2737	2057	1453
LDKT	3461	2888	2340	1799	1326	937

807	755	669	547	403	283
5580	4457	3527	2737	2057	1453
3461	2888	2340	1799	1326	937

a/ Overall kidney graft survival (%)
b/ Death censored kidney graft Survival (%)
PALK - pancreas after living kidney transplant,
SPKT - simultaneous pancreas kidney transplant,
LDKT - living donor kidney transplant.

Fig. 7. Kidney graft survival (Poommipanit et al., 2010).

Despite increased immunological risk, SPLK showed comparable results with SPK and PAK (Boggi et al., 2004). In a study from Maryland (Farney et al., 2000), it was reported that 1-year pancreas graft survival in the SPLK group was not significantly higher than in SPK and PAK (88% vs. 84% vs. 71%) Fig. 8,9,10 (Farney et al., 2000). The 1-year patient survivals were 95% (SPLK), 94% (SPK) and 100% (PAK). The SPLK group showed lower incidence of delay graft function and better kidney function.

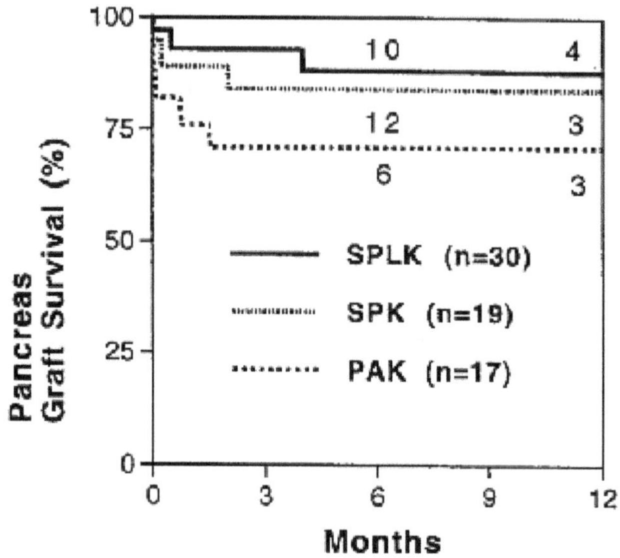

One-year pancreas graft survival rates were 88%, 84%, and 71%, respectively, for simultaneous cadaver-donor pancreas and living-donor kidney transplantation (SPLK), simultaneous cadaver kidney and pancreas transplantation (SPK) and living-donor kidney transplantation alone followed by a solitary cadaver-donor pancreas transplant (PAK)

Fig. 8. Pancreas graft survival rates (Farney et al., 2000).

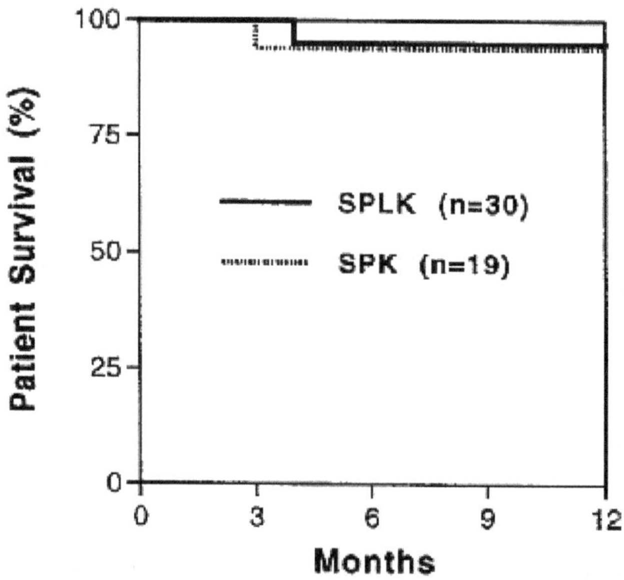

One-year patient survival rates were 95% and 94% for simultaneous cadaver-donor pancreas and living-donor kidney transplant (SPLK) and simultaneous cadaver kidney and pancreas transplant (SPK) recipients. The patient survival rate was 100% in living-donor kidney transplantation alone followed by a solitary cadaver-donor pancreas transplant (PAK) recipients (not shown).

Fig. 9. Patient survival rates (Farney et al., 2000).

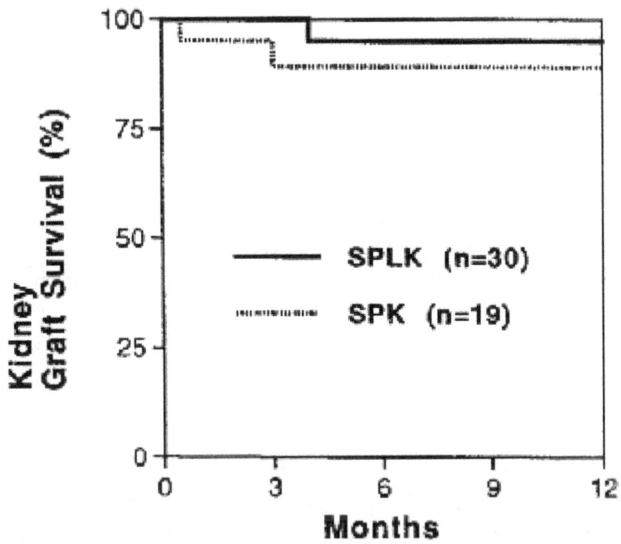

One-year kidney graft survival rates were 95% and 89% for simultaneous cadaver-donor pancreas and living-donor kidney transplant (SPLK) and simultaneous cadaver kidney and pancreas transplant (SPK) recipients. The only SPLK loss was death with function. No living-donor kidney transplantation alone followed by a solitary cadaver-donor pancreas transplant (PAK) kidney grafts were lost (not shown).

Fig. 10. Kidney graft survival rates (Farney et al., 2000).

7. Surgical complications

Despite worldwide growing experience with pancreas transplantation, this procedure is still associated with high incidence of pos-transplant complications; and compared with other solid organ transplants; it has the highest incidence of serious intrabdominal complications and reoperations. We know that up to 50% of pancreas recipients develop pos-transplant complication and around 32% of patients require further surgery to deal with these problems (Troppmann et al., 1998). According the United Network for Organ Sharing report, from 11% to 21% of all pancreas grafts are lost because of surgical complication (Gruessner & Sutherland, 2005).

There are recognised several factors that participate in development of postransplan complications. Diabetes was found to be the strongest independent risk factor. It is well documented that diabetics have significantly higher complication rate compared with non-diabetic population. Also, these patients receive strong immunosuppressive regiment, compared to other solid organ recipients. This makes patients more immunocompromised and vulnerable to infection. Open bowel or bladder, during pancreas implantation is other possible source of abdominal contamination and infection. Furthermore, SPK recipients are compromised by uraemia and PAK recipients are chronically immunosuppressed at the time of transplant. Additional risk factors include: older donors and recipients, long cold ischemia time and high BMI (UNOS & IPTR, 2008).

The most common surgical complication after pancreas transplantation is abdominal infection and graft pancreatitis (38%), followed by pancreas graft thrombosis (27%) and anastomotic leak (9%) (Troppmann et al., 1998).

7.1 Thrombosis

Vascular thrombosis is the second leading cause of pancreas graft failure after rejection. Incidence is reported between 2-20% and it can be either arterial or venous (Gruessner & Sutherland, 2000).

It is well known that pancreas is more susceptible to thrombosis than other organs. Pancreas has naturally low microvascular flow. Removing the spleen from pancreatic graft as a part of the pancreas bench-work, venous flow does reduce even more. The pancreas also requires vascular reconstruction because blood supply to the pancreas is divided during explantation. The donor iliac artery extension "Y" graft is joined to the superior mesenteric artery and the splenic artery to create a single arterial conduit (Fig. 11). The venous extension graft is an additional risk factor causing venous thrombosis. Furthermore, hyper-coagulable status in renal failure patients and endothelial damage are recognised as other negative factors in developing venous thrombosis (Muthusamy et al., 2010).

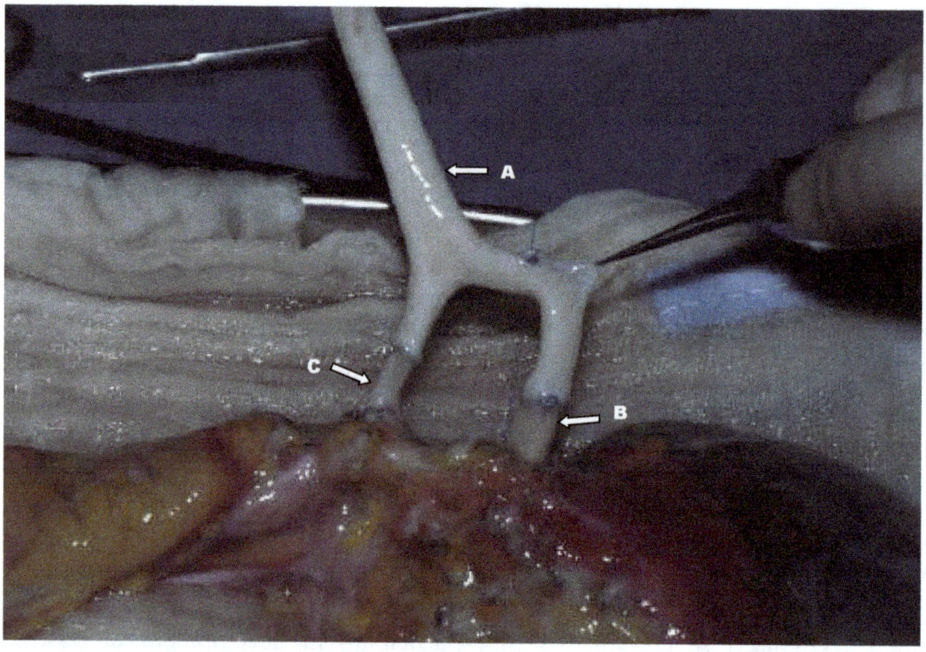

An end-to-end anastomosis between limb of internal iliac artery of the "Y" graft and stump of the splenic artery of the pancreas graft; and limb of external iliac artery and stump of the superior mesenteric artery.
A - "Y"graft, B- superior mesenteric artery, C - splenic artery

Fig. 11. Vascular reconstruction

If venous thrombosis occurs, often a patient develops abdominal pain due to organ swelling with an acute drop of haemoglobin levels. Raising levels of serum glucose are usually late sings of thrombosis. Arterial thrombosis is much less common with a less dramatic clinical picture. In the majority of cases, the pancreas graft is non-salvageable and requires urgent graftectomy. Some data report that in an early stage urgent radiological intervention with thrombectomy or thrombolysis can salvage a pancreas allograft (Stockland et al., 2009) (Fig. 12).

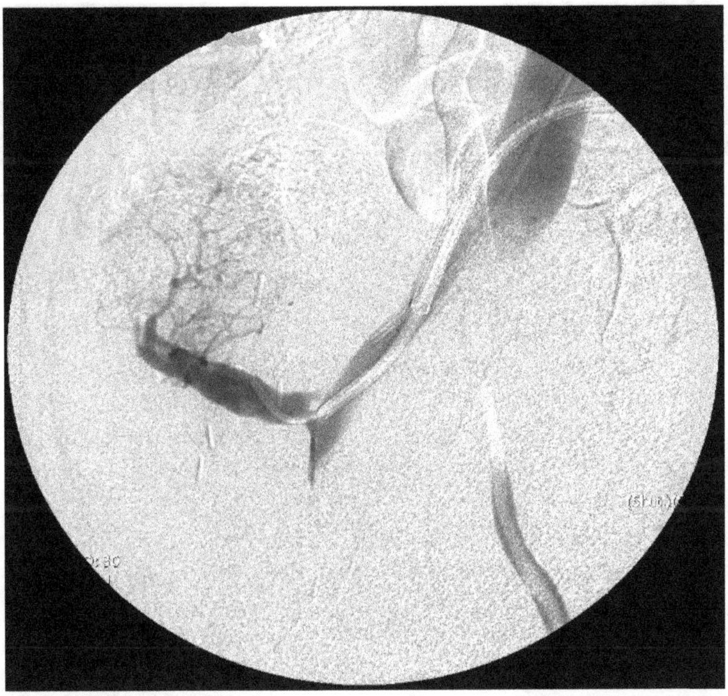

Fig. 12a

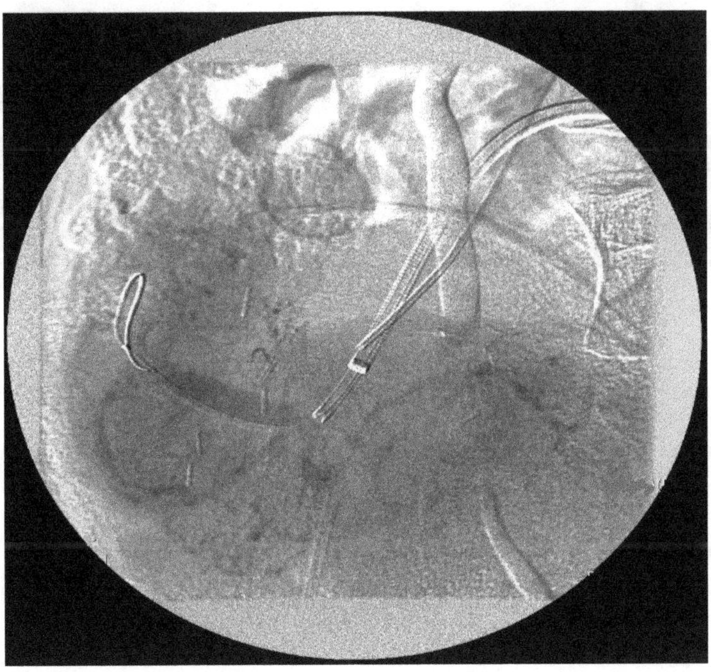

Fig. 12 b

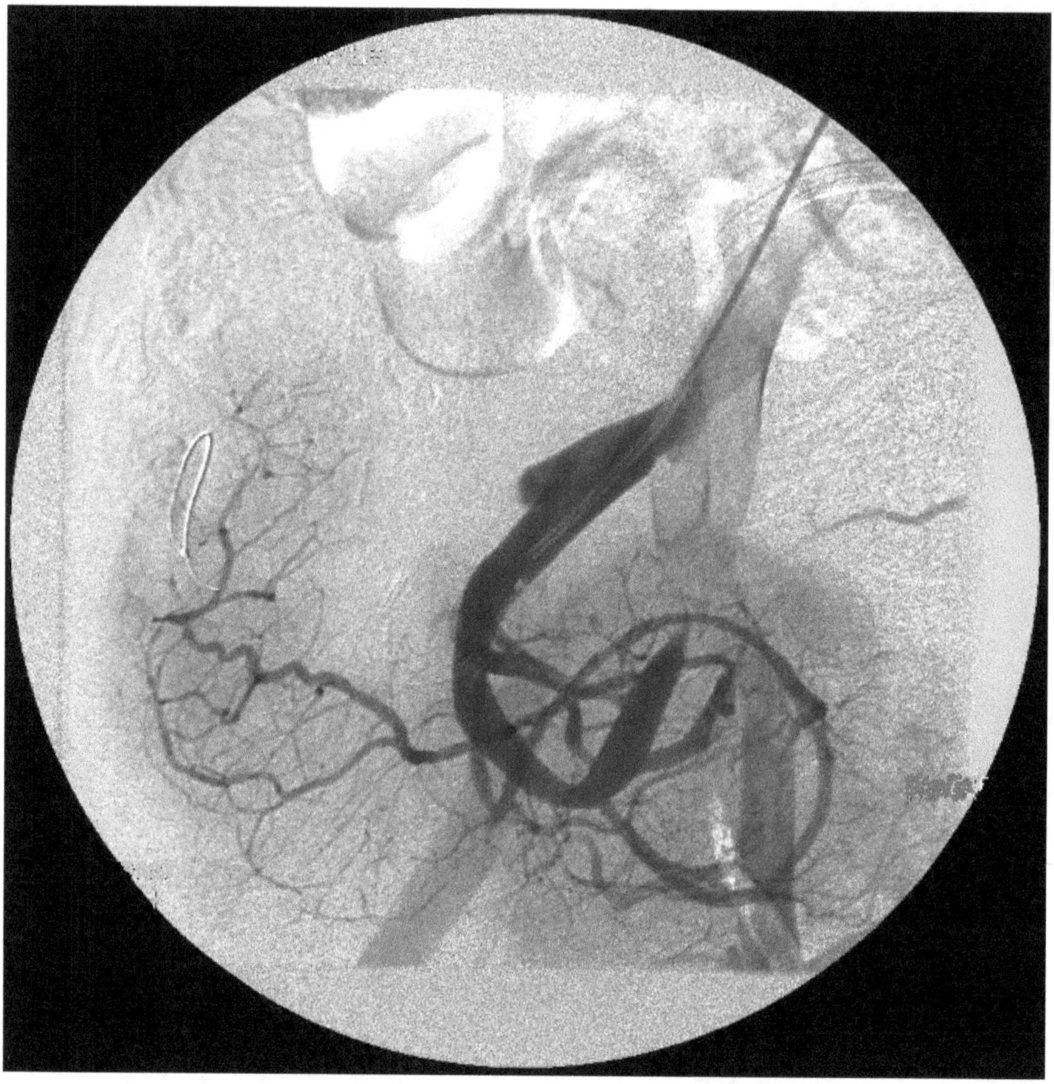

Fig. 12 c

a/ Thrombus in the portal vein of pancreas graft (black arrow points on filling defect, thrombus, in portal vein). A thrombectomy catheter is in the graft's portal vein via right external iliac vein by cannulation right femoral vein.
b/ Status after thrombectomy. Improvement in venous flow and full patency of portal vein without a thrombus.
c/ Normal angiogram of pancreas graft.

Fig. 12. Conventional angiography of pancreas graft.

A key part of the post-operative thrombosis management is prevention, close monitoring, early diagnosis and early intervention, but mainly meticulous vascular reconstruction, bench-work and refine implantation technique. Patients after transplantation receive a high dose of fractionated/continued infusion heparin to develop hypo-coagulable status to reduce clot formation. Sensitive markers for careful coagulation monitoring are APTT ratio (INR) and Thromboelastogram (TEG) (Burke et al., 2004). Several diagnostic methods are recommended for graft monitoring and diagnosis vascular complications: duplex ultrasound, CT-angiography or MR-angiography and formal angiography.

7.2 Bleeding

This vascular complication does mainly occur in combination with intra-abdominal infection or during sever hypo-coagulable status secondary to heparin treatment. Heparin induced bleeding usually has a slow progress and it is often managed conservatively; with antibiotics and blood transfusions. Bleeding secondary to infection is a serious event and it can be life-threatening. Clinical presentation is rapid, sudden hypotension, significant fall of haemoglobin levels and pulsative intra-abdominal mass. In that case urgent laparotomy is vital to control bleeding and abdominal sepsis. At presence of advanced abdominal sepsis or infection involving pancreas graft it is recommended to perform graftectomy to prevent fatal bleeding.

7.3 Pancreatitis

Graft pancreatitis usually occurs instantly after transplant as a result of excessive handling of an organ during retrieval, storage, bench-work and transplantation, as well as a consequence of ischemic-reperfusion injury. Most episodes of pancreatitis resolve uneventfully, however some may lead to secondary complications (fistula, pseudocyst, etc.). Also, Octreotide (synthetic somatostatin analog that inhibits exocrine pancreatic secretion) has been used to prevent and treat some pos-transplant complications (i.e. graft pancreatitis, pancreatic fistula). But data from published studies are controversial with no statistical difference in complication rate between recipients who received octreotide and patient treated by placebo (Stratta et al., 1993).

7.4 Miscellaneous

Other common early surgical complications involve anastomotic leak, pancreatic fistula, intra-abdominal sepsis, ileus, wound infection, etc. They may cause graft lost and recipients' mortality so it is important to actively search for them, to detect them early and to treat them.

8. Immunosuppression

The key role of immunosuppression in transplantation is to minimize graft lost due to rejection. Despite this major benefit, all immunosuppressive medication has some side effects. For that reason, a good immunosuppressive regiment should balance both aspects to deliver the best possible outcomes. The pancreas is a more immunogenic organ than the kidney, and precisely for that reason the majority of immunosuppressive regiments for pancreas transplantation are mainly based on quadruple drug therapy; including antibody agents for induction in combination with calcineurin inhibitors (CNI) and mycophenolate mofetil (MMF) or sirolimus and steroids (Singh & Stratta, 2008).

Initially, the IL-2 receptor antagonists (basiliximab, daclizumab) have been used as induction agents in pancreas transplantation for long period. In the PIVOT Study daclizumab induction was compared to no antibody induction in pancreas transplantation. The results showed that daclizumab significantly reduced the incidence of acute rejection. The 1-year rejection free interval in the daclizumab group was 68% compared to 51% in the non antibody induction group (Stratta et al., 2003). T-cells depleting antibody agents, such as antithymocyte globulin (ATG) and alemtuzumab (Campath), have gained great popularity these days. According to the United Network of Organ Sharing data, this type of induction significantly decreases incidence of immunologically related pancreas graft failure (Gruessner & Sutherland, 2003).

According to a review published in 1999 (Stratta, 1999), a combination of MMF and tacrolimus in primary immunosuppressive regiment resulted in an improved 2-years patient, kidney and pancreas survivals; 97.7%, 93.3% and 90%, respectively.

Lymphocyte-depleting antibody agents in combination with tacrolimus, and MMF or sirolimus, are effective in preventing acute rejection and allow corticosteroids elimination or even full avoidance (Heilman et al., 2010). The principle of the steroid sparing regiment is to avoid steroids related side effects (increased risk of hypertension, glucose intolerance, cholesterol, infection, cardiovascular events, anaemia, osteoporosis, etc.) in pancreas transplant recipients. There is strong evidence that steroid sparing/avoidance regiments are safe and effective with a positive impact on patient and graft survival. Also, we have seen significantly improved the short-term outcomes whereas the long-term outcomes are still insufficient (Mineo et al., 2009).

9. Monitoring pancreas function

The development of surgical techniques and immunosuppressive drugs has significantly improved short-term outcomes of pancreas transplantation (Fig. 13). So these days the main target is to improve long-term results and minimize late graft dysfunction.

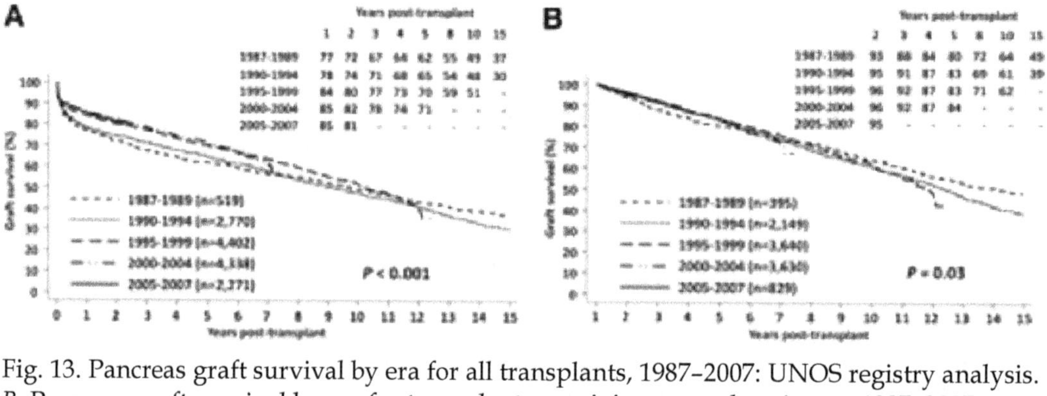

Fig. 13. Pancreas graft survival by era for all transplants, 1987–2007: UNOS registry analysis. *B*: Pancreas graft survival by era for transplants surviving more than 1 year, 1987–2007: UNOS registry analysis (UNOS, 2010).

Immunological graft loss still remains the main cause of graft failure; its rate in 1-year is significantly lower in SPK groups (2%) compared to solitary pancreas transplants (6% for PAK and PTA) (Fig 14) (Gruessner et al., 2008).

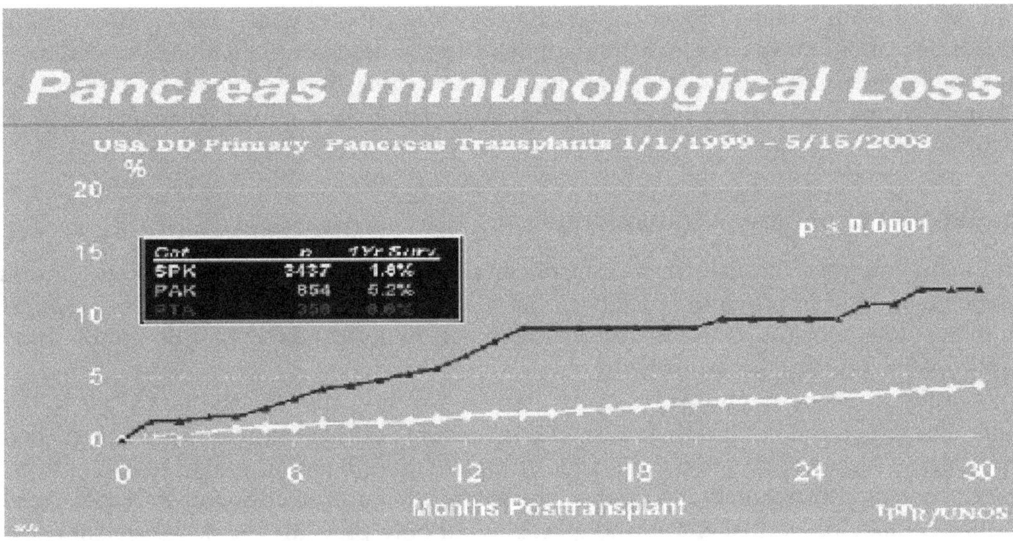

Fig. 14. Pancreas Immunological loss (Waiki et al., 2010).

The incidence of acute rejection is at its highest early after the transplantation. Induction regiments based on antibody depleting agents (i.e. ATG, Campath) delay the repopulation of lymphocytes; so the peak of rejection rate is around six to nine months after transplantation instead of three months as we see in regiments based on IL-2 receptor antagonists induction. A clinical picture of acute rejection is non-characteristic (fever, abdominal pain, ileus, tenderness, diarrhea, haematuria in bladder drained pancreas) or in the majority of cases absent.

Close monitoring of the pancreatic graft is a crucial part of pos-transplant surveillance. Unfortunately, there are not any biomarkers that can sensitively predict rejection yet. For that reason routinely are monitored the levels of fasting blood glucose, fasting C-peptide, HbA1c, serum amylase, serum lipase, oGTT and CRP; but with limited sensitivity and specificity. In SPK patients we do monitor serum creatinine as an indirect marker, too. Also, we know that islet function is resistant to pancreas damage so serum glucose elevation is a late manifestation of pancreas graft dysfunction and predicts poor prognosis; i.e. acute or chronic rejection, pancreatitis, thrombosis, etc.

The bladder-drained pancreas technique gives easy and convenient access to monitor pancreas graft function by measuring urine amylase. A low amylase level is a marker of graft dysfunction (rejection, pancreatitis, etc). Also, cystoscopy enables to perform repeated pancreas graft biopsies with a relatively low risk of complication rate.

The only objective way to diagnose rejection is a histological evaluation of the pancreas graft. Precise diagnoses help to tailor management and subsequently improve graft function. Despite a higher incidence of biopsy related complications pancreas graft biopsy is now widely employed (Gaber, 2007). SPK cases have a high incidence of synchronous pancreas and kidney rejection rate, around 62.5%. Kidney graft biopsy has lower risks of complications compared to pancreas biopsy. Also for that reason, kidney biopsy is routinely employed to diagnose pancreas graft rejection. On the other hand, there is a 25% occurrence of kidney only rejection; that usually correlates with elevation of serum creatinine. In 12.5% cases rejection involves only pancreas without involvement of renal graft (Kitada et al., 2009).

A successful Banff scheme of grading rejection in kidney (Solez et al., 2007) and liver (ICD, 1997) transplantation was subsequently applied in pancreas transplantation, too. On the 9th Banff conference on Allograft Pathology in 2007 (La Coruña, Spain) a final version (Tab. 4,5) of Banff Schema for Grading Pancreas Allograft Rejection was agreed (Drachenberg et al., 2008).

10. Benefits of pancreas transplantation

The main purpose of pancreas transplantation is to achieve eu-glycemia, insulin independence and improve the quality of life in diabetics. A number of studies examined the impact of successful pancreas transplantation also on secondary diabetic complications (nephropathy, retinopathy, neuropathy, etc).

Nephropathy: Diabetic nephropathy has a high recurrence rate, effects almost all kidney grafts and can lead to graft failure. Development of histological sings of diabetic nephropathy is seen within two years after transplantation (Bohman et al., 1984). It has been well documented that functioning pancreatic grafts have a protective role on kidney graft function. Achieving permanent normo-glycemia not only prevents the development of DN but it can also reverse histological lesions characteristic for DN (Fioretto et al., 1998).

Retinopathy: There is good evidence that pancreas transplantation and subsequent normoglycemia stabilizes and even improves retinopathy. However, patients with a high grade of retinal damage before a transplant may get a progression of retinopathy (Königsrainer et al., 1991).

1. Normal. Absent inflammation **or** inactive septal, mononuclear inflammation not involving ducts, veins, arteries or acini. There is no graft sclerosis. The fibrous component is limited to normal septa and its amount is proportional to the size of the enclosed structures (ducts and vessels). The acinar parenchyma shows no signs of atrophy or injury.
2. Indeterminate. Septal inflammation that appears active but the overall features do not fulfill the criteria for mild cell-mediated acute rejection.
3. Cell-mediated rejection
Acute cell-mediated rejection
- Grade I/Mild acute cell-mediated rejection
Active septal inflammation (activated, blastic lymphocytes, ± eosinophils) involving septal structures: venulitis (sub-endothelial accumulation of inflammatory cells and endothelial damage in septal veins, ductitis (epithelial inflammation and damage of ducts).
Neural/peri-neural inflammation.
and/or
Focal acinar inflammation. No more than two inflammatory foci^per lobule with absent or minimal acinar cell injury.
- Grade II/Moderate acute cell-mediated rejection
Multi-focal (but not confluent or diffuse) acinar inflammation (≥3 foci^per lobule) with spotty (individual) acinar cell injury and drop-out.
and/or
Minimal intimal arteritis

- Grade III/Severe acute cell-mediated rejection Diffuse, (widespread, extensive) acinar inflammation with focal or diffuse multi-cellular /confluent acinar cell necrosis. and/or Moderate- or severe-intimal arteritis and/or Transmural inflammation-Necrotizing arteritis Chronic active cell-mediated rejection. Chronic allograft arteriopathy (arterial intimal fibrosis with mononuclear cell infiltration in fibrosis, formation of neo-intima) **4. Antibody-mediated rejection** = C4d positivity[oo] + confirmed donor specific antibodies + graft dysfunction Hyperacute rejection. Immediate graft necrosis (≤1 h) due to preformed antibodies in recipient's blood Accelerated antibody-mediated rejection. Severe, fulminant form of antibody-mediated rejection with morphological similarities to hyperacute rejection but occurring later (within hours or days of transplantation). Acute antibody-mediated rejection. Specify percentage of biopsy surface (focal or diffuse). Associated histological findings: ranging from none to neutrophilic or mononuclear cell margination (capillaritis), thrombosis, vasculitis, parenchymal necrosis. Chronic active antibody-mediated rejection. Features of categories 4 and 5. **5. Chronic allograft rejection/graft sclerosis** - Stage I (mild graft sclerosis) Expansion of fibrous septa; the fibrosis occupies less than 30% of the core surface but the acinar lobules have eroded, irregular contours. The central lobular areas are normal. - Stage II (moderate graft sclerosis) The fibrosis occupies 30–60% of the core surface. The exocrine atrophy affects the majority of the lobules in their periphery (irregular contours) and in their central areas (thin fibrous strands criss-cross between individual acin). - Stage III (severe graft sclerosis) The fibrotic areas predominate and occupy more than 60% of the core surface with only isolated areas of residual acinar tissue and/or islets present. **6. Other histological diagnosis.** Pathological changes not considered to be due acute and/or chronic rejection. e.g. CMV pancreatitis, PTLD, etc.

[a] Categories from 2 to 6 may be diagnosed concurrently and should be listed in the diagnosis in the order of their clinico-pathological significance.

[o] See Table 2 for morphological definition of lesions.

[oo] If there are no donor-specific antibodies or these data are unknown, identification of histological features of antibody-mediated rejection may be diagnosed as 'suspicious for acute antibody- mediated rejection', particularly if there is graft dysfunction

Table 4. Diagnostic categories Banff working grading schema[a/o] (Drachenberg et al., 2008).

Diagnosis	Main histological findings	Clinical presentation
Posttransplant ischemic pancreatitis	Inflammation: neutrophils, foamy macrophages. Location: septal if mild or diffuse if severe Other features: fat necrosis, edema and interstitial hemorrhage. Patchy coagulation necrosis of clusters of acinar cells may be present. No fibrosis, the septa may be expanded due to edema/fat necrosis.	Increase in amylase and lipase in serum. Decrease in urinary amylase.* Hyperglycemia if there is extensive necrosis.
Peripancreatitis/peri - pancreatic fluid collection	Inflammation: mixed (lymphocytes, plasma cells, eosinophils, neutrophils). Location: septa and periphery of lobules Other features: dissecting bundles of active fibroblastic proliferation with obliteration of septal structures, relative preservation of the center of lobules ('cirrhotic appearance')	Local or systemic infectious symptoms, abdominal pain, peri-tonitis. Peripancreatic fluid accumulation.Increase in amylase and lipase in serum.
Cytomegalovirus pancreatitis	Inflammation: mostly mononuclear. Location: septal and acinar, patchy. Other features: cytomegalovirus cytopathic changes in acinar, endothelial or stromal cells.	Increase in serum amylase and lipase. Decrease in urinary amylase.* Systemic symptoms if generalized disease. Other: Duodenal cuff perforation.
Posttransplant lymphoproliferative disorder	Inflammation: ranging from polymorphic with lymphoblasts, plasma cells, eosinophils in low-grade disease, to monomorphic, predominantly lymphoid in high-grade disease (lymphoma). Other features: lymphoid proliferation is nodular, expansive. Necrosis may be present.	Asymptomatic, or increase in serum amylase and lipase. Lymphadenopathy. Tumor mass. May coexist with acute rejection.
Bacterial or fungal infection	Inflammation: variable; acute, chronic, purulent, necrotizing (abscess), granulomatous. Location: random. Other features: same as bacterial and fungal infections in other organs.	Systemic and/or localized infectious symptoms. Peritonitis, duodenal cuff perforation. Increase in serum amylase and lipase.
Recurrent autoimmune disease/diabetes mellitus	Inflammation: islet-centered lymphocytic inflammation (isletitis). No inflammation in late stages after disappearance of beta cells. Other features: immuno-histochemical stains for insulin and glucagon demonstrate absence of insulin producing beta cells in some or all islets depending if early or late disease.	Acute or chronic deterioration in glucose metabolism with increasing need for insulin. Although not pathognomonic, islet cell auto-antibodies typically present (i.e. GAD 65, IA-2, etc.).
Acute calcineurin inhibitor toxicity	Absence of inflammation. Variable degrees of islet cell injury (cytoplasmic swelling, vacuolization, islet cell drop-out. formation of empty spaces (lacunae), apoptotic fragments). Immuno-peroxidase stains: markedly diminished staining for insulin in comparison to controls and to glucagon stain. Electron microscopy: loss of insulin dense core granules with preservation of glucagon dense core granules.	Acute hyperglycemia. High levels of cyclosporine or tacrolimus with return to normoglycemia with adjustment of drug dose or discontinuation.

* In bladder-drained grafts.

Table 5. Pathological changes "other" than rejection in pancreas needle biopsies (Drachenberg et al., 2008).

Neuropathy: Initially after transplantation (SPK) neuropathy improves with correction of uraemia. Several studies reported improvement in motor and sensory nerve functions; confirmed by improved nerve conduction velocity. Less clear is the impact on autonomic function (arrhythmia, postural hypotension, diabetic diarrhoea, gastroparesis, neurogenic bladder, impotence, etc). Some data suggest that patients improve even with these symptoms but it is difficult to quantify (Nusser et al., 1991).

Cardio-vascular disease: Also, the positive impact of functioning pancreas graft on micro-vascular disease and cardiac function is well documented. This involve improvement in ventricular ejection function, reversal of diastolic function, and improved endothelial function.

Quality of Life: The main benefit of pancreas transplantation is the improved patients' quality of life. Sureshkumar, in his study (Sureshkumar et al., 2006), used three quality of life questionnaires (Diabetes Quality of Life Questionnaire, Medical Outcomes Questionnaire and Quality of Well-being Questionnaire) to compare outcomes of diabetics after SPK with patients on the Waiting List. He reports that SPK groups showed better diabetes-related quality of life.

Patient Survival: Results of SPK suggests that this group of patients do better over diabetics receiving cadaveric kidney transplants but there are no survival benefits compared to LRD recipients. The same study concludes that pancreas transplantation is not only life enhancing but also a life saving procedure (Reddy et al., 2003).

Algorithm of transplant alternatives in diabetics

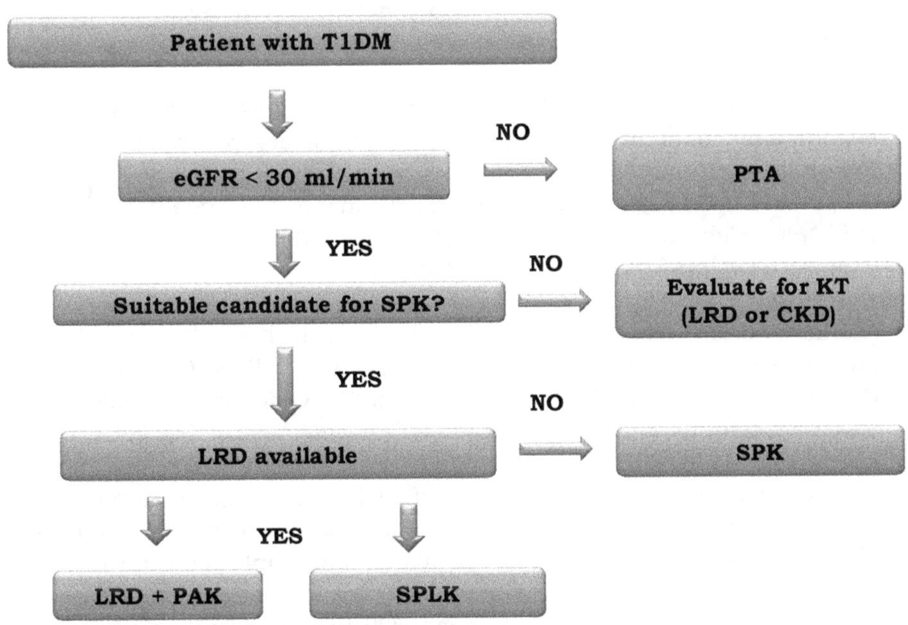

T1DM - type-1 diabetes mellitus, KT - kidney transplant, LRD - living related donor, CKD - cadaver kidney donor

Fig. 15. Algorithm to choose the best transplant alternatives for diabetics.

11. Summary

The outcomes following pancreas transplantation have significantly improved in the last decade. Careful patient selection, better organ procurement, refinements in surgical technique, new immunosuppressive drug regiments and better graft monitoring have all contributed to excellent outcomes. The available data provides strong evidence that pancreas transplantation not only improves diabetics' quality of life but also improves their medical conditions and prolongs their life expectancy.
Pancreas transplantation has become the option of choice to treat patients with type-1 diabetes. Currently several alternatives for these patients are available. The best option should be selected after careful patient assessment and individually weight pros and cons of each alternative (Fig. 15).

12. References

American Diabetes Association. (1999) Position statement: Diabetic nephropathy. *Diabetes Care*. Vol. 22, Suppl 1, pp. 66-69, ISSN 1935-5548

American Diabetes Association. Diabetes management in correctional institutions. *Diabetes Care*. Vol. 28, Suppl 1, (January 2005), pp. 53-60. ISSN 1935-5548

Bode BW. (2010) Comparison of pharmacokinetic properties, physiochemical stability and pump compatibility of three rapid-acting insulin analogs: aspart, lispro and glulisine. *Endocr Pract*. Vol. 6, (December 2010), pp. 1-36, ISSN 1530-891X

Boggi, U.; Pietrabissa, A.; Vistoli, F.; Del Chiaro, M.; Signori, S.; Coletti, L.; Morelli, L.; Moretto, C.; Barsotti, M.; Marchetti, P.; Del Prato, S.; Rizzo, G.; Mosca, F. Simultaneous pancreas-kidney transplantation is improved by living kidney donation program. *Transplant Proc*. Vol. 36, No. 4, (May 2004), pp. 1061-3, ISSN: 0041-1345

Bohman, S.O.; Wilczezck, H.; Jaremko, G.; Lundreg, G. (1984) Recurerance of diabetic nephropathy in human renal allografts: Preliminary report of a biopsy study. *Transplant proc*. Vol. 16, No. 3, (Jun 1984), pp. 649-53, ISSN 0041-1345

Braga, M.; Ljungqvist, O.; Soeters, P.; Fearon, K.; Weimann, A.; Bozzetti, F.; ESPEN. (2009) ESPEN Guidelines on Parenteral Nutrition: surgery. *Clin Nutr*. Vol. 28, No. 4, (August 2009), pp. 378-86, ISSN 1938-3207

Weimann, A.; Braga, M.; Harsanyi, L.; Laviano, A.; Ljungqvist, O.; Soeters, P.; DGEM (German Society for Nutritional Medicine); Jauch, K.W.; Kemen, M.; Hiesmayr, J.M.; Horbach, T.; Kuse, E.R.; Vestweber, K.H.; ESPEN (European Society for Parenteral and Enteral Nutrition). (2006) ESPEN Guidelines on Enteral Nutrition: Surgery including organ transplantation. *Clin Nutr*. Vol. 25, No. 2, (April 2006), pp. 224-44. ISSN 1938-3207

Burke, G.W. 3rd; Ciancio, G.; Figueiro, J.; Buigas, R.; Olson, L.; Roth, D.; Kupin, W.; Miller, J. Hypercoagulable state associated with kidney-pancreas transplantation. Thromboelastogram-directed anti-coagulation and implications for future therapy. *Clin Transplant*. Vol. 18, No. 4, (August 2004), pp. 423-8, ISSN 1399-0012

Cai, Q.; Serrano. R.; Kalyanasundaram, A.; Shirani. (2010) A preoperative echocardiographic predictive model for assessment of cardiovascular outcome after renal transplantation. *J Am Soc Echocardiogr*. Vol. 23, No. 5, (May 2010), pp. 560-6), ISSN 1532-2114

Calne, R.Y.; Rolles, K.; White, D.J.; et al. (1979) Cyclosporin A initially as the only immunosuppressant in 34 recipients of cadaveric organs: 32 kidneys, 2 pancreases, and 2 livers. *Lancet*. Vol. 314, No. 8151, (November 1979), pp. 1033-1036, ISSN 0140-6736.

Cecka, J.M. (1996) The UNOS Scientific Renal Transplant Registry. In: Clinical Transplants. Cecka, M.J.; Terasaki, P.I. eds. 1-14, UCLA Tissue Typing Laboratory, ISBN 0-7216-0409-9., Los Angeles, US

Cheung, CY., Cha, YH, Chan, HW., Chau, KF., Li CS. (2010) Optimal body mass index that can predict long term graft outcome in Asian renal transplant patients. *Nephrology*. Vol. 15, No. 2, (March 2010), pp. 359-65, ISSN 1533-3450

Collins, A.J.; Foley, R.; Herzog, C.; Chavers, B.; Gilbertson, D.; Ishani, A.; Kasiske, B.; Liu, J.; Mau, L.W.; McBean, M.; Murray, A.; St Peter, W.; Xue, J.; Fan, Q.; Guo, H.; Li, Q.; Li, S.; Li, S.; Peng, Y.; Qiu, Y.; Roberts, T.; Skeans, M.; Snyder, J.; Solid, C.; Wang, C.; Weinhandl, E.; Zaun, D.; Zhang, R.; Arko, C.; Chen, S.C.; Dalleska, F.; Daniels, F.; Dunning, S.; Ebben, J.; Frazier, E.; Hanzlik, C.; Johnson, R.; Sheets, D.; Wang, X.; Forrest, B.; Constantini, E.; Everson, S.; Eggers, P.; Agodoa, L.. Excerpts from the United States Renal Data System 2007 annual data report. Am J Kidney Dis. Vol. 51, Supplement 1, (January 2008), pp. 1-320

Corry RJ. Pancreatico-duodenal transplantation with urinary tract drainage. (1988) In: Groth, C.G., ed. Pancreatic Transplantation. 131-146, WB Saunders Company, ISBN 0. 7216 1614 3, Philadelphia, PA

Deferrari, G.; Repetto, M.; Calvi, C.; Ciabattoni, M.; Rossi, C.; Robaudo, C. (1998) Diabetic nephropathy: from micro- to macroalbuminuria. *Nephrol Dial Transplant*. Vol. 13, Suppl 8, (December 1998), pp. 11-15, ISSN 0931-0509

DiLandro, D.; Catalano, C.; Lambertini, D.; Bordin, V.; Fabbian, F.; Naso, A.; Romagnoli, G. (1998) The effect of metabolic control on development and progression of diabetic nephropathy. *Nephrol Dial Transplant*. Vol. 13, Suppl. 8, (1998), pp.35-43, ISSN 1460-2385

Document. (1997) Banff schema for grading liver allograft rejection. An international consensus document. *Hepatology*. Vol. 25, No. 3, (March 1997), pp. 658–663, ISSN 1527-3350

Drachenberg, C.B.; Odorico, J.; Demetris, A.J.; Arend, L.; Bajema, I.M.; Bruijn, J.A.; Cantarovich, D.; Cathro, H.P.; Chapman, J.; Dimosthenous, K.; Fyfe-Kirschner, B.; Gaber, L.; Gaber, O.; Goldberg, J.; Honsová, E.; Iskandar, S.S.; Klassen, D.K.; Nankivell, B.; Papadimitriou, J.C.; Racusen, L.C.; Randhawa, P.; Reinholt, F.P.; Renaudin, K.; Revelo, P.P.; Ruiz, P.; Torrealba, J.R.; Vazquez-Martul, E.; Voska, L.; Stratta, R.; Bartlett, S.T.; Sutherland, D.E. (2008) Banff schema for grading pancreas allograft rejection: working proposal by a multi-disciplinary international consensus panel. *Am J Transplant*. Vol. 8, No. 6, (April 2008), pp. 1237-49, ISSN 1600-6143

Farney, A.C.; Cho, E.; Schweitzer, E.J.; Dunkin, B.; Philosophe, B.; Colonna, J.; Jacobs, S.; Jarrell, B.; Flowers, J.L.; Bartlett, S.T. (2000) Simultaneous cadaver pancreas living-donor kidney transplantation: a new approach for the type 1 diabetic uremic patient Ann Surg. Vol. 232, No. 5, (November 2000), pp. 696-703, ISSN 1528-1140

Fioretto, P.; Steffes, M.W.; Sutherland, D.E.; Goetz, F.C.; Mauer, M. (1998) Reversal of lesions of diabetic nephropathy after pancreas transplantation. *N Engl J Med.* Vol. 339, No. 2, (Jul 1998), pp. 69-75. ISSN 1533-4406

Gaber, L.W. (2007) Pancreas allograft biopsies in the management of pancreas transplant recipients: histopathologic review and clinical correlations. Vol. 131, No. 8, (August 2007), pp. 1192-9, ISSN 1543-2165

Ganesh, SK., Stack, AG., Levin, N., Hulbert-Shearon, T., Part, F. (2001) Association of elevated serum phosphate, calcium x phosphate product and parathyroid hormone with cardiac mortality risk in chronic haemodialysis patients. *Journal of American society of nephrology.* Vol. 12, No. 10, (October 2001), pp. 2131-2138, ISSN 1533-3450

González-Posada, J.M.; Marrero, D.; Hernández, D.; Coll, E.; Tamajón, L.P.; Gutiérrez, P.; Martín, E.; Bravo, A.; Alarcó, A.; Matesanz, R. (2009) Pancreas transplantation: differences in activity between Europe and the United States. Nephrol *Dial Transplant.* Vol. 25, No. 3, (March 2010), pp. 952-9, ISSN 1460-2385

Gruessner, A.C.; Sutherland, D.E.R. Pancreas transplant outcomes from United States (US) cases reported to the United Network for Organ Sharing (UNOS) and non-US cases reported to the International Pancreas Transplant Registry (IPTR) as of October, 2000. In: Cecka JM, Terasaki PI, eds. Clinical Transplants. 45-72, UCLA Immunogenetics Center, ISBN 0965952207 Los Angeles, US

Gruessner, A.C.; Sutherland, D.E. (2005) Pancreas transplant outcomes for United States (US) and non-US cases as reported to the United Network for Organ Sharing (UNOS) and the International Pancreas Transplant Registry (IPTR) as of June 2004. *Clin Transplant.* . 19, No. 4, (August 2005), pp. 433-55, ISSN 1399-0012

Gruessner, A.C.; Sutherland, D.E. (2008) Pancreas transplant outcomes for United States (US) cases as reported to the United Network for Organ Sharing (UNOS) and the International Pancreas Transplant Registry (IPTR). *Clin Transpl.* Vol. 22, No.1, (January-February 2008), pp. 45-56, ISSN 0902-0063.

Grundy, S.M.; Benjamin, T.J.; Burke, G.L. et al. (1999) Diabetes and cardiovascular disease: a statement for healthcare professionals from the American Heart Association. *Circulation.* Vol. 100, No. 10, (September 1999), pp 1134-46, ISSN 0009-7322

Gu, Y.; Li, J.; Li, N. Insulin sensitivity after pancreaticoduodenal transplantation with systemic and portal venous drainage in inbred rats. *Chin Med J.* Vol. 115, No. 4, (April 2002), pp. 549-51, ISSN 0021-9738

Heilman, R.L.; Mazur, M.J.; Reddy, K.S. (2010) Immunosuppression in simultaneous pancreas-kidney transplantation: progress to date. *Drugs.* Vol. 70, No. 7, (May 2010), pp. 793-804, ISSN 0012-6667.

Herzog, C.A.; Marwick, T.H.; Pheley, A.M.; White, C.W.; Rao, V.K., Dick. C.D. Dobutamine stress echocardiography for the detection of significant coronary artery disease in renal transplant candidates. *Am J Kidney Dis.* Vol. 33, No. 6, (Jun 1999), pp. 1080-90, ISSN 0272-6386

Hoogeveen, E.K.; Aalten, J.; Rothman, K.; Roodnat, J.; Mallet, M.; Borm, G.; Weimer, W.; Haitsman, A.; de Fijter, J. (2011) Effect of obesity on the outcome of kidney transplant: A 20 year follow up. *Transplantation.* Published ahead of print, ISSN 1534-0608

Jiménez-Romero, C.; Manrique, A.; Morales, J.M.; López, R.M.; Morales, E.; Cambra, F.; Calvo, J.; García-Sesma, A.; Praga, M.; Moreno, E. (2009) Conversion from bladder to enteric drainage for complications after pancreas transplantation. *Transplant Proc.* Jul-Aug;Vol. 41, No. 6, (Jul-August 2009), pp. 2469-71, ISSN 0041-1345

Kashyap, P., Farrugia, G. (2010) Diabetic gastroperesis: what we have learned and had to unlearn in the past 5 years. *Gut.* Vol. 59, No. 12, (December 2010), pp. 1716-26, ISSN 1468-3288

Kelly, W.D.; Lillehei, R.C.; Merkel, F.K.; Idezuki, Y.; Goetz, F.C. (1967). Allotransplantation of the pancreas and duodenum along with the kidney in diabetic nephropathy. *Surgery.* Vol. 61, No. 6, (Jun 1967), pp. 827–37, ISSN 0002-9610

Kertes, PJ.; Johnson, TM. (Eds.) (2007). *Evidence Based Eye Care.*, Lippincott Williams & Wilkins. ISBN 0-7817-6964-7. Philadelphia, Ph

Kitada, H.; Sugitani, A.; Okabe, Y.; Doi, A.; Nishiki, T.; Miura, Y.; Kurihara, K.; Tanaka, M. (2009) Availability of pancreatic allograft biopsies via a laparotomy. *Transplant Proc.* Vol. 41, No. 10, (December 2009), pp. 4274-6, ISSN 0041-1345

Kleinclauss, F.; Fauda, M.; Sutherland, D.E.; Kleinclauss, C.; Gruessner, R.W.; Matas, A.J.; Kasiske, B.L.; Humar, A.; Kandaswamy, R.; Kaul, S.; Gruessner, A.C. (2009) Pancreas after living donor kidney transplants in diabetic patients: impact on long-term kidney graft function. *Clin Transplant.* Vol. 23, No. 4, (August-September 2009), pp. 437-46, ISSN 1399-0012

Königsrainer, A; Miller, K.; Steurer, W.; Kieselbach, G.; Aichberger, C.; Ofner, D.; Margreiter, R. (1991) Does pancreas transplantation influence the course of diabetic retinopathy? Diabetologia. Vol. 34, Suppl. 1, (Augusta 191), pp. 86-88, ISSN 1432-0428

Kuo, HT., Sampaio, MS., Vincenti, F., Bunnapradist, S. (2010) Association of post transplant diabetes mellitus, new onset diabetes after transplantation and acute rejection with transplant outcomes: an analysis of the organ procurement and transplant network/united network for organ sharing (OPTN/UNOS) database. *American Journal of Kidney Disease.* Vol. 56, No. 6, (December 2010), pp. 1127-39, ISSN 0272-6386

Larson, T.S.; Bohorquez, H.; Rea, D.J.; Nyberg, S.L.; Prieto, M.; Sterioff, S.; Textor, S.C.; Schwab, T.R.; Griffin, M.D.; Gloor, J.M.; Kudva, Y.C.; Kremers, W.K.; Stegall, M.D. (2004) Pancreas-after-kidney transplantation: an increasingly attractive alternative to simultaneous pancreas-kidney transplantation. *Transplantation.* Vol. 77, No. 6, (March 2004) pp. 838-43. ISSN 1534-0608

Lentine, K.L.; Hurst, F.P.; Jindal, R.M.; Villines, T.C.; Kunz, J.S.; Yuan, C.M.; Hauptman, P.J.; Abbott, K.C. (2010) Cardiovascular risk assessment among potential kidney transplant candidates: approaches and controversies. *Am J Kidney Dis.* Vol. 55, No. 1, (January 2010), pp. 152-67, ISSN 1523-6838

Lillehei, R.C.; Simmons, R.L.; Najarian, J.S.; Weil, R.; Uchida, H; Ruiz, J.O.; Kjellstrand, C.M.; Goetz, F.C. Pancreatico-duodenal allotransplantation: experimental and clinical experience. *Ann Surg.* Vol. 172, No. 3, (September 1970) , pp. 405-36, ISSN 1528-1140

Lo, A.; Stratta, R.J.; Hathaway, D.K.; Egidi, M.F.; Shokouh-Amiri, M.H.; Grewal, H.P., Winsett, R.; Trofe, J.; Alloway, R.R.; Gaber, A.O. (2001)Long-term outcomes in simultaneous kidney-pancreas transplant recipients with portal-enteric versus systemic-bladder drainage. *Transplant Proc.* Vol.33, No. 1-2, (February-March 2001), pp. 1684-6, ISSN 0041-1345

MacLeod, M.; McLay, J. Drug treatment of hypertension complicating diabetes mellitus. *Drugs*. Vol. 56, No. 2, (1998), pp. 189-202, ISSN 0012-6667

Matthew, D.D.; Thymothy, S.K.; Lawrence, I.R. (1997) Diabetic Retinopathy, In: Alberti, K.G.M.M.; Zimmet, P.; DeFronzo, R.A.; Keen, H. *International Textbook of Diabetes mellitus*, second edition, vol2, 1441-1446, John Wiley and Son, ISBN 0471939307, Canada

Meier-Kriesche, H.U., Arndarfer, J.A., Kaplan, B. (2002) The impact of BMI on renal transplant outcomes: A significant rick factor for graft failure and patient death. *Transplantation*. Vol. 73, No. 1, (January 2002), pp. 70-4, ISSN 1534-0608

Mineo, D.; Sageshima, J.; Burke, G.W.; Ricordi, C. (2008) Minimization and withdrawal of steroids in pancreas and islet transplantation. *Transpl Int*. Vol. 22, No. 1, (January 2009), pp. 20-37. ISSN 1432-2277.

Muthusamy, A.S.R.; Giangrande, P.L.F.; Friend, P.J. (2010) Pancreas Allograft Thrombosis. *Transplantation*. Vol. 90, No. 7, (October 2010), pp. 705-707, ISSN 1534-0608.

National Institutes of Health, National Institute of Diabetes, Digestive, and Kidney Diseases. United States Renal Data Systems. Digestive and Kidney Diseases. (April 1998), ISSN 1533-3450

http://www.usrds.org/download/1998/ch07.pdf

Noori, N., Kalantar-Zadeh, K., Kavesdy, CP., Murali, SB., Bross, R., Nissenson, AR., Kapple, JD. (2010) Dietary potassium intake and mortality in long term haemodialysis patients. *American Journal of Kidney Disease*. Vol. 56, No. 2, (August 2010), pp. 338-47, ISSN 0272-6386

Nusser, J.; Scheuer, R.; Abendroth, D.; Illner, W.D.; Land, W.; Landgraf, R. (1991) Effect of pancreatic and/or renal transplantation on diabetic autonomic neuropathy. *Diabetologia*. Vol. 34, Suppl. 1, (August 1991), pp. 118-20, ISSN 1432-0428.

Ojo, A.O.; Meier-Kriesche, H.U.; Hanson, J.A.; Leichtman, A.; Magee, J.C.; Cibrikm, D.; Wolfe, R.A.; Port, F.K.; Agodoa, L.; Kaufman, D.B.; Kaplan, B. (2001) The impact of simultaneous pancreas-kidney transplantation on long-term patient survival. *Transplantation*. Vol. 71, No. 1, (January 2001), pp. 82-90, ISSN 1534-0608

Orlando, G.; Stratta, R.J.; Light, J. (2010) Pancreas transplantation for type 2 diabetes mellitus. *Curr Opin Organ Tranplsnt*. Vol. No. , (December 2010), pp. ISSN 1531-7013

Pommipanit, N.; Sampaio, M.S.; Cho, Y.; Young, B.; Shah, T.; Pham, P.T.; Wilkinson, A.; Danovitch, G.; Bunnapradist, S. (2010) Pancreas after living donor kidney versus simultaneous pancreas-kidney transplant: an analysis of the organ procurement transplant network/united network of organ sharing database. *Transplantation*. Vol. 89, No. 12, (Jun 2010), pp. 1496-503, ISSN 1534-0608.

Rabbat, C.G.; Treleaven, D.J.; Russell, J.D.; Ludwin, D. Cook, D.J. (2003) Prognostic value of myocardial perfusion studies in patients with end-stage renal disease assessed for kidney or kidney-pancreas transplantation: a meta-analysis. J Am Soc Nephrol. Vol. 14, No. 2, (February 2003), pp. 431-9, ISSN 1533-3450

Radziuk, J.; Barron, P.; Najm, H.; Davies, K. (1993) The effect of systemic venous drainage of the pancreas on insulin sensitivity in dogs. *J Clin Invest*. Vol. 92, No. 4, (October 1993), pp. 1713-21, ISSN 0021-9738

Rayhill, S.C.; D'Alessandro, A.M.; Odorico, J.S.; Knechtle, S.J.; Pirsch, J.D.; Heisey, D.M.; Kirk, A.D.; Van der Werf, W.; Sollinger, H.W. (2000) Simultaneous pancreas-kidney transplantation and living related donor renal transplantation in patients with diabetes: is there a difference in survival? *Ann Surg*. Vol. 231, No. 3, (March 2000), pp. 417-23. ISSN 1528-1140.

Reddy, K.S.; Stablein, D.; Taranto, S.; Stratta, R.J.; Johnston, T.D.; Waid, T.H.; McKeown, J.W.; Lucas, B.A.; Ranjan, D. (2003) Long-term survival following simultaneous kidney-pancreas transplantation versus kidney transplantation alone in patients with type 1 diabetes mellitus and renal failure. *Am J Kidney Dis*. Vol. 41, No. 2, (February 2003), pp. 464-70, ISSN 0272-6386

Reddy, S., Ramsubeik, K., Vega, K., Frederico J., Palacio, C. (2010) Do HbA1c levels correlate with delayed gastric emptying in diabetic patients? *Journal of Neurogastroenterology and motility*. Vol. 16, No. 4, (October 2010), pp. 414-7, ISSN 1365-2982

Sato, H., Carvalho, G., Sato, T., Lattermann, R., Matsukawa, T., Schricker, T. (2010) The Association of preoperative glycaemic control, Intraoperative insulin sensitivity & outcomes after cardiac surgery. *Journal of Clinical Endocrinology & Metabolism*. Vol. 95, No. 9, (September 2010), pp. 4338-4344, ISSN 0021972X

Singh, R.P.; Stratta, R.J. (2008) Advances in immunosuppression for pancreas transplantation. *Curr Opin Organ Transplant*. Vol 13, No. 1, (February 2008), pp. 79-84, ISSN: 1531-7013.

Solez, K.; Colvin, RB.; Racusen, L.C. et al. (2007) Banff '05 Meeting Report: Differential diagnosis of chronic allograft injury and elimination of chronic allograft nephropathy ('CAN'). *Am J Transplant*. Vol. 7, No. 3, (March 2007), pp. 518–526. ISSN 1600-6143

Sollinger, H.W.; Belzer, F.O. Pancreas transplantation with urinary tract drainage. (1988) In: Groth, C.G., ed. Pancreatic Transplantation. 131-146, WB Saunders Company, ISBN 0. 7216 1614 3, Philadelphia, PA

Starzl, T.E.; Tzakis, A.G. (1988) Pancreatico-duodenal transplantation with enteric exocrine drainage. In: Groth CG, ed. Pancreatic Transplantation, (Ed.). pp. 119-129, WB Saunders Company, ISBN 0. 7216 1614 3 ,Philadelphia, PA

Stephanian, E.; Gruessner, R.W.; Brayman, K.L.; Gores, P.; Dunn, D.L.; Najarian, J.S.; Sutherland D.E. (1992) Conversion of exocrine secretions from bladder to enteric drainage in recipients of whole pancreaticoduodenal transplants. *Ann Surg*. Vol. 216, No. 6, (December 1992), 663-72, ISSN 1528-1140

Stockland, A.H.; Willingham, D.L.; Paz-Fumagalli, R.; Grewal, H.P.; McKinney, J.M.; Hughes, C.B.; Walser, E.M. (2009) Pancreas transplant venous thrombosis: role of endovascular interventions for graft salvage. *Cardiovasc Intervent Radiol*. Vol. 32, No. 2, (March 2009), pp. 279-83, ISSN: 1432-086

Stratta, R.J.; Taylor, R.J.; Lowell, J.A.; et al. (1993) Randomized trial of sandostatin prophylaxis for preservation

injury after pancreas transplantation. *Transplant Proc,* Vol. 25, No. 6, (December 1993), pp. 3190-2, ISSN: 0041-1345.

Stratta, R.J. (1999) Review of immunosuppressive usage in pancreas transplantation. *Clin Transplant*. Vol. 13, No. 1 (February 1999), p. 1-12, ISSN 1399-0012

Stratta, R.J.; Gaber, A.O.; Shokouh-Amiri, M.H. Reddy, K.S; Egidim, M.F.; Grewal, H.P.; Gaber, L.W. (2000) A prospective comparison of systemic-bladder versus portal-enteric drainage in vascularized pancreas transplantation. *Surgery*. Vol. 127, No. 2, pp. 217-26, (February 2000), ISSN 0002-9610

Stratta, R.J.; Alloway, R.R.; Lo, A.; Hodge, E.E. PIVOT Investigators. (2003) One year outcomes in simultaneous kidney-pancreas transplant recipients receiving an alternative regimen of daclizumab. Program and abstracts of American Transplant Congress 2003: The Fourth Joint American Transplant Meeting; May 30-June 4, 2003; Washington, DC. Abstract 662.

Sugitani A, Gritsch HA, Shapiro R, Bonham CA, Egidi MF, Corry RJ. (1998) Surgical complications in 123 consecutive pancreas transplant recipients: comparison of bladder and enteric drainage Transplant Proc. Vol. 30, No. 2, (March 1998), pp. 293-4, ISSN 0041-1345

Sutherland, D.E.R.; Goetz, F.C.; Najarian, J.S. (1988) Experience with single pancreatic transplantation compared with pancreas transplantation after kidney transplantation; and with transplantation with pancreas graft living related compared with cadaveric donors. In: Groth, C.G., ed. Pancreatic Transplantation. 175-189, WB Saunders Company, ISBN 0. 7216 1614 3 Philadelphia, Ph

Sureshkumar, K.K.; Patel, B.M.; Markatos, A.; Nghiem, D.D.; Marcus, R.J. (2006) Quality of life after organ transplantation in type 1 diabetics with end-stage renal disease. *Clin Transplant*. Vol. 20, No. 1, (January-February 2006), pp. 19-25, ISSN 0902-0063

The Diabetes Control and Complications Trial Research Group. (1993) The effect of intensive treatment of diabetes on the development andprogression of long-term complications in insulin-dependent diabetes mellitus. *N Engl J Med*. Vol. 30, No. 27, pp. 977–986, (September 1993), ISSN 1533-4406

Troppmann, C.; Gruessner, A.C.; Dunn, D.L.; Sutherland, D.E.; Gruessner, R.W. (1998) Surgical complications requiring early relaparotomy after pancreas transplantation: a multivariate risk factor and economic impact analysis of the cyclosporine era. *Ann Surg*. Vol. 227, No. 2, (February 1998), pp. 255-68, ISSN: 1528-1140

UK Transplant. September 2003. *National Protocol for assessment of kidney and pancreas transplant patients*. 28 February 2011, Available from: <http://www.uktransplant.org.uk/ukt/about_transplants/organ_allocation/pancreas/assessment_of_kidney_and_pancreas_tx_patients.doc>

United Network for Organ Sharing, 2010. Richmond, VA. Available from http://www.unos.org/Data/. Accessed 16 March 2010

Waki, K.; Terasaki, P.I.; Kadowaki, T. (2010) Long-Term Pancreas Allograft Survival in Simultaneous Pancreas-Kidney Transplantation by Era UNOS registry analysis. *Diabetes Care*. Vol. 33 , No. 8, (August 2010), pp. 1789-1791, ISSN 1935-5548

Ward, J.D. Diabetic Peripheral Neuropathy, In: Alberti, K.G.M.M.; Zimmet, P.; DeFronzo, R.A.; Keen, H. *International Textbook of Diabetes mellitus*, second edition, vol2, 1478-1496, John Wiley and Son, ISBN 0471939307, Canada

Watkins, P.J.; Edmonds, M.E.(1997) Autonomic Neuropathy, In: Alberti, K.G.M.M.; Zimmet, P.; DeFronzo, R.A.; Keen, H. *International Textbook of Diabetes mellitus*, second edition, vol. 2, pp. 1497-1506, John Wiley and Son, ISBN 0471939307, Canada

Watkins, P.J.; (2003) ABC of diabetes: Cardiovascular disease, hypertension, and lipids. *BMJ*. Vol. 326, No. 7405, (Jul 2003), pp. 874 , ISSN 0959-8138

Weimann, A.; Braga, M.; Harsanyi, L.; Laviano, A.; Ljungqvist, O.; Soeters, P.; DGEM (German Society for Nutritional Medicine); Jauch, K.W.; Kemen, M.; Hiesmayr, J.M.; Horbach, T.; Kuse, E.R.; Vestweber, K.H.; ESPEN (European Society for Parenteral and Enteral Nutrition). (2006) ESPEN Guidelines on Enteral Nutrition:

Surgery including organ transplantation. *Clin Nutr.* Vol. 25, No. 2, (April 2006), pp. 224-44. ISSN 1938-3207

Wiesbauer F, Heinze G, Regele H, Hörl WH, Schernthaner GH, Schwarz C, Kainz A, Kramar R, Oberbauer, R. (2010). Glucose control is associated with patient survival in diabetic patients after renal transplantation. *Transplantation,* Vol. 15, No. 5, (March 2010), pp. 612-619, ISSN 1534-0608

Wiseman, A.C. (2010) The role of kidney-pancreas transplantation in diabetic kidney disease. *Curr Diab Rep.* Vol. 10, No. 5, (October 2010), pp. 385-91, ISSN 1539-0829

Wong, T.Y.; Liew, G.; Tapp, R.J. *et al.* (2008). Relation between fasting glucose and retinopathy for diagnosis of diabetes: three population-based cross-sectional studies. *Lancet.* Vol. 371, No. 9614, (March 2008), pp. 736–43, ISSN 1474-547X.

Writing Team for the Diabetes Control and Complications Trial/ Epidemiology of Diabetes Interventions and Complications Research Group. (2003) Sustained effect of intensive treatment of type 1 diabetes mellitus on development and progression of diabetic nephropathy: the Epidemiology of Diabetes Interventions and Complications (EDIC) study. *JAMA* Vol. 22, No. 6, (October 2003), pp. 2159–2167, ISSN 00987484

Young, B.Y.; Gill, J.; Huang, E.; Takemoto, S.K.; Anastasi, B.; Shah, T.; Bunnapradist, S. (2009) Living donor kidney versus simultaneous pancreas-kidney transplant in type I diabetics: an analysis of the OPTN/UNOS database *Clin J Am Soc Nephrol.* Vol. 4, No. 4, (April 2009), pp. 845-52, ISSN 1555-905

5

Pathogenesis and Preventive Strategies of Chronic Dysfunction of Renal Allograft

Wenqian Huo, Keqin Zhang, Chengguo Ge, Gang Wu,
Fengshuo Jin, Gang Yuan and Qiansheng Li
*Department of Urology, Institute of Surgery Research, Daping Hospital,
Third Military Medical University, Chongqing,
China*

1. Introduction

Novel immunosuppressants have decreased the incidence rate of acute rejection significantly, but fail to prevent chronic allograft dysfunction (CAD). Around 40% patients develop CAD gradually in several months or several years after renal transplantation. They present with progressive deterioration of long-term allograft function and allograft failure, and end up with resuming dialysis. It has also been demonstrated that CAD may increase the cardiovascular mortality after renal transplantation. Therefore, it is crucial for promoting long-term allograft survival to investigate the pathogenesis and preventive and therapeutic strategies of CAD. CAD, formerly termed chronic rejection (CR), is also known as late graft loss (LGI) or chronic allograft nephropathy (CAN), since it involves both immune factors (transplantation antigen dependent) and non-immune factors (transplantation antigen independent).

CAD refers to progressive functional impairment of allograft, with pathologic changes including tubular atrophy, interstitial fibrosis, progressive glomerulosclerosis, and arterial fibrous intimal thickening and arteriole hyalinosis. These pathologic changes include immune and non-immune injury to allograft. Chronic rejection is usually associated with acute rejection or subclinical rejection, HLA mismatch, panel reactive antibodies (PRA), and donor specific antibodies (DSA). In contrast, non-immune allograft injury is usually associated with calcineurin inhibitors (CNI), preexisting delayed graft function (DGF), hypertension, hyperlipidemia, proteinuria, viral infection, chronic obstruction and chronic pyelonephritis. In addition, CAD includes recurrent kidney disease, de novo nephritis, posttransplantation lymphoproliferative diseases (PTLD). Many of the above-mentioned factors that lead to CAD usually exist simultaneously; thus, the pathologic manifestations of CAD are complex and not specific, making the treatment of CAD difficult. In short, there are many factors influencing the incidence and development of CAD, and the pathogenesis of CAD remains largely unclear. Microcirculation injury mediated by donor specific antibodies is thought to be the major cause for long-term allograft dysfunction.

2. Risk factors for CAD

2.1 Transplantation antigen dependent risk factors

Epidemiologic study indicated that patients with acute rejection are more likely to develop chronic rejection than those without. The frequency, histologic type and time of onset of acute rejection are closely associated with allograft dysfunction. In particular, frequent and delayed (more than one year) acute rejection is likely to result in allograft dysfunction. Gulanikar et al. reported that the risk for CAD was 9% in patients developing acute rejection once after renal transplantation, was 38% in those developing acute rejection twice, and was 50% in those developing acute rejection thrice, and that early-stage acute vascular rejection was more harmful than acute interstitial rejection. Van et al. reported that the the 5-year kidney survival rates were 34%, 71%, and 74% in patients developing acute vascular rejection, acute interstitial rejection, and without acute rejection in the 3 months after transplantation. It was reported that acute rejection may increase the expression of platelet-derived growth factor (PDGF) and its receptor on arterial smooth muscle cells. PDGF is one of the main stimulators for interstitial cell proliferation in CAD. Hence, PDGF may play a role in acute rejection and CAD.

1. HLA match

Major Histocompability Complex (MHC) mismatch is a crucial risk factor for CAD. The long-term allograft survival rate is the highest for cadaveric renal transplantation with perfect MHC match, and CAD does not occur following homogenic transplantation. Among HLA-A, B, and DR, group A is not so important as groups B and D. Mismatch of both loci of group B is likely to lead to acute rejection and subsequent chronic rejection. In the presence of mismatch of one locus of group B and one locus of group DR, 82% of type I helper T cells proliferate; in the absence of mismatch, only 6% proliferate. Meanwhile, in the presence of mismatch, the release of allogenic antigen peptide increases by 10 folds. The long-term allograft survival rates differ significantly with different number of mismatching MHC sites, suggesting the importance of transplantation antigen dependent factors in the development of CAD.

2. Antibodies

The main mechanism for CAD is believed to relate to allograft stimulated production of anti-donor specific circulating antibodies. As currently available immunosuppressants mainly suppress T cells, antibodies might be a main factor for chronic rejection. In chronic allograft rejection, there are many antibody-secreting plasma cells in the kidney, and these antibodies are against mesenterial cells, focal adhesion plaques, molecules synthesized and secreted by activated mesenterial cells or basement membrane antigen. Interfering recombination activation gene 2(RAG-2) will lead to T and B cell defect, and immunoglobin transmembrane domain-encoding gene defect will preclude the production of mature B cells and antibodies. In both cases, allograft atherosclerosis will not occur. In addition, macrophage dysfunction and defect of MHC class II antigen mitigate atherosclerosis, and defects of MHC class I antigen, CD8 positive cells and NK cells exacerbate atherosclerosis.

Hypersensitivity to panel reactive antibodies (PRA) correlates highly to acute rejection. PRA or the reaction rate of donor lymphocytes to recipient serum is frequently used to predict the risk for acute rejection. Preoperative PRA being more than 10% correlates significantly to the three-year allograft survival rate. Anti-lymphocyte antibody was detected in 28.2% patients with chronic rejection, and of them, 57% were found to have anti-HLA antibody. In vitro study confirmed that monoclonal antibody against type I HLA molecule induced the expression of fibroblast growth factors receptor on endothelial cells and smooth muscle cells. Allogenic antibodies exhibit the same effect, and they promote glomerulosclerosis and fibrosis. Antibodies against occult epitopes may cause chronic damage, and elevated levels of antibodies against molecules contributing to tissue injury will lead to excessive fibrosis during tissue repair.

3. TGF-β1 pathway

It was demonstrated that molecules recognized by antibodies following transplantation, biglycans and modified molecules also bind to TGF-β1. TGF-β1 is the main cytokine regulating CAD fibrosis. Sharma et al. reported that TGF-β1 mRNA expression correlates significantly to kidney allograft interstitial fibrosis and CAD. Angiotensin II receptor antagonists were shown to reduce plasma TGF-β1 level by 50%, suggesting the potential of angiotensin II receptor antagonists to prevent CAD. Meanwhile, urine TGF-β1 secretion is obviously higher in CAD patients than in patients with stable renal function.

2.2 Transplantation antigen independent risk factors

Non-immune factors and multiple risk factors jointly lead to chronic rejection-like changes of allograft. Rats survived for long term following homogenic renal transplantation. In case of renal function damage, macrophage infiltration and cytokine upregulation were observed in the allograft, just like chronic rejection changes following allogenic renal transplantation. After an allograft with functional impairment was transplanted back into the donor, early-stage renal damage may restore normal, but late-stage damage will continue to deteriorate, demonstrating that early-stage chronic rejection depends on allogenic antigens and is reversible, while late-stage injury does not depend on allogenic antigens and is irreversible.

1. Early-stage ischemia /reperfusion injury

Renal allografts will undergo a series of ischemic events during organ harvesting, preservation, and transplantation. The longer the ischemia time, the more serious the reperfusion related injury. During 2- 5 d of ischemia/reperfusion injury, the expression of leukocyte and endothelial cell adhesion molecules, endothelin, MHC class II molecules, interferin γ and TNF-α is upregulated in kidney tissue, which is complicated by increased oxyradical production and T cells and macrophages in the allograft. Connolly et al. reported that prolonged cold ischemia affected the short-term and long-term survival of cadaveric renal allograft adversely, and that the benefit of HLA match for allograft survival was offset by prolonged cold ischemia. Ischemia /reperfusion injury damages the kidney through the following mechanisms: ① microcirculation disturbance, early-stage renal function loss or delayed renal function, tubular necrosis, TGF-p increase, interstitial fibrosis; ② oxyradical caused acute vascular endothelial cell injury and arterial sclerosis; ③ activation of T lymphocytes, causing subclinical immune reaction, arteritis, nephron reduction, monocyte/macrophage infiltration and interstitial fibrosis.

2. Cytomegalovirus

CMV infection of allograft endothelial cells will lead to chronic rejection quickly. CMV may enhance MHC expression, which leads to the production of anti-endothelial cell antibody and endothelial cell damage. In clinical practice, if acute rejection is refractory to immunosuppressants, and if there are a number of memory CD8+T cells in peripheral blood and evidence of asymptomatic CMV infection, anti-CMV treatment is usually effective to improve renal function. The mechanism is as follows: the immediate early gene of CMV encodes homologous protein, which cross-reacts to HLA-DR-β chain, thus enhancing the recipient's immune reaction to donor antigens. CMV encodes a glycoprotein, which is homologous to the heavy chain of MHC class I antigen and can react to the light chain of MHC class I antigen. Active CMV infection, along with VCAM-1 expression enhancement and leukocyte adhesion and infiltration on capillary endothelial cells will influence allograft function for long term. In addition, in CMV infection, inflammatory cytokines aggavate endothelial cell damage and vascular pathologic changes.

3. Drug toxicity

Cyclosporin (CsA) and Tacrolimus (FK-506) are both CNI-type immunosuppressants. When they relieve early-stage acute rejection significantly, CNI induced long-term kidney toxicity may be an important cause for accelerating CAD progress. As a result, the long-term survival of allograft may decrease. Chronic nephrotoxicity of CNI is characterized by interstitial fibrosis, hyalinization of small artery and tubular vacuolar degeneration in the kidney. The causes of nephrotoxicity include kidney vasospasm, release of endothelin–β, and excessive expression of transforming growth factor-β (TGF-β) and vascular endothelial growth factor (VEGF). It has been demonstrated recently that allograft function may be protected and allograft survival be prolonged by early reduction or withdrawal of CNIs and administration of Sirolimus (SRL) following renal transplantation, without the risk of increasing acute rejection (AR). In addition, the combination of nephrotoxicity-free immunosuppressants, e.g., SRL and Mycophenolate mofetil helps to delay the incidence of CAD.

4. Nephron reduction

Nephron reduction due to various causes leads to glomerular hyperfiltration, early-stage compensated glomerular hypertrophy and increased exudation, kidney dysmetabolism, and allograft failure. Nephron reduction may be associated with the following factors: ① donor/recipient mismatch of body size, or inappropriate ratio of kidney weight /body weight. For instance, an allograft from a donor weighing 50kg is transplanted into a recipients weighing more than 90kg, which means nephron reduction and may result in renal functional impairment; ② the donor is too young (less than three years) or too old (more than 60 years). If the donor is too young, the nephron is immature and cannot tolerate the perfusion pressure for adult kidneys. If the donor is too old, there may be vascular sclerosis and nephron reduction in the kidney; ③ sex difference. The three-year survival rate of allografts from female donors is 5% lower than from male donors.

5. Hyperlipidemia

Food rich in cholesterol and hyperlipidemia synergize in kidney injury, and they change macrophage function, and lead to secretion of vasoactive substances and cell proliferation, thus aggravating kidney damage. Controlled intake of protein can temporarily stabilize allograft function in patients with chronic rejection. Cholesterol-rich apoprotein B and triglyceride are independent risk factors for chronic rejection, and they induce arterial sclerosis and enhance oxidization. Oxidized low-density lipoprotein may lead to proliferation and migration of smooth muscle cells and aggravate vasculopathy.

6. Other risk factors

The following factors are shown to associate with chronic rejection: ① blood pressure elevation is associated with allograft failure. However, which occurs first is still unclear; ② smoking may promote allograft vasculopathy and CAD. Little investigational work has been done in this regard; ③ epidemiologic survey has revealed that continuous proteinuria occurs in approximately 20% of patients following transplantation, and two thirds of these patients suffer from CAD. Chronic allograft damage resulting from proteinuria is an important risk factor for CAD, possibly because of persistent protein loss, failure of epithelial cell repair, and epithelial atrophy and secondary tissue fibrosis.

3. Pathologic classification of CAD

Allograft fibrosis and sclerosis are main pathologic changes in CAD, which can be observed in any anatomical structures of allograft. There may also be progressive proliferation and focal sclerosis of glomerular matrix, and intimal thickening of small artery and capillary in the kidney due to fibrosis and hyaline substance aggregation. Peritubular capillaries may develop multilayered basal lamina, and there may be thickening of glomerular capillary walls with reduplication of basement membrane and mesangial interposition. Gradual accumulation of interstitial matrix leads to interstitial fibrosis (IF), collagen scars, interstitial capillary loss and tubular atrophy (TA).

Allograft fibrosis is the final common pathway of multi-factorial injury. Therefore, chronic rejection alone cannot explain the pathogenesis of fibrosis. Chronic allograft nephropathy (CAN) was used to describe chronic allograft fibrosis. Nevertheless, CAN is not an etiologic diagnosis. Thus, in 2005, the Banff consensus conference recommended adopting need-based diagnosis and abandoning the concept of 'CAN'. According to the Banff 2005 meeting report, possible causes of IF/TA include drug toxicity (especially calcineurin inhibitor toxicity), bacterial or viral infection, hypertension, obstruction, recurrent and de novo glomerular and tubulointerstitial diseases, as well as chronic rejection. Pathologic changes vary depending on different etiologic factors, and they should be discriminated.

Macroscopic examination reveals no obvious allograft changes at the early-stage of CAD, but obvious shrinkage, thickening and adhesion of renal capsule, with scars of various sizes on the uneven, pale surface of kidney at the late-stage of CAD. Small scarring kidney is hard and has a thin cortex. Histopathologic changes include glomerular, interstitial, tubular and vascular changes.

1. Transplant glomerulopathy

Transplant glomerulopathy is mainly characterized by glomerular basement membrane thickening, glomerular mesenterial lysis, and accumulation of mesenterial matrix, mesenterial sclerosis, and glomerulosclerosis. However, it usually does not present with obvious proliferative reaction or dense substance deposition. In this way, it can be differentiated from membranoproliferative glomerulonephritis (Figure 1). Immune injury is generally thought to be the main cause for transplant glomerulopathy, because it correlates obviously to endothelial cell C4d deposition.

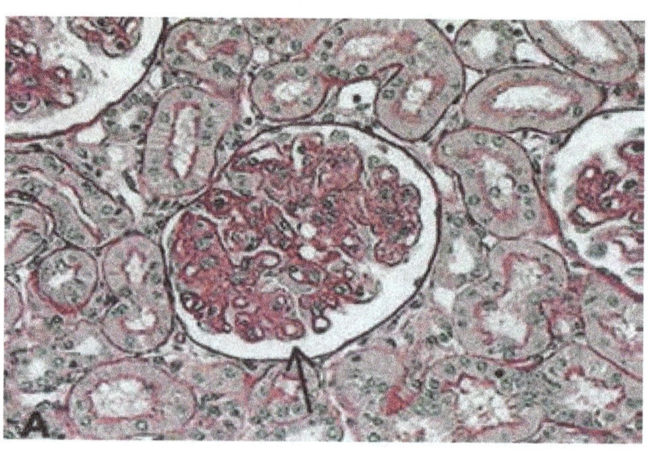

Fig. 1.

2. Interstitial fibrosis

Interstitial fibrosis is not specific to CAD, but is the final outcome of various kidney diseases. Various immune, hemodynamic and metabolic factors may lead to interstitial fibrosis. Tubular cell atrophy, diffuse interstitial infiltration of monocytes and lymphocytes, laminin and fibronectin expression increase, and gradual interstitial fibrosis may be observed (Figure 2). A number of proinflammatory and fibrogenic cytokines expressed in renal allografts may accelerate renal fibrosis, including tumor necrosis factor-α, transforming growth factor-β, platelet-derived growth factor, interferon-γ, and basic fibroblast growth factor. These factors are usually deemed early-stage markers for fibrosis.

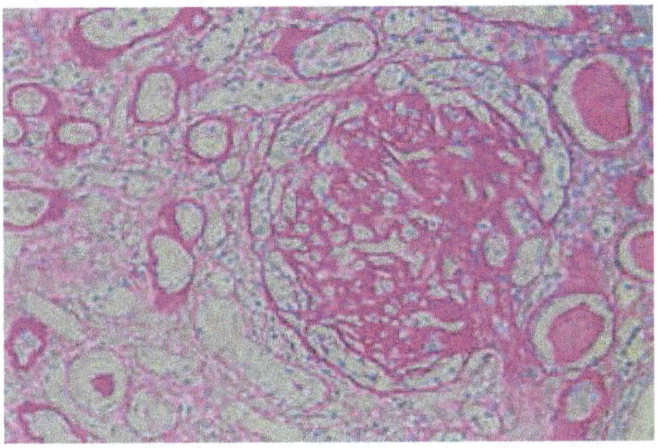

Fig. 2.

3. Tubular atrophy

Tubular atrophy (TA) is also a non-specific manifestation of various chronic kidney injuries. Ischemia/reperfusion injury, drug nephrotoxicity and immune injury may lead to TA. Generally, tubulitis is characteristics of acute cell-mediated rejection; however, whether tubulitis is the sole cause for tubular atrophy is uncertain. Tubular basement membrane loss due to acute rejection may cause late-stage tubular atrophy. At 2-3 weeks following transplantation, persistent peritubular granulomatous reaction, infiltration of tubular basement membrane by multinucleated giant cells, and partial or complete tubular atrophy can be observed (Figure 3). Therefore, immune injury may be an important factor for TA.

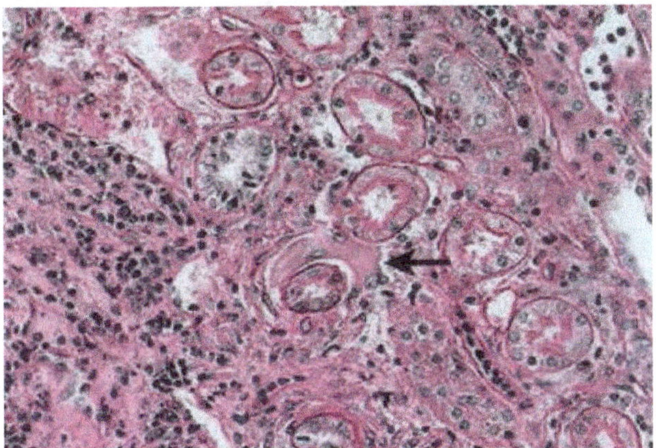

Fig. 3.

4. Transplant vasculopathy

Transplant Atherosclerosis

Transplant atherosclerosis may result from donor factors, non-immune injury (e.g., CNI nephrotoxicity) and chronic rejection. However, there are T cells or macrophages that infiltrate the affected vascular intima, which usually means vascular endothelitis (Figure 4). The incidence rate of systemic atherosclerosis increases in patients with chronic rejection, while renal failure per se does not influence the incidence of atherosclerosis greatly. Moreover, graft atherosclerosis occurs mostly in young, hypersensitive recipients or those with late-stage acute rejection. This suggests that transplant atherosclerosis is closely associated with immune injury. The specification of diagnostic criteria for chronic rejection and other entities by the Banff 2005 conference was an important achievement, and the positive staining for C4d in peritubular capillaries is thought to correlate to AMR (antibody mediated rejection).

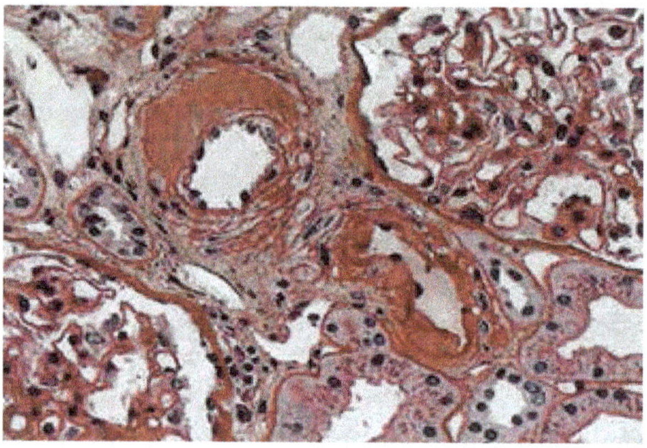

Fig. 4.

Arteriolar hyalinosis

Arteriolar hyalinosis is a characteristic feature of hypertensive nephrosclerosis, diabetic nephropathy, and chronic calcineurin renal toxicity. Hyaline change in the media of the arteriole, which may represent a consequence of myocyte necrosis, is a characteristic feature of cyclosporine-associated arteriolopathy (Figure 5). In many circumstances, such pathologic changes are not direct evidence of diagnosis, and diagnosis should be made with reference to previous pathologic findings obtained by biopsy.

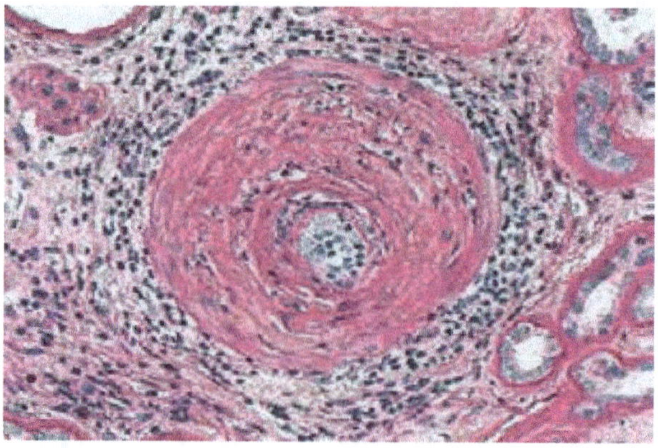

Fig. 5.

In summary, allograft fibrosis and sclerosis are caused by multiple factors, and they are the final manifestations of various acute and chronic kidney injuries. Interstitial fibrosis and tubular atrophy are non-specific. Therefore, a range of diagnostic criteria of CAD should be further investigated, and these diagnostic criteria can and should define specific lesions, thus enabling identification of pathogenic processes that affect the allograft, such as drug toxicity, bacterial or viral infection, hypertension, obstruction, recurrent or de novo renal diseases, and acute and chronic cell and/or antibody-mediated rejection.

4. Injury mechanism for CAD

4.1 Humoral immunity-mediated injury

Antibodies can contribute to transplant rejection through the classical pathways, such as activation of complements and ADCC. After antibody binding to transplantation antigens, complements are activated, followed by activation of the complement-coagulation system, which directly leads to destruction of target cells, vasodilatation, and thrombosis, resulting in allograft rejection. Athough such injury is typical for hyperacute rejection, vascular intimal thickening and presence of complements, immunoglobin and anti-endothelial cell antibody in the necrotic vascular wall have been observed in allografts with chronic rejection. There is another pathway through which T lymphocytes recognize transplantation antigens, i.e., the indirect pathway. In this indirect pathway, TCR on CD4+ T cells can recognize donor's MHC molecule allogenic antigen peptide treated and presented by APCs, also called type II helper T cell (CD4+Th2) reaction. CD4+ T cell activation by the indirect pathway reveals the priming of the rejection effector mechanism, which includes delayed hypersensitivity, cell-mediated toxicty and production of allogenic antibodies. This mechanism exacerbates acute rejection, and plays a major role in CAD. IL-4 and IL-10 produced by Th2 cells are involved in humoral immunity. Activation of helper T cell surface antigen specific TCR triggers intracellular reaction to synthesize specific new antibodies, and this plays an important role in chronic rejection. Early-stage ischemia /reperfusion injury can also activate immunity and upregulate proinflammatory mediators to produce antibodies in the recipients. For instance, in ischemic tissues, vascular endothelial cell phenotype is activated, triggering new antigen expression and leading to immune complex deposition.

4.2 Cellular immunity-mediated injury

In transplant rejection, antigen presenting cells, e.g., dendritic cells, monocytes, and macrophages are crucial for triggering immune response through: ① acquiring, processing and presentating antigens to TH/TDTH and B cells, thus activating first messengers; ② secreting second messengers, e.g., IL-1, thus leading to TH cell activation and release of IL-2, IL-4, IL-5, IL-6 and IFN-γ. Under the action of these cytokines, TDTH, Tc, and B cells that have recognized transplantation antigens begin to proliferate and differentiate into effector Tc, TDTH and antibody secreting cells, leading to transplant rejection. Tc cells directly kill target cells, and TDTH cells contribute to rejection through inducing delayed hypersensitive inflammation. At early-stage acute rejection following renal transplantation, CD4+T cells directly recognize MHC class II antigens in the allograft, and CD8+T cells directly recognize MHC class I antigens in the allograft, producing strong cell- and cytokine-mediated reactions and clinical manifestations of acute rejection. In chronic rejection, weak reactions occur through CD4+Th2 (indirect presentation as mentioned above). Donor MHC may peel from the parenchymal cells of allograft, enter blood circulation, and be phagocytized and processed by recipient's APCs, and be presented by recipient's MHC, or be taken up and processed in situ by macrophages. The recipient's APCs interalize exogenous proteins derived from the allograft, and process and present polypeptides to T cells, thus providing essential signals for lymphocyte activation. This is the classical pathway for antigen processing and presentation by the immune system. In animals immunized with donor's MHC class II antigens, allograft rejection is accelerated significantly, including serious vascular and cellular rejection, which demonstrates the role of the allogenic recognition based indirect pathway in transplant rejection. Nevertheless, immunosuppressants prevent acute rejection and induce CD4+Th2 reaction, leading to development of chronic rejection.

The intimal plaques of allograft artery in chronic rejection comprise mainly macrophages. Macrophages upregulate the expression of fibrosis factors, interleukin-1(IL-1), IL-6, TNF-a and membrane cofactor protein -1(MCP-1) and growth factors, particularly, fibroblast growth factors (bFGF) and transforming growth factors around glomeruli and vessels, thus promoting vascular wall hypertrophy, glomerulosclerosis and kidney fibrosis. Platelet derived growth factors (PDGF), intracellular adhesion molecule (ICAM) and vascular adhesion molecule -1(VCAM-1) are also present on glomerular capillary endothelial cells and other structures. Upregulation of lymphocytes function associated antigen -1(LFA-1) and very late appearing antigen -4(VLA-4), as well as infiltrating cells and cytokines in the allograft promote the waterfall effect of adhesion molecules.

In triggering immune reactions, multiple cytokines such as TNF and IFN-γ promote lymphocytes to mature and helper T cells Th1 to synthesize IL-2, IFN-γ and IL-12. Anti-inflammatory cytokines, e.g., TGF-β, lead Th2 cytokines IL-4 and IL-10 to mature, and suppress immune reactions against allogenic antigens. During rejection, all these cytokines are present in the allograft. However, in case of immune tolerance, Th1 cytokines reduce, and Th2 cytokines increase. CD4+Th2 cytokines, particularly, IL-4, IL-10 and TGF-β, suppress the synthesis of matrix metalloproteinases (MMPs) on smooth muscle and macrophages. MMPs regulate cellular matrix deposition and degradation. Hence, MMPs suppression causes vascular endothelial cell matrix to accumulate, gradually resulting in arterial sclerosis.

Although CD4+Th2 reactions dominate in chronic rejection, other cells, including endothelial cells, CD8+ T cells, NK cells and macrophages, are required to maintain chronic rejection. For instance, CD8+T cells can activate allogenic class I antigens crosslinking on endothelial cells to produce IL-4, IL-10 and TGF-β. Crosslinking of allogenic antibodies to class I antigen molecules on endothelial cell surface will lead to activation and synthesis of TGF-β, PDGF and FGF.

4.3 Allograft structural component reactivity

Various structural components of allograft exhibit different reactivity at early-stage and late-stage following transplantation. In chronic rejection, vascular obstruction results from repeated activation, injury, proliferation and repair of endothelial cells and deposition of extracellular matrix proteins. Vascular wall injury is caused by homogeneous immune reactions because early-stage antigens or proinflammatory factors (e.g., leukotriene, oxyradicals) upregulate complements and adhesion molecules. Allograft arteriosclerosis is associated with autoimmune reactions induced by heat shock protein produced by activated endothelial cells. Changes in the phenotype of activated endothelial cells cause cell denudation and exposure of subendothelial collagen to platelets and plasma proteins, which promotes focal coagulation and thrombosis. Ischemic tissues produce various coagulants, and injured or activated endothelial cells release cytokines, chemical inducers, mediators, thromboxanes, leukotriene and growth factors, including PDGF, platelet-activating factor, NOSi and elastin. Chemical inducers and adhesion molecules promote circulating leukocytes to migrate to the site of injury, and then to vascular wall and perivascular space. Inflammatory reactions caused by cytokines and growth factors result in vascular smooth muscle proliferation and migration, tissue deformation, and vascular involvement. In chronic rejection, there are focal or diffuse glomerular changes, and macrophage infiltration may accelerate early-stage glomerular injury to develop into glomerulosclerosis. Glomerulosclerosis and vascular luminal narrowing lead to gradual renal functional impairment and systemic hypertension. As a result, remnant nephrons are subject to glomerular hyperfiltration and fibrosis, and finally lose function. Non-specific interstitial fibrosis and tubular atrophy stem from organ injury. Therefore, in the presence of early-stage injury following organ transplantation, despite persistent administration of immunosuppressants, renal function may be impaired gradually over several months to several years, and these changes correlate to the reactivity of various structural components of allograft.

4.4 Recurrent and de novo allograft disease

Recurrent glomerulonephritis posttransplantation refers to glomerulonephritis of allograft following renal transplantation, which is pathologically identical to glomerulonephritis of autologous kidney. De novo glomerulonephritis posttransplantation refers to glomerulonephritis of allograft following renal transplantation, which is pathologically different from glomerulonephritis of autologous kidney or the pathology of allograft prior to transplantation. The key to diagnose recurrent and de novo glomerulonephritis lies in the availability of biopsy findings of the autologous kidney and allograft prior to transplantation. In effect, glomerulonephritis is virtually recurrent in all cases. The incidence of recurrent nephropathy of allograft correlates obviously to the histologic type of kidney before transplantation and the time following transplantation. Some glomerular diseases are likely to recur, e.g., mesenterial capillary nephritis, and IgA nephropathy, with the incidence rate of 50-90%. However, these recurrent diseases are unnecessarily influence allograft function seriously. Generally, renal function impairment progresses slowly, with long stable periods. Tables 1-2 list common recurrent and de novo allograft diseases. Currently, most investigations focus on the incidence rate, risk factors and clinical manifestations of recurrent allograft nephritis. Clinically, large doses of immunosuppressants are administered to prevent allograft rejection, but allografts may develop recurrent nephritis, demonstrating that currently available immunosuppressants cannot suppress the incidence of preexisting glomerular diseases. Novel immunosuppressants e.g., MMF and Rapamycin, can suppress cell proliferation in vitro, but their efficacy for recurrent glomerular disease has not been established. Therefore, further investigating the treatment of recurrent and de novo nephritis will deepen the understanding of the pathophysiology of autologous glomerulonephritis and immune pathogenesis of allograft rejection.

Pathologic classification	Recurrent rate (%)	Allograft loss rate (%)
FSGS	20~40	25
IgA nephropathy	50	5~10
Membranous nephropathy	20	5~10
MPGN-I	25	5~10
MPGN-II	90	20
HUS	10~50	10~50
HSPN	30~80	10
Wegener's granuloma	5~20	5~20
Anti-GBM disease	<10	<1
Lupus nephritis	5~10	<5

FSGS: focal segmental glomerulosclerosis, MPGN: membranoproliferative nephritis, HUS: hemolytic uremic syndrome, HSPN: anaphylactoid purpura nephritis

Table 1. Recurrent rate and allograft loss rate of allograft nephritis

Pathologic classification Incidence rate (%)
Etiologies
Allograft nephropathy 5 Rejection? T cell mediated endothelial cell injury? viral infection?
De novo membranous nephropathy 2 Rejection related? de novo antigens produced after allograft injury form immune complexes in situ
De novo HUS 1~3 Calcium channel blockers, allograft ischemia, transplant rejection
De novo MPGN ? 2 HCV, cryoglobulin? deposition of HCV antigens in glomeruli
Alport syndrome
Anti-GBM disease Rare IgG product related to type IV collagen α chain

Table 2. Common de novo allograft diseases

4.5 Posttransplantation lymphoproliferative disease

PTLD is one of the serious complications after organ and marrow transplantation, which presents with lymphocyte proliferation disorder and formation of lymphoma. The probability of PTLD in renal transplantation patients is 20 times that in normal populations. Nevertheless, the incidence rate of PTLD is relatively low (1 %-10%) in renal transplantation patients. PTLD usually affects lymph nodes, the allograft, small intestine and central nervous system, and it occurs mostly in the 2 years following transplantation. PTLD localized to the allograft usually occurs earlier than that outside the allograft. PTLD occurs earlier in patients positive for EB virus than in those negative for EB virus. PTLD mostly stems from B lymphocytes (approximately 87%), and sometimes from T lymphocytes (12%). PTLD stemming from B lymphocytes is mostly complicated by EB virus positivity, while only 38% of PTLD stemming from T lymphocytes is complicated by EB virus positivity. Although PTLD may originate from the donor's cells or the recipient's cells, it mainly originates from the donor's cells. PTLD originating from the donor's cells has a better prognosis than that originating from the recipient's cells. PTLD has varied clinical manifestations, which relate mainly to the affected site and severity of pathologic changes. Common clinical manifestations include ardent fever, neutrocytopenia, anemia, anorexia, diarrhea, and stomachache. Imaging examinations are not specific for the diagnosis of

PTLD. A definite diagnosis depends on pathologic examination. When PTLD is localized to the allograft, with diffuse infiltration, but without obvious masses, it resembles allograft rejection with gradual function loss.

5. Diagnosis of CAD

5.1 Clinical manifestations

Chronic allograft rejection mostly occurs at 2 months to several years following transplantation, with clinical manifestations such as progressive impairment of allograft function, proteinuria and /or anuria, slow increase in blood creatinine (clinically termed "climbing creatinine"), hypertension, progressive anemia and allograft shrinkage.

5.2 Imaging examinations

1. Color Doppler ultrasonography

Since the allograft is shallow, ultrasonic imaging of the allograft will not be influenced substantially by organs and muscle tissue. In addition, due to great acoustic impedance difference between the kidney and surrounding tissues, allograft structures, kidney vessels, ureters and adjacent tissues are shown distinctly. Ultrasonography is able to reveal the allograft size, kidney structures, and various complications of renal transplantation. With the use of color Doppler flow imaging (CDFI) and color Doppler energy (CDE) techniques, blood flow and blood supply to the allograft, and vascular complications following transplantation can be shown clearly. In addition, under ultrasonic guide, biopsy, puncturation and drainage, and visualization are accurate, simple, safe, and non-radioactive, and unlikely to cause complications. Hence, ultrasonography is the preferred imaging modality for allograft. Under ultrasonography, CAD exhibits the following manifestations: the allograft size increases first and then decreases gradually, with a long diameter usually less than 9cm; the kidney parenchyma has enhanced and thickened echoes; the cortex becomes thinner, with indistinct borderline between the kidney parenchyma and renal sinus; at late-stage, the kidney structure is deranged. CDFI frequency spectrum indicates reduced vessels. At late-stage in serious cases, in absence of blood flow in interlobar and arcuate arteries, acute rejection cannot be excluded by ultrasonography. The renal vascular systolic peak flow rate decreases, and the end-diastolic flow rate also decreases. The renal vascular resistance differs significantly between various orders of vessels, particularly between the renal artery and arculate artery. However, the renal vascular resistance is lower than that in hyperacute rejection, accelerated rejection, and acute rejection, but higher than normal. Interstitial vascular resistance is thought to be small; hence, it may be insensitive to Doppler ultrasonography. In contrast, vascular resistance is obvious; hence, it may be sensitive to Doppler ultrasonography. If the RI is normal or less than0.7, CAD cannot be ruled out by ultrasonography. CDE indicates decreased renal vascular perfusion, particularly, in the cortex.

2. Radionuclide imaging

In CAD, the allograft is diminished, and its perfusion and excretion, particularly, uptake, are impaired. Isotope nephrogram indicates perfusion reduction.

3. Digital subtraction angiography (DSA)

In CAD, kidney arteries reduce, and they are thin and bead-like. The kidney parenchyma presents with nonuniform density and patchy changes.

4. CT and MRI
CT and MRI are atraumatic, and have high resolution for soft tissues; hence, they are complementary to other imaging methods for allograft.

5.3 Pathologic study

Currently, biopsy is the most direct, reliable tool for rejection diagnosis. In clinical practice, biopsy findings should be considered in combination with various clinical manifestations and other immunologic, biochemical and imaging findings. Percutaneous thick needle aspiration biopsy or fine needle aspiration biopsy (FNAB) are frequently adopted. If they fail to establish a diagnosis, open biopsy may be considered.

1. Fine needle aspiration biopsy (FNAB)
This method is safe, fast, highly sensitive and specific, and allows continuous observation. Under the guide by ultrasonography or palpation, a 0.7-0.8mm needle with core is inserted into the cortex of the shallower kidney pole, and 10-15tB kidney parenchyma is aspirated and mixed with 5ml heparinized RPMI 1640. The cells are harvested by centrifugation and smeared onto slides. May-Grunlvcald-Giemsa or Wright staining is performed, and cells are counted under an immersion objective. Meanwhile, blood is sampled from the fingers and cells are counted as described above. In typical specimens, there are at least 7 kidney parenchymal cells (endothelial cells, basophilic small tubular epithelial cells, large transparent tubular epithelial cells, large granular tubular epithelial cells or glomerular mesenterial cells) out of 100 inflammatory cells, or there is at least 0.25 parenchymal cell per high power field. The number of a kind of inflammatory cells in the peripheral blood is subtracted from the number of the same kind of inflammatory cells in the allograft to obtain the increament (I). The negative values are discarded. Then, the I values that represent various types of inflammatory cells multiply with a correction coefficient that reflects the contribution of the inflammatory cell type to obtain the corrected I (CI). The CI for each type of inflammatory cells is cumulated to get the total CI (TCI), which represents the extent of inflammatory reactions. Meanwhile, kidney parenchymal cells are graded according to their morphology: 0, morphologically normal; 1, swelling; 2, swelling and vacuolar degeneration; 3, swelling, vacuolization and presence of inclusion materials; 4, necrosis. FNAB specimens can also be investigated by immunocytochemical staining, e.g., peroxide-anti-peroxydase (PAP) staining, indirect immunofluorescence staining, double immunofluorescence staining, immunogold or immunosilver staining, and biotin-avidin immunostaining. FNAB is accurate for diagnosing acute cell-mediated rejection, but is useless for diagnosing CAD and vascular rejection.

2. Percutaneous thick needle aspiration biopsy
This method is the most determinant and reliable tool for differentiating allograft rejection, cyclosporin A toxicity or acute tubular necrosis. In China, the most frequently used needles are Menghini, Franklin-Vim-Silverman, Tru-Cut and Jamshidi types, which are all fit for allograft puncturation. Specimens can be aspirated from the outer edge of the midpoint of the upper and lower kidney poles or the upper kidney pole. For shallow allografts, the needle can be inserted under the guide of palpation. However, in obese patients, ultrasonography or fluoroscopy (with or without intravenous pyelography) may be adopted to guide needle insertion. In case that all these methods failed, CT guide may be considered. The complications are mainly hematuria, perirenal hematoma, arteriovenous fistula, lymphatic fistula and infection.

3. Pathologic diagnosis
   a. The allograft is slightly enlarged or normal at early-stage, and is diminished obviously at late stage. At late stage, the allograft is light and pale, with uneven surface and scars; hence, it is called "small scarring kidney". The renal capsule is obviously thickened and adhered, and cortex atrophy can be observed on the cross-section. Renal function deteriorates progressively, which is proportional to the degree of interstitial fibrosis and glomerulotubular atrophy.
   b. Histologic changes include intimal proliferation dominated proliferating vasculitis, capillary basement membrane thickening and mesenterial matrix increase. There are several pathologic types.

1. Occlusive vasculitis Small artery and arteriole are affected seriously, and interlobar and arcuate arteries may also be affected. In small interlobar artery, afferent glomerular artery and larger artery, smooth muscle and fibroblast proliferation and fibrosis of intima, intima thickening, and luminal narrowing and even obstruction can be observed. Proliferating cells are mostly intimal fibroblasts, and smooth muscle cells originate from the intima. Both cell types produce collagen fibers ultimately. In some cases, subendothelial smooth muscle cells proliferate obviously around the lumen axis, and take on a cyclic, onion-like shape, forming so-called "second tunica media". Serious arterial lesions may influence blood supply to the kidney, lead to multiple infarction, ischemic renal parenchymal atrophy, and renal interstitial sclerosis.

2. Renal interstitial sclerosis Diffuse or focal renal interstitial fibrous proliferation is the major change, which involves the cortex to the medulla. Renal interstitial matrix proliferates, with rare cells and infiltration by lymphocytes and monocytes. Tubular changes are varied, including basement membrane thickening and tubular epithelial cell regeneration. Regenerated tubular epithelial cells are large and may have multiple nuclei. Occasionally, there are single or groups of necrotic epithelial cells. Some tubules are dilated in compensation, resembling mesenchyme. Rejection glomerulonephritis or recurrent glomerulonephritis may be observed. Some patients present with obvious proliferative glomerulonephritis, with obvious increase of glomerular matrix or crescent formation.

   c. Immunofluorescence assay: IgG, IgM and C3 deposit on the glomerular capillary wall and interstitial vascular wall. In particular, in occlusive vasculitis, infiltrating inflammatory cells contain strong fluorescence-emitting IgM.
   d. Electron microscopy: The space between endothelial cells and basement membrane is widened obviously in capillary loop and electron dense substance deposits in a linear or granular manner, with obvious basement membrane thickening. There is a lot of linear and granular electron dense substance deposition along the tubular basement membrane. Mesenterial matrix and surrounding basement membrane are thickened obviously, and are curved. Collagen increases in small artery wall, and smooth muscle cells and fibroblasts proliferate. Lipid droplets increase and myofilaments decrease in the cytoplasm of smooth muscle cells, which may become fibroblasts or foam cells.
   e. Oligonucleotide microarray hybridization assay: B cell chemokine (CXCL13) and mast cells may be determined as predictors for CAD.

4. Differential diagnosis

CAD presents with glomerulosclerosis, recurrent or rejection related glomerulonephritis. Recurrent glomerulonephritis refers recurrence of preexisting nephritis in the allograft, which can be recognized through examining the recipient's original kidney specimens.

Rejection related glomerulonephritis and focal glomerulonephritis can be differentiated by vasculopathy. In serious rejection-related glomerulonephritis, glomerular capillary basement membrane is thickened obviously, which should be differentiated from membranous glomerulonephritis through PAS or PASM staining. In rejection-related glomerulonephritis, there are no spike-like deposits on the epithelial surface of basement membrane, but bilayer basement membrane. In CAD, vascular sclerosis of the allograft should be differentiated from atherosclerosis. Vascular sclerosis is characterized by typical concentric proliferation of smooth muscle and breach of internal elastic layer, but no cholesterol crystals. In contrast, atherosclerosis is characterized by deranged intimal fibers and obvious cholesterol crystals. In CAD, interstitial sclerosis is obvious sometimes, which should be differentiated from chronic interstitial nephritis. In CAD, there are renal interstitial sclerosis, rare nuclei, spare fibers, and few inflammatory cells; hence, the tissue resembles mesenchyme. In chronic interstitial nephritis, fibers are usually dense in scar tissues, with abundant nuclei and a certain number of inflammatory cells.

6. Prevention and treatment of CAD

CAD treatment

No effective treatments for CAD are available yet. The main therapeutic options include controlling blood pressure, administering immunosuppressants, stosstherapy with Methyllprednisolone (MP), intermittent intravenous infusion of Cyclophosphamide (CTX), and use of antithymocyte globulin (ATG), antilymphocyte globulin (ALG), OKT3 and OKT4 monoclonal antibodies, tripterygium glycosides, Bailing capsule, and Niaoduqing granules. The overall therapeutic effect is not good. Over recent years, many treatments have been reported. However, the overall strategy involves the rational use of immunosuppressants, preventing and treating risk factors, and prolonging the functioning life of remnant nephrons. Below are some treatments that are effective for CAD:

1. Dietary therapy Dietary therapy is one of the fundamental measures to delay renal failure in CAD. It has been established both clinically and experimentally that low protein diet and essential amino acid therapy can delay chronic renal failure in most patients. Dietary therapy is mainly aimed to minimize metabolic waste, while providing nutrients to meet basic physiologic needs. By correcting dysmetabolism of nutrients, dietary therapy can relieve the burden on remnant nephrons, correct hemodynamic disturbances, and delay the progress of kidney disease. The measures include ① low protein diet: It is generally thought that low protein diet should be prescribed for patients with chronic renal failure once the endogenous creatinine clearance rate (Ccr) falls to 55ml/min. Meanwhile, sufficient energy should be supplied. This is because high protein diet will increase kidney blood flow and the glomerular filtration rate drastically. Long-term high protein diet will result in persistent high glomerular filtration and glomerulosclerosis through cumulative effect. ② essential amino acids (EAAs): It has been demonstrated that EAAs can improve the nutritional status of patients with chronic renal failure, and can reduce the adverse effect of proteins and common amino acids on the hemodynamics of kidney, thus effectively delaying renal functional impairment. Generally EAAs should be given at week 2 of low protein diet. ⑨ low phosphorus diet and calcium supplementation: Strict control of dietary phosphorus will prevent hyperphosphatemia and secondary

hyperparathyroidism, and relieve tubular interstitial damage. Calcium supplementation should be considered for patients with hypocalcemia and controlled hyperphosphatemia. ④ Supplementation of vitamins and trace elements: Proper supplementatin of water soluble vitamins and trace elements may benefit CAD patients.

2. Cyclosporin A (CsA) The efficacy for CsA is still controversial. According to a retrospective study following up 435 cases for 14 years in the United States, the median allograft survival rate is 3 years. Compared to Azathioprine, CsA showed non-inferiority in relieving renal functional impairment. The median allograft survival rate was 11.6 years in CsA treated patients, and was 9.7 years in Aza treated patients. In animal models, CsA cannot prevent the emergence of pathologic characteristics of CAD after heart, kidney or aorta transplantation. It was also demonstrated that the use of CsA can increase the early-stage success rate obviously and the long-term survival rate as well. Long-term use of CsA is especially superior to Aza. Nevertheless, CsA may increase angiotensin and TGF-β, which is not desirable for CAD treatment. A few scholars hold that low doses of cyclosporin A (CsA) in combination with other immunosuppressants e.g., Mycophenolate mofetil (MMF), is somewhat effective for CAD.
3. FK506 Ji et al. reported that FK506 may delay the progress of CAD safely and effectively. Wang et al. reported that FK506, in place of CsA, was effective for early-stage CAD, particularly, in cases with Scr less than 400umo/L. After FK506 treatment, the Scr level decreased substantially, and hypertension and renal dysfunction improved obviously. One-year follow-up indicated that the patients' condition was stable. Nevertheless, FK506 treatment is less effective in cases with Scr more than 400umol/L. Hence, it is concluded that FK506, in place of CsA is effective for early-stage CAD. Theruvath et al. reported that the FK506+MMF immunosuppressant regimen can reduce anti-donor HLA antibody in recipients, which is of significance to prevent and treat CAD. A US-based, multi-center study primarily on renal transplantation showed that in comparison with CsA, FK506 can effectively prevent acute or glucocorticosteroids or antibody resistant allograft rejection, with increasing side effects. Among 77 patients with acute rejection, 74% of them healed after the combined use of CsA and FK506. 20 patients had obvious vasculopathy, which was refractory to antibody treatment. However, whether FK506 stabilizes allograft function for long is still unclear.
4. Mycophenolate mofetil (MMF) MMF is superior to azathioprine in the treatment of CAD. It was reported that three large clinical trials were undergoing to investigate the efficacy of MMF plus CsA plus prednisone. The dose of MMF to prevent acute rejection is 2g/d or 3g/d. Compared to the control group or the Aza treatment group, the incidence rate of acute rejection decreased obviously at 6 months postoperatively, as confirmed by biopsy. The dose of 3g/d was more effective than 2g/d. MMF may lead to abdominal discomfort, leukopenia and infection. It is now thought that MMF can reduce the incidence of acute rejection and irreversible CAD. MMF in combination with low doses of cyclosporin A (CsA) and prednisone decreased blood creatinine, cured proteinuria and improved renal function in patients with CAD. MMF was found to ameliorate CAD caused chronic renal dysfunction, particularly, mild to moderate renal dysfunction that develops in the first three years after renal transplantation. Nevertheless, long-term follow-ups should be carried out. With the use of MMF, the dose of CsA and glucocorticosteroids can be decreased to reduce the toxic or side effects

of CsA and glucocorticosteroids. The toxic or side effects of MMF are acceptable. With accumulating experience with the clinical use of MMF, the incidence rate of MMF's adverse reactions may be further decreased. CAD patients may benefit from the replacement of Azathioprine with MMF.

5. Sirolimus Sirolimus is a macrolide antibiotic produced by Streptomyces (an actinomycete). As an immunosuppressant, it resembles FK506 structurally. It is not nephrotoxic, and can reduce chronic CsA toxicity. Sirolimus suppresses vascular proliferation, and fibroblast proliferation in vitro; hence, it may prevent CAD. Sirolimus prevents allogenic CAD also through downregulation of adhesion molecule and growth factor encoding gene expression. Replacing calcineurin inhibitors with Sirolimus may delay the incidence of CAD and relieve its clinical symptoms.
6. Lelfunomide In rodent models of heart transplantation with chronic vascular rejection, Lelfunomide exhibited very significant efficacy, and it can reduce and reverse chronic vasculopathy in the allograft. Unlike other immunosuppressants, Lelfunomide will not induce diabetes. Lelfunomide has not been approved for clinical use, but it may become a new treatment for CAD.
7. Polyunsaturated fatty acids Experimental and clinical studies have demonstrated that fish oil treatment can regulate immune reaction. In rat models of heart transplantation, ω-3 polyunsaturated fatty acid can prolong the survival time of allograft obviously. However, allograft survival prolongation correlated to and the reduction of the ω-3 fatty acid content. It is possible that the ratio of dietary ω-3/ω-6 fatty acids is more important than the level of certain fatty acids. ω-3 polyunsaturated fatty acids may regulate immunity via multiple mechanisms: to suppress the effects of IL-1/TNF, to change DR antigen expression, and to reduce vascular smooth muscle cell proliferation and vascular permeability. Another study demonstrated that ω-3 polyunsaturated fatty acids (e.g., fish oil) in combination with 3-hydroxy-3-methyl-glutaryl-CoA (HMG-CoA) reductase inhibitors can reduce the incidence rate of allograft rejection, and they have no obvious toxic and adverse effects.
8. Hypolipidemic treatment HMG-CoA reductase inhibitors (e.g., Statins) are commonly used hypolipidemic agents. Regardless of the blood lipid level in patients, these drugs exhibit good protective effect. In addition to decreasing cholesterol, these drugs can stimulate vascular endothelial cells to release monoxide nitrogen, restore endothelial cell function, and improve kidney hemodynamics. They can also suppress platelet aggregation and thrombosis. It was reported that Simvastatin can reduce the incidence rate of coronary heart disease in rat models for heart transplantation, possibly through reducing the production of 7FXAz. Statins reduce the incidence rate of CAD indirectly, through protecting allograft vessels. CsA, glucocorticosteroids and rapamycin can lead to blood lipid increase. However, it is still unclear to what extent blood lipid should be increased for long. Large multicenter randomized controlled trials or systematic appraisals should be carried out to address this issue.
9. Control of hypertension It has been demonstrated that 90% of CAD patients present with various degrees of hypertension, and require antihypertensive treatment. Hypertension leads to CAD, possibly through increasing renal vascular shear stress, leading to vascular sclerosis, increasing renal vascular resistance, and finally leading to renal ischemia. CAD treatments include control of hypertension and hyperlipidemia. Angiotensin converting enzyme inhibitors or angiotensin receptor blockers can change

intraglomerular pressure and slow down renal functional impairment. Angiotensin suppression can relieve vascular fibrosis and injury in CAD.

10. Anticoagulant therapy As most patients with chronic renal failure have disturbances of blood coagulation, anticoagulant therapy can delay the progress of kidney disease. It has been demonstrated recently [39] that low molecule weight heparin can effectively improve the functional and morphologic status of CAD; however, the precise mechanism is to be elucidated. In addition, traditional Chinese medicines that can promote blood flow and remove blood stasis, e.g., Danshen and Szechwan Lovage Rhizome, exhibit certain therapeutic effects on CAD. However, these therapies need further experimental investigation and clinical observation.
11. Hyperbaric oxygen treatment Pang et al. demonstrated in animals that hyperbaric oxygen is important to prevent or relieve CAD. It was found that proteinuria was milder and the creatinine clearance rate was higher in the hyperbaric oxygen treatment group than the control group. Renal interstitial fibrosis, glomerulosclerosis, artery intimal thickening and T cell, monocyte/macrophage infiltration were milder in the hyperbaric oxygen treatment group than the control group. Therefore, it is concluded that hyperbaric oxygen is useful for CAD treatment. However, further clinical trials should be carried out in larger sample sizes.
12. Traditional Chinese medicines Glucosidorum Tripterygll Totorum and Bailing capsules are effective for CAD, and they help protect remnant nephrons and improve renal function in CAD. However, their mechanisms of action remain unclear. Further studies should be carried out to determine the pharmacokinetics, optimal medication regimen and dosage of traditional Chinese medicines.
13. Excision of renal allograft When CAD develops to renal failure and uremia, the patient needs dialysis to sustain life. The renal allograft is excised prior to discontinuation of immunosuppressants, so as to avoid the production of antibody in allograft and allow a second renal transplantation.
14. Gene therapy It may be one of the important directions in the management of CAD.

In summary, CAD should be treated comprehensively and individually.

CAD prevention

1. To optimize allograft quality Damage should be avoided during harvesting, preserving and trimming allografts. It has been demonstrated that the older the donor is, the earlier and more serious allograft glomerulosclerosis and renal interstitial fibrosis occur. Therefore, allografts should better be harvested from young donors.
2. Preoperative HLA match CAD is mainly caused by immunologic injury. Preoperative HLA match is critical to reduce CAD. It is currently thought that the UNOS six-antigen matching program is a useful tool to achieve optimal HLA match. Allografts with perfect match on the HI, A-A, B and DR loci should better be chosen.
3. To reduce ischemia /reperfusion injury The cold ischemia time should better be less than 20h. High quality vascular anastomosis and avoidance of vascular restenosis are important to reduce ischemia /reperfusion injury. In cadaveric renal transplantation, the use of 200mg recombinant human-superoxide dismutase (RH-SOD) can suppress radical-induced injury, allograft immunity, and MHCII antigen and adhesion molecule upregulation, thus relieving acute and chronic rejection.
4. To reduce acute rejection The severity, frequency and time of onset of acute rejection correlate closely to CAD, and acute rejection is the major immune factor for CAD.

Immunosuppressants have certain toxicity to allografts. Therefore, acute rejection should be prevented with most effective immunosuppressants at the smallest possible dose.

5. To improve the patient's compliance Poor compliance is found to be an important factor for allograft failure. Hence, the patient's compliance should be improved by minimizing the drug dose, educating the patient about the unwanted outcomes of irregular medication, helping the patient to schedule the medication, and establishing a close relationship with the patient.
6. To closely monitor renal function To monitor renal function closely can help physicians to supervise patients taking immunosuppressants, and to find acute rejection promptly. Both patients and physicians must bear in mind that CAD following transplantation seldom has symptoms and physical signs. Therefore, regular monitoring of blood creatinine is feasible for monitoring long-term CAD.
7. To perform biopsy regularly It has been demonstrated that low-grade tubulitis or critical acute rejection can increase the risk for CAD. If biopsy was performed regularly in the first several months following transplantation and rejection was detected and managed promptly, the creatinine level remained low in the first two years. In contrast, in the control group without receiving regular biopsy, the creatinine level was found high upon biopsy and treatment. Therefore, it is concluded that it is crucial to caution against acute and chronic rejection and prescribe kidney biopsy for more patients.
8. To manage hyperlipidemia Hyperlipidemia can promote arteriosclerosis and damage renal function. Pravastatin decreases lowly oxidized low density lipoprotein-cholesterol and triglyceride, and suppress growth factor expression and vascular smooth muscle proliferation. Therefore, to manage hyperlipidemia proactively may exert certain effect on renal arteriosclerosis.
9. To treat hypertension Cardiovascular complications are the second leading cause for death one year after renal transplantation. Both CsA and FK506 can cause hypertension. If the systolic pressure exceeds 150mmg, autoregulation of afferent glomerular artery fails, and the glomerular artery dilates, which results in the production of angiotensin-2 peptide and TGF-β. TGF-β promotes renin secretion. Various factors may reduce nephrons of the allograft, and remnant nephrons are subject to high perfusion pressure, high filtration and high secretion, thus causing glomerulosclerosis. At the early-stage of CAD, if the systolic pressure is controlled below 140mmHg, and the urine protein at 0.25-1g/d, the renal function may not deteriorate for three years. If the urine protein is kept at 1-3g/d, blood pressure may be controlled with higher doses of drugs or more drugs. If the urine protein exceeds 3g/d, blood pressure must be controlled strictly to prevent renal functional deterioration for long. In addition to antihypertensive action, Carvedil suppresses smooth muscle proliferation.
10. To prevent cytomegalovirus infection The CMV infection rate is 70% -100% in the population. Following cadaveric renal transplantation, 8% patients develops symptomatic CMV disease, and the mortality rate is 20%. When CMV disease leads to interstitial pneumonia which requires machine ventilation, the mortality rate is 90%. In the CMV infection group, the three-year allograft survival rate reduced by 30%. Active CMV replication can be detected by CMV antigen assay, LSAB assay, and monoclonal antibody determination of CMV encoded PP65 antige as early as 1-6 days prior to onset of CMV disease. CMV disease can be prevented and treated with Ganciclovir in the first three postoperative months in patients positive for CMV infection.

7. References

Najafian B, Kasiske BL. Chronic allograft nephropathy. Curr Opin Nephrol Hypertens. 2008;17(2):149-55.

Jevnikar AM, Mannon RB. Late kidney allograft loss: what we know about it, and what we can do about it. Clin J Am Soc Nephrol. 2008;3 Suppl 2:S56-67.

Solez K, Colvin RB, Racusen LC, Sis B, Halloran PF, Birk PE, Campbell PM, Cascalho M, Collins AB, Demetris AJ, Drachenberg CB, Gibson IW, Grimm PC, Haas M, Lerut E, Liapis H, Mannon RB, Marcus PB, Mengel M, Mihatsch MJ, Nankivell BJ, Nickeleit V, Papadimitriou JC, Platt JL, Randhawa P, Roberts I, Salinas-Madriga L, Salomon DR, Seron D, Sheaff M, Weening JJ. Banff'05 Meeting Report: differential diagnosis of chronic allograft injury and elimination of chronic allograft nephropathy ('CAN') Am J Transplant. 2007;7(3):518-26.

Gulanikar AC, MacDonald AS, Sungurtekin U, Belitsky P. The incidence and impact of early rejection episodes on graft outcome in recipients of first cadaver kidney transplants. Transplantation 1992;53:323–8.

Issa N, Cosio FG, Gloor JM et al. Transplant glomerulopathy: risk and prognosis related to anti-human leukocyte class II antibody levels.Transplantation 2008; 86: 681–685.

Jindra PT, Hsueh A, Hong L et al. Anti-MHC class I antibody activation of proliferation and survival signaling in murine cardiac allografts. J Immunol.2008; 180: 2214– 2224.

Haas M, Rahman MH, Racusen LC et al. C4d and C3d staining in biopsies of ABO and HLA-incompatible renal allografts: correlation with histological findings. Am J Transplant 2006; 6: 1829–1840.

Lemst rom K, Koskinen P, Hayry P, et al. Molecular mechanisms of chronic renal allograft rejection. Kidney Int, 1995, (Suppl 52):2 - 10.

Factors Influencing Outcome After Deceased Heart Beating Renal allograft Transplantation in the United Kingdom: An Evidence Base for a New National Kidney Allocation Policy.Transplantation: 2010, 89(4):379-386.

Kaija Inkinen, Anu Soots, Leena Krogerus , Cathrien Bruggeman, Juhani Ahonen and Irmeli Lautenschlager.Cytomegalovirus increases collagen synthesis in chronic rejection in the rat.Nephrology Dialysis Transplantation, 2001, 17(5):772-779.

Abramowicz D, Manas D, Lao M, et al. Cyclosporine withdrawal from a mycophenolate mofetil-containing immunosuppressive regimen in stable kidney transplant recipients: a randomized, controlled study. Transplantation. 2002;74:1725-1734.

Ahmed F Hamdy, Mohamed A Bakr and Mohamed A Ghoneim. Long-term Efficacy and Safety of a Calcineurin Inhibitor-free Regimen in Live-Donor Renal Transplant Recipients. J Am Soc Nephrol.2008, 19: 1225-1232.

Malek, Sayeed K.Chronic Allograft Dysfunction: A Multifactorial Problem with an Elusive Solution. Nephrology Times, 2010, 3 (6):18-19.

Li C, Yang CW. The pathogenesis and treatment of chronic allograft nephropathy. Nat Rev Nephrol 2009; 5: 513–519.

Lorraine C. Racusen and Heinz Regele.The pathology of CAD. Kidney International.2010, 78 (Suppl 119), 27–32.

Tan JC, Workeneh B, Busque S et al. Glomerular function, structure, and number in renal allografts from older deceased donors. J Am Soc Nephrol 2009; 20: 181–188.

Kambham N, Nagarajan S, Shah S et al. A novel, semiquantitative, clinically correlated calcineurin inhibitor toxicity score for renal allograft biopsies. Clin J Am Soc Nephrol 2007; 2: 135–142.

Mengel M, Gwinner W, Schwarz A et al. Infiltrates in protocol biopsies from renal allografts. Am J Transplant 2007; 7: 356–365.

Sis B, Jhangri GS, Bunnag S et al. Endothelial gene expression in kidney transplants with allo antibody indicates antibody-mediated damage despite lack of C4d staining. Am J Transplant.2009; 9: 2312–2323.

Solez K, Colvin RB, Rcusen LC et al. Banff meeting report: differential diagnosis of chronic allograft injury and elimination of chronic allograft nephropathy (CAN) Am J Transplant, 2007; 7: 518–526.

Hallgrimur Benediktsson. Histopathology of Chronic Renal Allograft Dysfunction. Transplantation Reviews. 2004, 18, (2): 80-85.

Nagase H, Woessner JF Jr. Matrix metalloproteinases.J Biol Chem. 1999;274(31):21491-21494.

Bigg HF, Morrison CJ, Butler CS, et al.Tissue inhibitor of metalloproteinases-4 inhibits but does not support the activation of gelatinase A via efficient inhibition of membrane type 1-matrix metalloproteinase.Cancer Res.2001;61(9):3610.

Galina Pizov, Michael M Friedlaender.Immunohistochemical Staining for Proliferation Antigen as a Predictor of Chronic Graft Dysfunction and Renal Graft Loss. Nephron 2002;92:738-742.

Helen Robertson, Simi Ali, Benjamin J McDonnell, Alastair D Burt and John A Kirby. Chronic Renal Allograft Dysfunction: The Role of T Cell–Mediated Tubular Epithelial to Mesenchymal Cell Transition. J Am Soc Nephrol. 2004, 15:390-397.

Anthony M Jevnikar and Roslyn B Mannon, Late Kidney Allograft Loss: What We Know about It, and What We Can Do about It? CJASN, 2008, 3: 56-67.

Michael Zeisberg and Eric G Neilson.Mechanisms of Tubulointerstitial Fibrosis. J Am Soc Nephrol, 2010, 21: 1819-1834.

B Y Choy, T M Chan and K N Lai. Recurrent Glomerulonephritis After Kidney Transplantation. American Journal of Transplantation 2006; 6: 2535–2542.

Denton MD, Singh AK. Recurrent and de novo glomerulonephritis in the renal allograft.Semin Nephrol. 2000;20(2):164-75.

Claudio Ponticelli, and Richard J Glassock.Posttransplant Recurrence of Primary Glomerulonephritis. CJASN, 2010, 5 (12): 2363-2372.

Worawon Chailimpamontree, Svetlana Dmitrienko, Guiyun Li, Robert Balshaw, Alexander Magil, R Jean Shapiro, David Landsberg, John Gill, Paul A Keown and the Genome Canada Biomarkers in Transplantation Group. Probability, Predictors, and Prognosis of Posttransplantation Glomerulonephritis. JASN, 2009;20 (4): 843-851.

Birkeland S A, Hamilton-Dutoit S. Is posttransplant lymphoproliferative disorder (PTLD) caused by any specific immunosuppressive drug or by the transplantation per se?Transplantation. 2003, 76(6):984-988.

Fellstrom B. Impact and management of hyperlipidem ia post-transplantation. Transplantation, 2000; 70 (11 supp l):SS51.

Ferreira A.C., Viana H., Carvalho F., Pinto J.R., Galvão M.J., Nolasco F., andSantos J.R.Chronic Allograft Dysfunction-Is There a Treatment? Transplantation Proceedings, 2009, 41(3):874-876.

Afzali B, Taylor AL, Goldsmith JA: What can we do about chronic allograft nephropathy: role of immunosuppressive modulations. Kidney Int. 2005, 1:145,

Chapman JR, O'Connel PJ, Nankivell BJ: Chronic renal allograft dysfunction. J Am Soc Nephrol. 2005, 16:3015.

Johnson RW, Kreis H, Oberbauer R, et al: Sirolimus allows early cyclosporine withdrawl in renal transplantation resulting in improved renal function and lower blood pressure. Transplantation. 2001, 72:777.

Kruger B, Fischereder M, Jauch KW, et al:Five-year follow up after late conversion from calcineurin inhibitors to sirolimus in patients with chronic renal allograft dysfunction. Transplant Proc.2007, 39:518.

Kaplan B. Overcoming barriers to long-term graft survival. Am J Kidney Dis.2006;47:S52-64.

Dikow R, Becker LE, Schaier M, Waldherr R, Gross ML, Zeier M. In renal transplants with delayed graft function chemokines and chemokine receptor expression predict long-term allograft function.Transplantation. 2010, 15;90(7):771-776.

Sandovici M, Deelman LE, Benigni A, Henning RH. Towards graft-specific immunosuppressantion: Gene therapy of the transplanted kidney.Adv Drug Deliv Rev. 2010, 30;62(14):1358-1368.

John PV, Mohamed HS. Diagnosis and Management of Renal Allograft Dysfunction. Therapy in Nephrology & Hypertension (Third Edition), 2007, Pages 994-1008.

Krüger B, Fischereder M, Jauch KW, Graeb C, Hoffmann U, Böger CA, Banas B, Obed A, Schlitt HJ, Krämer BK. Five-Year Follow-up After Late Conversion From Calcineurin Inhibitors to Sirolimus in Patients With Chronic Renal Allograft Dysfunction. Transplantation Proceedings, 2007, 39(2):518-521.

Fischereder M, Graeb C, Krüger B, Kammerl MC, Zülke C, Jauch KW, Krämer BK.Conversion From Calcineurin Inhibitors to Sirolimus in Patients With Chronic Renal Allograft Dysfunction.Transplantation Proceedings, 2006, 38(5):1295-1297.

Garcia R, Pinheiro-Machado PG, Felipe CR, Park SI, Silva LA, Franco MF, Tedesco- Silva H Jr, Medina-Pestana JO.Conversion From Azathioprine to Mycophenolate Mofetil Followed by Calcineurin Inhibitor Minimization or Elimination in Patients With Chronic Allograft Dysfunction.Transplantation Proceedings, 2006, 38(9):2872- 2878.

6

Vascular Complications in Kidney Transplantation

Alexandros Giakoustidis, Nikolaos Antoniadis and Dimitrios Giakoustidis
Division of Transplantation, Department of Surgery, Medical School
Aristotle University of Thessaloniki and Hippokration General Hospital, Thessaloniki
Greece

1. Introduction

Kidney transplantation evolved as the treatment of choice for end-stage renal disease. Accumulated expertise and experience along with refined surgical techniques resulted in excellent patient and graft survival. Despite the improvements in surgical techniques vascular complications consists a significant and sometimes life-threatening problem that occurs in 10-20% of patients. Vascular complication can be divided in general in three main categories. Graft renal artery thrombosis and stenosis, graft renal vein thrombosis and stenosis and arterial injury.

2. Transplant renal artery stenosis

Transplant renal artery stenosis (TRAS) is a very common vascular complication following kidney transplantations. It is reported in a wide range of frequency occurring in 3-12% of patients (in some reports even up to 20% depending on the awareness and the available imaging means especially MDCT-angiography) (Akbar 2005, Sebastia, 2001)]. It is very difficult to have the definitive true incidence of TRAS by looking at the literature and this discrepancy is due to the different definitions, the surgeon's experience and technical skills in avoiding or preventing the TRAS and different peri-operative management. If we try to classify all arterial stenosis in kidney transplantation, we could divide it into two main categories; TRAS and proximal or pseudo-TRAS. TRAS can be categorised by the level of stenoses and this includes anastomotic stenoses, stenoses of the proper transplant renal artery and finally segmental renal artery stenoses. Proximal-TRAS refers to pre-existing or developing atherosclerotic inflow stenoses in the native iliac arteries of the transplant recipient. The incidence of proximal-TRAS has been reported to be 0%-2.4% and may become more prevalent with increasing age. Predisposing factors for transplant renal artery stenosis, are cadaveric transplant, end-to-end anastomosis, surgical clamp injury, intimal dissection, and inadequate suturing technique, long or kinking artery, prolonged cold ischemia time, acute cellular rejection, and cytomegalovirus (CMV) infection (Audard, 2006).

Patients with TRAS in the immediate post-transplant period, present oliguria or anuria and are dialysis dependent. After the first week, patients with TRAS usually present with severe renovascular hypertension. Even though severe renovascular hypertension could be attributed to TRAS we should always keep in mind and all other causes like chronic rejection, steroid use, cyclosporine toxicity, recurrent glomerulonephritis and disease of native kidneys (Mangray, 2011, Tutone, 2005). If TRAS is not managed properly in due time, it could lead to renal dysfunction and graft deterioration. Non-invasive imaging is mandatory in the immediate post-transplant period to evaluate for possible transplant renal artery stenosis. Doppler ultrasound should be the initial diagnostic modality used because of its ability to reveal the location, length, and gross appearance of a stenosis. In addition, it is widely available, cost-effective, and does not use ionizing radiation and the nature of the transplanted renal arteries makes Doppler ultrasound an ideal screening modality (Baxter, 1995, Irshad, 2008, 2009). Whilst Doppler ultrasound is ideal in recognizing a possible lesion, categorisation and better characterisation of TRAS would be using magnetic resonance angiography with or without contrast medium (especially gadolinium-enhanced), MDCT-angiography, Radionuclide imaging that includes the administration of an angiotensin-converting enzyme inhibitor (captopril scan) shows findings similar to those of renovascular hypertension in native kidneys (Sebastia, 2001). Catheter-based angiography is the gold standard technique for diagnosing TRAS. The use of low- or iso-osmolar contrast material is recommended to reduce the risk of contrast material–induced nephropathy. When renal insufficiency is present, carbon dioxide may be substituted for an iodinated contrast agent during preliminary angiography to minimize the use of iodinated agents.

2.1 Definition and natural history

Unfortunately there is no consensus definition of TRAS and it would be difficult to have one in the future. Usually there is the classic presentation with refractory hypertension, deteriorating renal function, and congestive cardiac failure secondary to fluid retention. It is very impressive that marked reversal of symptoms occurs when stenosis is successfully treated (Garovic, 2005, Mangray, 2011). The timeline of TRAS usually begins at 2 months to 2 years after transplantation and hypertension is due to activation of the renin-angiotensin system (Basso, 2001, Mangray, 2011). Another important issue concerns asymptomatic normotensive patients with Doppler examination of at least 50% without evident graft dysfunction. The problem with those patients is the potential risk carrying from a procedure to treat a clinically insignificant TRAS in the short to medium term. It is unclear whether treating a non-clinically significant TRAS would have an impact in long term survival of renal grafts but since hypertension is an independent risk factor for long term renal graft survival, anything that could contribute to this direction would be beneficial. Close follow up of those patients, with significant expertise and experience of the transplant centre, along with availability of vascular interventional techniques is of paramount importance in decision making. Nevertheless, there are no reports of the long-term safety of this line of management, and the natural history of a 50% TRAS is unknown, and that conservative treatment is safe provided that there is no deterioration of kidney function (Audard, 2006, Buturovic-Ponikvar, 2003). This may not be the case for other causes, such as intimal hyperplasia, and the indication for angiography is strong when graft deterioration is revealed in the absence of other causes of graft dysfunction or chronic allograft nephropathy (CAN). Increased awareness with follow up observation should be in case of a stenosis of 80% on ultrasound examination, even in cases without suspicion of a hemodynamically significant TRAS. Due to increased susceptibility to occlusion in the presence of dehydration or cardiovascular instability, and in this case intervention should be considered.

2.2 Pathophysiology

Since Goldplatt et al published their study on the hypertensive role of partial reduced renal perfusion of the kidney back in 1934; there has been subsequent identification by various investigators of the role of the renin-angiotensin system, with renin being the hormone released in elevated blood levels from the ischemic kidney (Goldplatt, 1934). Angiotensin is being released enzymatically from angiotensinogen, and has various properties, including vasoconstriction, aldosterone secretion, renal sodium retention, and myocardium hypertrophy (Brewster, 2003). There is evidence that when there are two kidneys the above theory has been proven probably right, however it has been showed that this is not the case for the sole kidney or the transplanted kidney. Hypertension is also present but predominantly as a balance between volume regulation depending on salt and water retention and the renin-angiotensin dependent mechanism. It is the highly circulating volume and not the pressor effect from the renin-angiotensin system that is capable to keep a normal GFR rate with normal renin blood levels. In case that ACE inhibitors are prescribed there is a subsequent reduction in kidney perfusion and finally renal function deterioration. In patients with kidney transplantation, and in order to control hypertension, it is not uncommon to establish a diagnosis of TRAS, when an ACE inhibitor is introduced.

2.3 Diagnosis

Doppler ultrasonography is considered as the best screening test TRAS assessment. There are many advantages in the use of Doppler ultrasound as initial approach over other imaging methods, especially iodine contrast media. The fact that Doppler ultrasound is a noninvasive method, does not expose the recipient to the risk of iodine contrast examination, is widely and promptly available in all hospital settings makes it an excellent first choice for TRAS evaluation. The most significant limitation of the method, as in other conditions, is the fact that ultrasonography is operator dependent.

Digital subtractive angiography (DSA), used to be the gold standard technique for establishing the diagnosis, but today tends to be replaced by MRI angiography and more recently Multi Detector CT-angiography. DSA is an invasive technique and potential complications are groin hematoma, renal artery dissection, thrombosis, perforation, and acute kidney injury caused by contrast-induced nephropathy. Doppler ultrasound can also be used to evaluate the hemodynamic changes due to TRAS. Doppler findings in TRAS include peak systolic velocity 2.0-2.5 m/s, low pulsatility index, and a parvus et tardus waveform with a systolic acceleration time of ≥ to 0.1 seconds (Snider, 1989, Irshad, 2009, Baxter, 1995). Snider et al compared Doppler ultrasonography with conventional angiography and showed 94% sensitivity and 87% specificity on US (Snider, 1989). A velocity ratio of the stenotic to pre-stenotic segments of greater than 2:1 is considered supportive of the diagnosis.

Multidetectors helical CT gives accurate assessment of the site and degree of TRAS and provides accurate and valuable imaging, requires less volume of iodinated contrast medium than DSA (Sebastia, 2001). The nature of the vascular contrast medium may be of consideration, rather than the volume. Risk of contrast nephropathy is probably not related to the volume of contrast medium or the degree of renal failure (Birck, 2003, Pannu, 2004). Protection of the allograft with sufficient volume and N-acetylcysteine is recommended when intravenous contrast medium is injected, regardless of renal function and contrast volume. The alternative is to perform MRI with gadolinium, a non-iodinated contrast medium even though there have been reports of nephrogenic systemic sclerosis.

2.4 Treatment

Treatment options for TRAS include both surgical and endoluminal options. Primary treatment for TRAS involves Percutaneous transluminal angioplasty (PTA) with or without stent placement (Audard, 2006, Bruno, 2004). The type of arterial anastomosis that is present is the deciding factor in determining the angiographic approach utilized. The technical success rate of PTA has been reported to be as high as 94%, with a clinical success rate of 82% (Patel, 2001). Recurrent stenosis may occur in more than 10%, and allograft loss has been reported in up to 30% of cases (Fervenza, 1998). There have been reports correlating TRAS with acute cellular rejection and that long term survival is significantly higher in non-TRAS patients compared with the TRAS. Surgical revascularization is now considered rescue therapy and generally has been reserved for patients with disease unsuitable for PTA

2.5 Endoluminal Interventions

Since the introduction and the evolution of the endovascular interventions there has been a shift in TRAS treatment option with Percutaneous Transluminal Angioplasty (PTA) with or without the use of stent (Beecroft, 2004) being now the gold standard and the initial option of treatment. The method is considered very efficient especially in experienced hands and technical success has been reported to be greater than 90%. However when we consider the clinical impact that has on hypertension or improvement of allograft function, this is significantly lower.

As we have already pointed out, the results in clinically insignificant TRAS can be evaluated only on the degree of the radiological success. PTA with or without stenting, is carrying a significant risk for the allograft and unless a significant pressure decrease exists across the TRAS, PTA should not be undertaken. Unfortunately there is no consensus as to the appropriate value of stenosis measurement beyond which intervention is warranted, and it would be very difficult to obtain one in the future since radiological success does not always results in clinical improvement. A cut off point proposed by Schoenberg et al (Schoenberg, 2000), could be pressure decrease at least 10 mm Hg across the stenosis.

The type of arterial anastomosis that is present is the deciding factor in determining the angiographic approach utilized. If there is an end-to-end anastomosis with the internal iliac artery, commonly done in living donor allografts, then a contralateral femoral approach is utilized to make access to the downward sloping artery as easy as possible. However, if there is an end-to-side anastomosis with the external iliac artery, then an ipsilateral femoral approach is preferred by some authors to access the cephalad sloping artery (Bruno, 2004).

Results after PTA depend largely on the radiologists or vascular surgeons experience and expertise, and should have smooth cooperation with the transplant surgeons. Most of the complications relate to puncture site, but there could be also more severe complication like hemorrhage, rupture of transplant renal artery, iliac artery and loss of the allograft, in those case there could be a need for "salvage" operation. Evolution in endovascular technology, with newer pre-mounted stents, has minimised complications especially the life threatening ones and the risk for allograft loss. Rate of re-stenosis are reported to be 10% to 50% and depends on the primary cause of the stenosis, length of follow-up, and use of stents (Voiculescu A 2005). Even though there are several reports on the topic, there are limitations provided by the retrospective nature of those manuscripts and the limited number of patients. In a french study of 29 patients with TRAS treated with PTA, the technical success rate was 93.1%, and there was 27.5% re-stenosis (Audard, 2006). In other study from the US, TRAS was found in 26 (3.1%) renal allografts, and 17 were treated with PTA with a success rate of 94%. Re-stenosis occurred in 12% of the patients [Patel NH 2001] In case of segmental branches, there is a lower success rate and the success rate is even lower for anastomotic strictures, and even though the incidence of stenosis is similar between end-to-side anastomosis to the external iliac artery and end-to-end anastomosis to the internal iliac artery, PTA in the latter situation is technically more difficult and results in a higher complication rate and more graft loss (Voiculescu, 2005).

2.6 Surgical correction

Surgical correction of TRAS is regarded as a difficult operation with graft loss rates exceeding 20% (Bruno, 2004). A couple of risks existing; to the recipient and to the allograft, the latter is not a contraindication to surgery, since severe TRAS could deteriorate the transplanted kidney, the patient proceeds to renal failure, and finally to end up in heamodialysis. Surgery is now considered as rescue therapy for cases unsuitable for PTA.

In general indications for surgery include: TRAS caused by kinking, anastomotic strictures and complex atherosclerotic disease. There are several options to treat TRAS; mostly excision of the stenosis with direct anastomosis to the external iliac artery and grafting with saphenous vein, recipient internal iliac artery, and preserved ABO blood group compatible deceased donor artery. Reported surgical success rates range from 63% to 92%, with recurrence in 12% of patients (Roberts, 1989). A study comparing PTA vs. surgical repair of TRAS showed an immediate and long-term success rate of 92.1% and 81.5% and 69% and 40.5% for surgical repair and PTA respectively [Benoit G 1990]. Limitations of surgical procedure are access to the artery and most importantly the subsequent warm ischemia time. A warm ischemia of 60 minutes might be tolerated by a kidney allograft that has been heparinised even though the risk for Acute Tubular Necrosis (ATN) and cortical necrosis is increased due to diminished blood flow. An alternative option even though rarely used, is back table reconstruction of a complex arterial problem and autotransplantation of the allograft.

3. Transplant renal artery kinks and allograft torsion

Positioning the allograft is sometimes tricky and the source of pitfalls in kidney transplantation and can result in allograft torsion. Allograft torsion can be an early or late complication. One of the main problems caused by improper positioning or torsion is the arterial kinking. Usually arterial kinks are formed due to long renal graft artery when there is a shift in the graft and/or pelvic contents that causes turn of the artery. Even though the differential diagnosis between TRAS and arterial kinking is often difficult to have, it is of paramount importance to identify an arterial narrowing due to a kink and not TRAS. Prompt diagnosis permits graft detorsion and possible salvage. The most suggestive imaging finding is a change in the axis of the transplanted kidney. CT and MR imaging can show changes in renal graft orientation and vascular pedicle kinking. Surgery remains the primary treatment for arterial kinks and only in cases where surgery is contraindicated or patients refuses surgery, we should proceed with endovascular treatment. TPA with or without stents, may increase the risk of arterial vasospasm and dissection and in addition, placing stents across kinks usually can be technically demanding.

4. Thrombophilias

The thrombophilias, also referred to as hypercoagulable states, comprise hereditary or acquired conditions that predispose individuals to thrombosis. It was the third factor of

Virchow's triad that suggested that systemic alterations in the coagulability of blood, is a critical factor in thrombogenesis (Virchow, 1856). Thrombophilias are classified as congenital (inherited), acquired (secondary), or both (mixed) conditions (Schafer, 2007).

Congenital hypercoagulable states are caused by inherited thrombotic disorders due to mutations in genes encoding plasma proteins involved in coagulation mechanisms. They can be broadly classified into two categories: 1) quantitative deficiencies or qualitative defects of the physiologic anticoagulants: antithrombin, protein C and protein S deficiency, and 2) increased levels or function of the coagulation factors: factor V Leiden, prothrombin gene mutation, elevated levels of specific coagulation factors (Schafer, 2003). Congenital abnormalities of anticoagulant or procoagulant proteins result in an increased risk for venous thromboembolism (VTE) as well as arterial thrombosis with the risk to be higher in cases with decreased levels of antithrombotic proteins than in those with increased levels of prothrombotic proteins. The overall incidence of venous thromboembolism (per 100 patient-years) is found to be 1.07 for antithrombin deficiency, 0.54 for protein C deficiency, 0.50 for protein S deficiency, and 0.30 for activated protein C resistance or factor V Leiden (Bucciarelli, 1999). Half of the patients with inherited hypercoagulable state present with venous thromboembolism before the age of 45 years, particularly in the absence of well recognized risk factors, and often have a family history of thrombosis (Anderson, 2010). The secondary hypercoagulable states encompass a variety of heterogeneous disorders that have been associated with an increased risk of thrombotic complications (Schafer, 2003). Acquired hypercoagulable states include antiphospholipid antibody syndrome, cancer, heparin-induced thrombocytopenia, pregnancy and estrogen therapy, and a prior history of venous thromboembolism. Acquired coagulation defects are particularly common in patients with endstage renal disease (Wagenknecht, 1999). The prevalence of antiphospholipid antibodies in patients awaiting renal transplantation is more than 10%, but the rate of clinical events is far less than the frequency of thrombophilic states. Hyperhomocysteinemia is the typical hypercoagulable state that occurs due to a combination of inherited and acquired factors. Elevated serum levels of homocysteine have been associated with an increased risk of arterial thrombosis (myocardial infarction, stroke, and peripheral arterial disease) and venous thromboembolism (Cattaneo, 1999).

After renal transplantation the donor kidney endothelium is conditioned to exhibit a prothrombotic state as a consequence of reperfusion injury, tissue trauma, inflammation and expression of tissue factor, in addition to the recipient immune response (Key, 1992, Irish, 1999). The combination of a conditioned endothelium and a genetic or acquired predisposition to a hypercoagulable state increase the risk of thrombosis. Factors specific for the renal transplant patients that have been suggested to contribute to this thrombotic risk include the use of calcineurin-inhibiting drugs, high levels of homocysteine, diabetic nephropathy, antiphospholipid syndrome, cytomegalovirus infection, and the presence of proteinuria or nephrotic syndrome (Kujovich, 2004).

It has been proposed that inherited risk factors of venous thromboembolism, such as factor V-Leiden, prothrombin G20210A, and methylenetetrahydrofolate reductase (MTHFR) C677T, might be associated with poorer survival rates of transplanted kidneys, attributed to the context of graft perfusion defects, venous thromboembolic complications, and acute graft loss by vascular rejection, possibly reflecting immunological injury upon the vascular wall exacerbated or induced by the prothrombotic state (Heidenreich, 2003, Wuthrich, 2001). Later study with larger number of patients, did not find a statistically significant association of polymorphisms factor V-Leiden G1691A and MTHFR C677T with renal graft survival Meyer, 2007).

Factor V-Leiden mutation or activated protein C resistance is the most common inherited thrombophilic disorder, found in 5% to 8% of the general population, in 20% of patients with a first venous thrombosis, and in up to 50% of patients with a personal or family history of recurrent thrombosis (Kujovich, 2004). In renal transplant recipients, factor V Leiden has been associated with a variety of complications after renal transplantation and a significantly higher incidence of venous thromboembolism which occurred in up to 39% of FVL carriers (Wuthrich, 2001, Irish, 1997). Also FVL carriers had 12-fold higher risk of an early graft perfusion defect (Wuthrich, 2001). A higher risk of vascular rejection was found in FVL carriers, which was linked to the presence of endotheliolitis or fibrinoid necrosis on histopathology of renal grafts lost within the first year after transplant (Ekberg, 2000).

The reported prevalence of prothrombin gene heterozygous mutation in renal transplant recipients is 3.7%, similar to that in the general population. The mutation was associated with a nearly threefold increased risk of graft failure, which was attributable to arterial, venous, or microvascular thrombosis in the majority of carriers (Fischereder, 2001, Kujovich, 2004).

A polymorphism of the methylenetetrahydrofolate reductase (MTHFR) gene coding for an enzyme that degrades the endothelium toxic product homocysteine have been associated with ESRD (Girndt, 2007). This mutation occurs in 50% to 90% of chronic dialysis patients presenting with mild hyperhomocysteinemia and have been associated with cardiovascular disease and vascular access thrombosis in this population (Mallamaci, 2005, Mallamaci, 2002). Additionally hyperhomocysteinemia can be acquired, such as in renal failure and in deficiencies of folate, vitamin B12, or vitamin B6. Even though many studies found that hyperhomocysteinemia is an independent risk factor for both first and recurrent venous thromboembolism (den Heijer, 1996, Cattaneo, 1999) and that hyperhomocysteinemia is an independent risk factor for cardiovascular disease (Ducloux D et al 2000), the effect of hyperhomocysteinemia on the risk of graft thrombosis is unknown. Antiphospholipid syndrome is the most common acquired blood protein defect associated with either venous or arterial thrombosis or both (Koniari, 2010). Antiphospholipid antibodies (APLA) are found in approximately 10% of patients awaiting renal transplantation. Since only a fraction of patients with antiphospholipid antibodies experience thrombotic complications, the description of antiphospholipid antibody syndrome (APAS), defines by the presence of antiphospholipid antibodies and a clinical history of thrombosis. Antiphospholipid antibodies include not only the lupus anticoagulant (LA) and anticardiolipin antibodies (ACLAs) but also more recently recognized subgroups of antiphospholipid antibodies (antibodies against beta-2-glycoprotein-I [B-2-GP-I]) and antibodies to phosphatidylserine, phosphatidylethanolamine, phosphatidylglycerol, phosphatidylinositol, phosphatidylcholine, and anti-annexin-V (Bick, 2003). Patients with antiphospholipid antibodies in association with other autoimmune disease, most commonly lupus, are classified as having secondary antiphospholipid syndrome. Approximately 40% of patients with SLE have an antiphospholipid (anticardiolipin) antibody (lupus anticoagulant). The presence of antiphospholipid antibodies has been recognized as an important risk factor for early allograft failure (Wagenknecht, 1999. Patients with APAS are at high risk for renovascular thrombosis and renal allograft loss was reported to be universal in the absence of anticoagulation (Vaidya, 2000). Whereas, and despite the lack of anticoagulation, no allografts were lost to thrombosis, in patients with detectable anticardiolipin antibodies but no prior history of thrombosis. In a later report all patients with antiphospholipid antibodies were successfully transplanted using postoperative anticoagulation (Morrissey, 2002).

Other prothrombotic changes that have been reported in renal transplant recipients include decreases in antithrombin, protein C and protein S levels, markedly elevated factor VIII levels and over-expression of plasminogen activator inhibitor-1 by donor epithelium (suggestive of impaired regional fibrinolysis) (Irish, 1999).

In vitro data suggest that immunosuppressive drugs like cyclosporine and OKT3 may increase the risk of thrombosis but an independent clinical association with allograft thrombosis is unproven (Gruber, 1989, Abramowicz, 1992). Specifically, the prothrombotic effects of cyclosporine include activation of monocytes to express tissue factor, increased platelet aggregation, endothelial dysfunction and activation of the intrinsic coagulation pathway, impaired fibrinolysis and impaired activation of protein C (Carlsen, 1988, Fishman, 1991, Bombeli, 1996, Evans, 1997, Levi, 1992).

Thrombotic complications after renal transplantation are usually catastrophic. Inherited and acquired hypercoagulable states have to be considered prior to kidney transplantation and proper prophylactic treatment initiated for the purpose to improve transplant outcome. Andrassy et al. provided specified screening recommendations for thrombophilia prior to kidney transplantation (Andrassy, 2004). A general screening for thrombophilia, to include factor V Leiden, prothrombin gene G20210A polymorphism, antithrombin III, protein C and S activity, antiphospholipid antibodies and lupus anticoagulant, should be performed in all children and adolescents because they have the highest risk for thrombotic complications. Adults only with history of thrombotic events should be thoroughly screened (recurrent AVC fistula thrombosis should be taken into account). When risk factors are absent, screening only for antiphospholipid antibodies and lupus anticoagulant is recommended.

There is also no consensus on the optimal management of renal transplant patients with thrombophilic disorders. Treatment strategies to reduce thrombotic risk including heparin, warfarin, and aspirin have been evaluated in several reports. While inadequate anticoagulation may place the patient at risk for thrombosis, preemptive or intense perioperative anticoagulation can result in postoperative bleeding (Morrissey, 2002, Murashima, 2010, Friedman, 2001). Morissey et al. (Morrissey, 2002) recommended management approach for renal transplant patients with thrombophilia. Patients with diagnosis or suspected to have thrombophilia is suspected, the risk for thrombotic complications should be stratified as low, intermediate or high. In high risk are patients with inherited thrombotic disorder and history of at least two thrombotic episodes. For the high risk patients indefinite oral anticoagulation has been advocated. In intermediate risk are patients with a known inherited thrombotic disorder who are asymptomatic or have experienced a single thrombotic event. They should receive adequate prophylaxis in high-risk situations such as surgery for a minimum of 6 months. For patients with no suspicion of thrombophilia, no anticoagulation or a short term postoperative anticoagulation may be given.

5. Renal vein and artery thrombosis

Renal transplantation is established as the preferred treatment for most cases of end-stage renal disease. Postoperative vascular complications include thrombosis of renal vein and artery, with a delay in the diagnosis and management of these complications leading to significant morbidity for the recipient, with a high risk of graft loss and mortality (Akbar, 2005). It consists of a rare complication that often results in graft loss, with reported incidence ranging from 0.4% to 6% (Rouviere, 2002, Giustacchini, 2002). Bakir et al reported that thrombosis represented 45% and 37% of renal allograft loss at 3 and 12 months (Bakir, 1996).

5.1 Renal vein thrombosis

Renal vein thrombosis (RVT), although an unusual event, most often has graft loss as a result (Figure 1). The causes that may lead to this serious complication include compression due to hematomas or lymphoceles, angulation or kinking of the vein, anastomotic strictures, or an underlying state of deep venous thrombosis or hypercoaguability (Penny, 1994). RVT usually occurs suddenly and towards the end of the first week of an otherwise uncomplicated kidney transplantation. Specifically it occurs in the first 2 weeks post transplant, with 80% occurring in the first month and 93% within the first year (Kobayashi, 2007). Clinical presentation is initiated by oliguria and hematuria with a tender swollen graft, which if ruptured, is accompanied by life-treatening bleeding (Kobayashi, 2007).

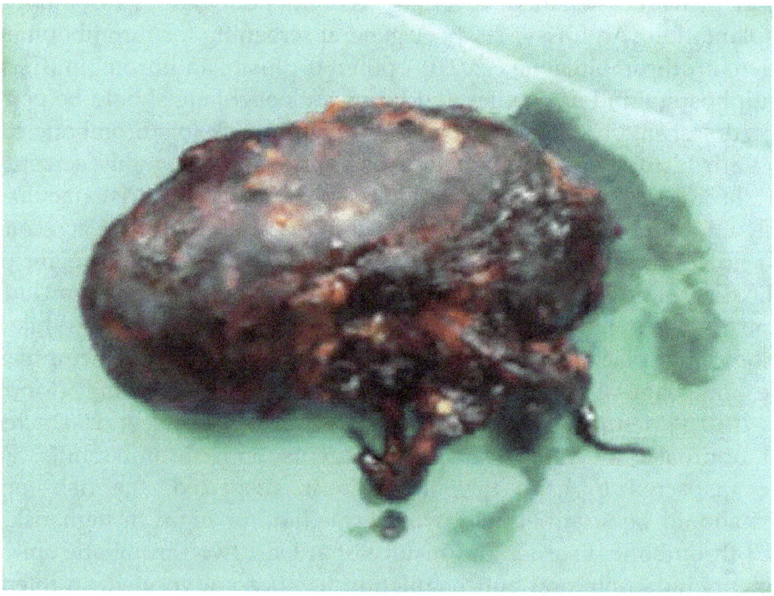

Fig. 1. Specimen of renal allograft nephrectomy due to renal vein trhrombosis

5.2 Renal artery thrombosis

This uncommon complication which may occur most often as an early but also as a late event after kidney transplantation consists a devastating clinical condition leading frequently to graft loss. Renal artery thrombosis (RAT) onset most often follows a technical problem such as intimal dissection, kinking or torsion of the vessels. Risk factors include poor cardiac output, hyperacute rejection, unresponsive acute rejection, and a hypercoagulable state. It presents with a rapid onset of oliguria. In cases of segmental infarct, there can be lack of symptomatology or a presentation of renal dysfunction and increased blood pressure. When RAT occurs as a late event, it could be attributed to renal artery stricture or its manipulation post-operatively e.g. during angiography, or usually due to graft rejection.

5.3 Diagnosis

An early clinical diagnosis is very important for both RVT and RAT, even during the morning ward round. Diagnosis of these complications is established by colour flow Doppler studies, demonstrating in RVT a swollen graft with a crescent of clot along the convex margin of the kidney. In this case it is essential that the patient is taken immediately to theatre. Under normal clinical conditions, the spectral Doppler renal arterial waveform shows high resistive index with reversal of diastolic flow. On the contrary, in RAT a lack of flow in the renal artery is demonstrated, with the presence of intraluminal filling defects. In RAT, diagnosis is set by Doppler studies or at time of surgical exploration, however by that time it is not possible for the graft to be saved due to the kidney's low tolerance to warm ischemia (Rouviere, 2002).

5.4 Treatment

Following establishment of diagnosis for RVT, the treatment of choice is urgent thrombectomy. However graft salvage may not be possible, in which case graft nephrectomy is usually required. In case thrombectomy is applied early, within 1 hour following the event, graft salvage can be achieved. The increased risk of swelling, edema and also a possible rupture of the kidney graft in such a condition, makes urgent exploration essential. Systemic anticoagulants can be applied as treatment only in cases of partial vein thrombosis.

The surgical treatment for renal graft thrombosis includes laparotomy, thrombectomy and ultimately a possible graft nephrectomy. Several authors describe endoluminal therapy for renal graft thrombosis; however the exact role of interventional radiologic treatment is not yet well-defined (Obed, 2008). The technique for percutaneous treatment involves placing the tip of a catheter within the thrombus, 1 cm distal to the surgical anastomosis, with infusion of a thrombolytic agent (Rouviere, 2002). Because transcatheter thrombolysis revascularizes arteries at a slower rate than surgical thrombectomy, patients with a heavy clot burden should be primarily offered surgical treatment (Hedegard, 2009). Transcatheter thrombolysis should be limited to low clot burden, segmental artery thrombosis, or high-risk surgical candidates. Additionally catheter-directed thrombolytics should be avoided in the first 2 weeks following kidney transplant due to the immature anastomotic suture line. On the other hand RAT can be determined as a terminal event, which can be averted only if poor graft function can be attributed to arterial inflow and in this case intervention should be immediate. By the time the diagnosis is set, the transplanted kidney is lost.

5.5 Prevention

Although in many cases of renal allograft vascular thrombosis, no cause can be identified, epidemiological studies have attempted to categorise risk factors as modifiable, including drugs and the surgical procedure among others, and nonmodifiable, including age, diabetes mellitus and vascular anomalies. Additionally studies have identified changes in coagulation or fibrinolysis promoting a more thrombotic state, as risk factors as well.

Prevention may hold an important role in avoiding the formation of vascular thrombosis. This requires of course a combination of different measures such as avoiding prolonged cold and warm ischemia. Attention to precise surgical technique, use of preservation solution such as University of Wisconsin solution and an immediate and effective management of rejection, should all be outlined as important in the prevention strategy.

Additionally identification and management of thrombophilic states could act as a preventive measure against renal vascular thrombosis, with a possible need for routine screening and directed therapy to reduce the risk of thrombosis and graft loss, however no consensus for either strategy have been introduced. Previous reports indicate a possible laboratory investigation to potential recipients with a previous history or family history of thrombotic events, such as deep and superficial vein thromboses, pulmonary emboli, fistulas having been thrombosed or incidents of multiple occlusions of central venous dialysis catheters, as well as patients undergoing preemptive transplantation with a living donor kidney (Andrassy, 2004).

The risk of thrombosis must be balanced against that of bleeding. For known thrombophilia and a history of clinical events, perioperative heparinization followed by long-term anticoagulation with warfarin has shown good results, including successful retransplantation. However since results of the few available, prospective randomized studies on heparin use in renal transplant patients, show conflicting conclusions, one understands that there is a great need for a preoperative classification of thrombotic and hemorrhagic risk among renal transplant candidates and for establishment of consensus guidelines.

6. Extrarenal pseudoaneurysm

Extrarenal arterial pseudoaneurysms in renal transplantation are rare, and their prevalence is less than 1% (Bracale, 2009). Extrarenal pseudoaneurysms are directly related to arterial anastomosis, percutaneous nephrostomy placement and infectious causes. It is usually asymptomatic and rarely can cause renal dysfunction or compression of adjacent structures (Bracale, 2009). When extrarenal pseudoaneurysms become large, there is a strong indication to be surgically removed to avoid spontaneous rupture and loss of the allograft (Figure 2).

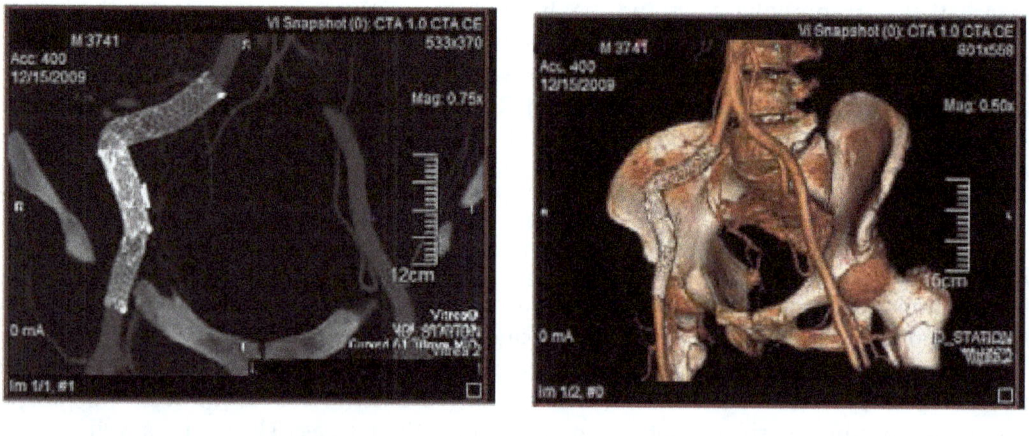

Fig. 2. External iliac artery pseudoaneurysm presented as a complication of renal vein thrombosis and allograph nephrectomy. The pseudoanurysm was formed at the stump of the arterial anastomosis due to inflammation. Preemptive treatment with double stent placement was successfully performed.

7. Arteriovenous fistula

Arteriovenous fistula (AVF) is a well-recognized vascular complication of percutaneous biopsy. The reported incidence of AVF ranges between 0.5 and 16% (Martinez, 1998). An arteriovenous fistula (AVF) may be formed when both arterial and venous walls are punched by the biopsy needle. Mostly they are asymptomatic, rarely may cause persistent hematuria or recurrence of hematuria, hypertension and deterioration of renal function. Rarely, renal graft ischemia may be the result of steal phenomenon from a large AVF (Harrison, 1994, Matsell, 1992, Cruzado, 19990. Factors that may predispose to the development of arteriovenous fistula include early postransplant period, the presence of hypertension, sclerosis and interstitial fibrosis, the formation of intrarenal hematoma (Schwarz, 2008). About 70% of AVF cases resolve spontaneously within weeks or months (Matsell, 1992).

Doppler sonography allowing noninvasive diagnosis of AVFs is the diagnostic examination of choice (Ozbek, 1995). Angiography is the reference standard as it confirms the presence of the AVF, accurately assesses its size and location, and permits endovascular treatment (Loffroy, 2008). On Doppler, the AVF shows a focal area of turbulent flow and a localized region of disorganized color that extends outside the normal vessels on color Doppler. In the area of AVF, the duplex US shows a very high velocity with low resistive index in the feeding artery with arterialization of the flow in the draining vein (Irshad, 2009).

In most cases AVFs close spontaneously within a few months, but they warrant observation to exclude the need for therapeutic intervention. The likelihood of and time to spontaneous closure in renal allografts, and the optimal time for therapeutic intervention are not predictable (Loffroy, 2008). Treatment has been recommended when bleeding persists for more than 72 h, renal function deteriorates markedly, lesion enlarges and there is suspicion of steal phenomenon. Endovascular superselective embolization is the therapeutic procedure of choice, as loss of normal parenchyma is minimal, with success rate of approximately 88% with no significant loss of allograft function (Loffroy, 2008, Tarif, 2002). In the majority of cases, successful embolization can be achieved using coils or microcoils. Schwarz et al (Schwarz,2008) proposed a hemodynamic prognostic test to predict which AVF would probably profit from AVF coiling, by comparing Doppler sonographic resistive indices of the main renal artery and the non-AVF associated segmental arteries (Schwarz, 2008). The resistive index of the main renal artery should be at least 0.05 less than that of the non-AVF-associated segmental renal arteries indicating under-perfusion of the rest renal parenchyma.

8. Conclusions

Renal transplantation is regarded as an optimal treatment for End-stage renal disease. Improvements in surgical techniques and advanced immunosuppressive drugs have resulted in remarkable survival of patients and renal grafts. However complications occur in both the immediate postoperative period and later. Awareness for early post-operative complications, like renal vein and artery thrombosis could save allografts and patients. Cardiovascular disease remains the most frequent cause of death and transplant loss after kidney transplantation, with hypertension present in vast majority of kidney transplant recipients and a risk factor for cardiovascular disease. Improvements in imagining modalities and interventional techniques resulted in earlier identification and management of TRAS. It is of paramount importance for the transplant surgeon to keep in mind that early and late vascular complications after renal transplantation could be very challenging and potentially allograft and/or life threatening

9. References

Akbar SA, Jafri SZ, Amendola MA, Madrazo BL, Salem R, Bis KG. (2005). Complications of renal transplantation. *Radiographics,*Vol. 25, No. 5, (Sep-Oct 2005), p:1335-1356,.Anderson JA, Weitz JI (2010). Hypercoagulable states. *Clinics in Chest Medine,* Vol. 31. No. 4 (December 2010), p;31:659-73.

Andrassy J, Zeier M, Andrassy K. (2004). Do we need screening for thrombophilia prior to kidney transplantation? Nephrology Dialysis Transplantation, Vol. 19, Suppl 4, p:iv-64-iv-68.

Audard V, Matignon M, Hemery F, Snanoudj R, Desgranges P, Anglade MC, Kobeiter H, Durrbach A, Charpentier B, Lang P, Grimbert P. (2006). Risk factors and long-term outcome of transplant renal artery stenosis in adult recipients after treatment by percutaneous transluminal angioplasty. *American Journal of Transplantation* Vol. 6, No. 1, (January 2006), p:95-99.

Bakir N, Sluiter WJ, Ploeg RJ, van Son WJ, Tegzess AM. (1996). Primary renal graft thrombosis. *Nephrology Dialysis Transplantation,* Vol. 11, No. 1, (January 1996), p:140-147, 1996

Basso N, Terragno NA (2001). History about the discovery of the rennin angiotensin system. *Hypertension,* Vol. 38, No 6, (December 2001) p: 1246-1249.

Baxter GM, Ireland H, Moss JG, Harden PN, Junor BJ, Rodger RS, Briggs JD. (1995). Colour Doppler ultrasound in renal transplant artery stenosis: which Doppler index? *Clinical Radiology,* Vol. 50, No. 9, (September 1995), p: 618-622.

Beecroft JR, Rajan DK, Clark TW, Robinette M, Stavropoulos SW. (2004): Transplant renal artery stenosis: outcome after percutaneous intervention. *Journal of Vascular Interventional Radiology,* Vol. 15, No 12, (December 2004), p: 1407-1413, 2004.

Benoit G, Moukarzel M, Hiesse C, Verdelli G, Charpentier B, Fries D. (1990): Transplant renal artery stenosis: Experience and comparative results between surgery and angioplasty. *Transplant International,* Vol. 3, No. 3, (October 1990), p:137-140.

Birck R, Krzossok S, Markowetz F, Schnülle P, van der Woude FJ, Braun C. (2003). Acetylcysteine for prevention of contrast nephropathy: meta-analysis. *Lancet,* Vol. 362, No. 9384, (August2003), p:598-603, 2003.

Bick RL (2003). Antiphospholipid thrombosis syndromes. *Hematology Oncology Clinics of North America,* Vol. 17, No. 1,(February 2003), p:115-47.

Bracale UM, Carbone F, del Guercio L, Viola D, D'Armiento FP, Maurea S, Porcellini M, Bracale G. (2009). External iliac artery pseudoaneurysm complicating renal transplantation. *Interactive Cardiovascular Thoracic Surgery,* Vol. 8, No. 6, (June 2009), p:654-60.

Brewster UC, Setaro JF, Perazella MA. (2003). The renin-angiotensin-aldosterone system: cardiorenal effects and implications for renal and cardiovascular disease states. *The American Journal of Medical Sciences,* Vol. 326, No. 1 (July 2003):15-24.

Bruno S, Remuzzi G, Ruggenenti P. (2004). Transplant renal artery stenosis. *Journal of the American Society of Nephrology*, Vol. 15, No. 1, (January 2004), p:134-141.

Bucciarelli P, Rosendaal FR, Tripodi A, Mannucci PM, De Stefano V, Palareti G, Finazzi G, Baudo F, Quintavalla R (1999). Risk of venous thromboembolism and clinical manifestations in carriers of antithrombin, protein C, protein S deficiency, or activated protein C resistance: a multicenter collaborative family study. *Arteriosclerosis Thrombosis and Vascular Biology*, Vol. 19, No. 4, (April 1999), p:1026-33.

Buturovic-Ponikvar J. (2003). Renal transplant artery stenosis. *Nephrology Dialysis Transplantation*, Vol. 18, No. S5, (July 2003), p:v-74-v-77.

Cattaneo M (1999). Hyperhomocysteinemia, atherosclerosis and thrombosis. *Thrombosis and Haemostasis*, Vol. 81, No. 2, (February 1999), p:165-76.

den Heijer M, Koster T, Blom HJ, Bos GM, Briet E, Reitsma PH, Vandenbroucke JP, Rosendaal FR (1996). Hyperhomocysteinemia as a risk factor for deep-vein thrombosis. *The New England Journal of Medicine*, Vol. 21, No. 334, (March 1996), p:759-62.

Cruzado JM, Torras J, Domínguez J, Sancho C, Alsina J, Grinyó JM. (1999). An unusual cause of post-biopsy oliguria in an allograft. *Nephrology Dialysis Transplantation*, Vol. 14, No. 8, (August 1999), p:2022-4.

Ducloux D, Motte G, Challier B, Gibey R, Chalopin JM (2000). Serum total homocysteine and cardiovascular disease occurrence in chronic, stable renal transplant recipients: a prospective study. *Journal of the American Society of Nephrology*, Vol. 11, No. 1, (January 2000), p:134-7.

Ekberg H, Svensson PJ, Simanaitis M, Dahlbäck B (2000). Factor V R506Q mutation (activated protein C resistance) is an additional risk factor for early renal graft loss associated with acute vascular rejection. *Transplantation*, Vol. 27, No. 69, (April 2000), p:1577-81.

Fervenza FC, Lafayette RA, Alfrey EJ, Petersen J. (1998). Renal artery stenosis in kidney transplants. American Journal of Kidney Disease, Vol. 31, No. 1, (January 1998), p:142-8.

Fischereder M, Schneeberger H, Lohse P, Krämer BK, Schlöndorff D, Land W (2001). Increased rate of renal transplant failure in patients with the G20210A mutation of the prothrombin gene. *American Journal of Kidney Diseases*, Vol. 38, No. 5, (November 2001), p:1061-4.

Friedman GS, Meier-Kriesche HU, Kaplan B, Mathis AS, Bonomini L, Shah N, DeFranco P, Jacobs M, Mulgaonkar S, Geffner S, Lyman N, Paraan C, Walsh C, Belizaire W, Tshibaka M.(2001). Hypercoagulable states in renal transplant candidates: impact of anticoagulation upon incidence of renal allograft thrombosis. *Transplantation*, Vol27, No. 72, (September 2001), p:1073-8

Garovic VD, Textor SC. (2005): Renovascular hypertension and ischemic nephropathy. *Circulation*, Vol. 112, No. 9, (August 2005), p:1362-1374.

Girndt M, Heine GH, Ulrich C, Köhler H. DialGene Consortium. (2007). Gene polymorphism association studies in dialysis: vascular access. *Seminars in Dialysis*, Vol. 20, No. 1, (Jan-Feb 2007), p:63-67.

Giustacchini P, Pisanti F, Citterio F, De Gaetano AM, Castagneto M, Nanni G. (2002). Renal vein thrombosis after renal transplantation: An important cause of graft loss. *Transplantation Proceedings*, Vol. 34, No. 6, (September 2002), p:2126-2127

Goldblatt H, Lynch J, Hanzal RE, Summerville WW. (1934). Studies on experimental hypertension, I: the production of persistent elevation of systolic blood pressure by means of renal ischaemia. *The Journal of Experimental Medicine*, Vol. 59, No. 3, (February 1934), p:347-379.

Harrison KL, Nghiem HV, Coldwell DM, Davis CL. (1994). Renal dysfunction due to an arteriovenous fistula in a transplant recipient. *Journal of the American Society of Nephrolology*, Vol. 5, No. 6, (December 1994), p:1300-6.

Hedegard W, Saad WE, Davies MG. (2009). Management of vascular and nonvascular complications after renal transplantation. *Techniques in Vascular Interventional Radiology*, Vol, 12, No. 4, (December 2009), p:240-62

Heidenreich S, Junker R, Wolters H, Lang D, Hessing S, Nitsche G, Nowak-Göttl U. (2003). Outcome of kidney transplantation in patients with inherited thrombophilia: data of a prospective study. *Journal of the American Society of Nephrology*, Vol. 14, No. 1, (January 2003), p:234-9.

Irish AB, Green FR, Gray DW, Morris PJ. (1997). The factor V Leiden (R506Q) mutation and risk of thrombosis in renal transplant recipients. *Transplantation*, Vol. 64, No. 4, (August 1997), p:604-7.

Irish A. (1999). Renal allograft thrombosis: can thrombophilia explain the inexplicable? *Nephrology Dialysis Transplantation*, Vol. 14, No. 10, (October 1999), p:2297-303.

Irshad A, Ackerman S, Sosnouski D, Anis M, Chavin K, and Baliga P. (2008). A Review of Sonographic Evaluation of Renal Transplant Complications. *Current Problems in Diagnostic Radiology*, Vol. 37, No. 2 (Mar-Apr 2008), p:67-79

Irshad A, Ackerman SJ, Campbell AS, Anis M. (2009). An overview of renal transplantation: current practice and use of ultrasound. *Seminars in Ultrasound CT and MR*, Vol. 30, No. 4, (August 2009), p:298-314.

Key NS (1992). Scratching the surface: endothelium as a regulator of thrombosis, fibrinolysis, and inflammation. *The Journal of Laboratory Clinical Medicine*, Vol. 120, No. 2, (August 1992), p:184-6.

Kobayashi K, Censullo ML, Rossman LL, Kyriakides PN, Kahan BD, Cohen AM. (2007). Interventional radiologic management of renal transplant dysfunction: Indications, limitations, and technical considerations. *Radiographics*, Vol. 27, No. 4, (Jul-Aug 2007), p:1109-30

Koniari I, Siminelakis SN, Baikoussis NG, Papadopoulos G, Goudevenos J, Apostolakis E. (2010). Antiphospholipid syndrome; its implication in cardiovascular diseases: a review. *Journal of Cardiothoracic Surgery*, Vol. 3, No. 5, (November 2010), p:101-10.

Kujovich JL. (2004). Thrombophilia and thrombotic problems in renal transplant patients. *Transplantation*, Vol. 15, No. 77, (April 2004), p:959-64.

Loffroy R, Guiu B, Lambert A, Mousson C, Tanter Y, Martin L, Cercueil JP, Krausé D. (2009). Management of post-biopsy renal allograft arteriovenous fistulas with selective arterial embolization: immediate and long-term outcomes. Clinical *Radiology*, Vol. 63, No. 6, (June 2008), p:657-65.

Mallamaci F, Zoccali C, Tripepi G, Fermo I, Benedetto FA, Cataliotti A, Bellanuova I, Malatino LS, Soldarini A. CREED Investigators. (2002). Hyperhomocysteinemia predicts cardiovascular outcomes in hemodialysis patients. *Kidney International*, Vol. 61, No. 2, (February 2002), p:609-14.

Mallamaci F, Bonanno G, Seminara G, Rapisarda F, Fatuzzo P, Candela V, Scudo P, Spoto B, Testa A, Tripepi G, Tech S, Zoccali C. (2005). Hyperhomocysteinemia and arteriovenous fistula thrombosis in hemodialysis patients. *American Journal of Kidney Diseases*, Vol. 45, No. 4, (April 2005), p:702-7.

Mangray M, and Vella JP. (2011). Hypertension After Kidney Transplant. *American Journal of Kidney Diseases*, Vol. 57, No. 2, (February 2011), p:331-341

Martinez T, Palomares M, Bravo JA, Alvarez G, Galindo P, Entrena AG, Osuma A, Asensio C. (1998). Biopsy-induced arteriovenous fistula and venous aneurysm in a renal transplant. *Nephrology Dialysis Transplantation*, Vol. 13, No. 11, (November 1998), p:2937-9.

Matsell DG, Jones DP, Boulden TF, Burton EM, Baum SL, Tonkin IL. (1992). Arteriovenous fistula after biopsy of renal transplant kidney: diagnosis and treatment. *Pediatric Nephrology*, Vol. 6, No. 6, (November 1992), p:562-4.

Meyer M, Laux G, Scherer S, Tran TH, Opelz G, Mytilineos J. (2007). No association of factor V Leiden, prothrombin G20210A, and MTHFR C677T gene polymorphisms with kidney allograft survival: a multicenter study. *Transplantation*, Vol 27, No. 83, (April 2007), p:1055-8.

Morrissey PE, Ramirez PJ, Gohh RY, Yango AY, Kestin A, Madras PN, Monaco AP. (2002). Management of thrombophilia in renal transplant patients. American Journal of *Transplantation*, Vol 2, No. 9, (October 2002), p:872-6.

Murashima M, Konkle BA, Bloom RD, Sood SL, Grossman RA, Brunelli SM, Stein SH. (2010). A single-center experience of preemptive anticoagulation for patients with risk factors for allograft thrombosis in renal transplantation. *Clinical Nephrology*, Vol. 74, No. 5, (November 2010), p:351-7

Obed A, Uihlein DC, Zorger N, Farkas S, Scherer MN, Krüger B, Banas B, Krämer BK. (2008). Severe renal vein stenosis of a kidney transplant with beneficial clinical course after successful percutaneous stenting. American Journal Transplantation, Vol. 8, No. 10, (October 2008), p:2173-2176

Pannu N, Manns B, Lee H, Tonelli M. (2004). Systematic review of the impact of Nacetylcysteine on contrast nephropathy. *Kidney International*, Vol. 65, No, 4, April 2004), p:1366-1374.

Patel NH, Jindal RM, Wilkin T, Rose S, Johnson MS, Shah H, Namyslowski J, Moresco KP, Trerotola SO. (2001). Renal arterial stenosis in renal allografts: retrospective study of predisposing factors and outcome after percutaneous transluminal angioplasty. *Radiology*, Vol. 219, No. 3, (June 2001), p:663-667.

Penny MJ, Nankivell BJ, Disney AP, Byth K, Chapman JR. (1994). Renal graft thrombosis: a survey of 134 consecutive cases. *Transplantation*, Vol. 58, No. 5, (September 1994), p:565-569.

Roberts JP, Ascher NL, Fryd DS, Hunter DW, Dunn DL, Payne WD, Sutherland DE, Castaneda-Zuniga W, Najarian JS. (1989). Transplant renal artery stenosis. *Transplantation*, Vol. 48, No. 4, (October 1989), p:580-583.

Rouvière O, Berger P, Béziat C, Garnier JL, Lefrançois N, Martin X, Lyonnet D. (2002). Acute thrombosis of renal transplant artery: Graft salvage by means of intra-arterial fibrinolysis. *Transplantation*, Vol. 73, No. 3, (February 2002), p:403-409

Sebastià C, Quiroga S, Boyé R, Cantarell C, Fernandez-Planas M, Alvarez A. (2001). Helical CT in Renal Transplantation: Normal Findings and Early and Late Complications. *RadioGraphics*, Vol. 21, No. 5, (Sep-Oct 2001), p:1103–1117

Schafer AI, Levine MN, Konkle BA, Kearon C. (2003). Thrombotic disorders: diagnosis and treatment. *Hematology American Society of Hematology Educational Program*, p:520–539

Schafer, AI. (2007). Hypercoagulable State. In *Cardiovascular Medicine,* Willerson JT, Wellens HJ, Cohn JN, Holmes DR, pp:2423-2438, Springer-Verlag, London.

Schwarz A, Hiss M, Gwinner W, Becker T, Haller H, Keberle M. (2008). Course and relevance of arteriovenous fistulas after renal transplant biopsies. *American Journal of Transplantation*, Vol. 8, No. 4, (April. 2008), p:826-31.

Snider JF, Hunter DW, Moradian GP, Castaneda-Zuniga WR, Letourneau JG. (1989). Transplant renal artery stenosis: Evaluation with duplex sonography. *Radiology*, Vol. 172, (September 1989), p:1027-30.

Schoenberg SO, Bock M, Kallinowski F, Just A. (2000). Correlation of hemodynamic impact and morphologic degree of renal artery stenosis in a canine model. *Journal American Society Nephrology*, Vol. 11, No 12, (December 2000), p:2190-2198

Tarif N, Mitwalli AH, Al Samayer SA, Abu-Aisha H, Memon NA, Sulaimani F, Alam A, Al Wakeel JS. (2002). Congenital renal arteriovenous malformation presenting as severe hypertension. *Nephrology Dialysis Transplantation*, Vol. 17, No. 2, (February 2002), p:291-4.

Tutone VK, Mark PB, Stewart GA, Tan CC, Rodger RS, Geddes CC, Jardine AG. (2005). Hypertension, antihypertensive agents and outcomes following renal transplantation *Clinical Transplantation*, Vol 19, No. 2, (April 2005), p: 181–192

Virchow R. Gesammalte Abhandlungen zur Wissenschaftlichen Medtzin. Frankfurt, Germany: *Medinger Sohn*, 1856:219– 732.

Vaidya S, Sellers R, Kimball P, Shanahan T, Gitomer J, Gugliuzza K, Fish JC. (2000). Frequency, potential risk and therapeutic intervention in end-stage renal disease patients with antiphospholipid antibody syndrome: a multicenter study. *Transplantation*, Vol. 69, No. 7, (April 2000), p:1348-52.

Voiculescu A, Schmitz M, Hollenbeck M, Braasch S, Luther B, Sandmann W, Jung G, Mödder U, Grabensee B. (2005). Management of arterial stenosis affecting kidney graft perfusion: a single-centre study in 53 patients. *American Journal of Transplantation*, Vol. 5, No. 7, (July 2005), p:1731-1738.

Wagenknecht DR, Becker DG, LeFor WM, McIntyre JA. (1999). Antiphospholipid antibodies are a risk factor for early renal allograft failure. *Transplantation*, Vol. 68, No. 2, (July 1999), p: 241–246.

Wuthrich RP, Cicvara-Muzar S, Booy C, Maly FE. (2001). Heterozygosity for the factor V Leiden (G1691A) mutation predisposes renal transplant recipients to thrombotic complications and graft loss. *Transplantation*, Vol. 72, No. 3, (August 2001), p: 549-50.

7

Delayed Graft Function

Qiansheng Li, Wenqian Huo, Keqin Zhang, Gang Wu,
Fengshuo Jin, Xi Lin, Xiaojiang Jiang and Dong Gao
*Department of Urology, Institute of Surgery Research, Daping Hospital,
Third Military Medical University, Chongqing,
China*

1. Introduction

Delayed graft function (DGF) is a common complication of renal transplantation. According to a clinical data analysis of 34,647 cases of cadaveric renal transplantation documented by the Renal Transplantation Registry of the United Network Sharing (UNOS), graft function did not recover instantly after transplantation and for ever in some cases; the 1-year rate of graft loss was up to 20% in cases with poor renal function recovery; the long-term loss rate of graft was higher in cases with poor renal function recovery than those with instant graft function. The half-life time of graft is 7 years in cases with delayed graft function, and is 12 years in cases with instant graft function. Based on our 30 years of experience in renal transplantation and the literature, we reviewed the diagnosis and management of DGF.

2. Diagnostic criteria

Currently, graft function recovery is defined as follows.

1. Instant graft function (IGF): postoperative urine output >7000ml, serum creatinine recovery to normal in 3-7 days.
2. Slow graft function (SGF): postoperative urine output is normal, but serum creatinine decreases slowly, and not to normal in one week. Nevertheless, dialysis is not needed.
3. Delayed graft function (DGF): DGF can be diagnosed according to the three aspects below.
    i. **Need for postoperative dialysis:** Need for dialysis in the first week after transplant once hyperacute rejection, vascular and urinary tract complications and hyperkalemia are ruled out.
    ii. **Urine output and serum creatinine:** ① Rise in serum Cr at 6–8 h post-operatively or <300 ml of urine despite adequate volume and diuretics. ② Urine output <1 L in 24 h and <25% fall in serum creatinine from baseline in first 24 h post-transplant. ③ Urine output <75 mL/h in first 48 h or failure of serum Cr to decrease by 10% in the first 48 h. ④ Serum creatinine increases or remains unchanged or decreases <10%/day during 3 consecutive days postoperatively. ⑤ Serum creatinine >2.5 mg/dL on Day 7 or need for post-transplant hemodialysis. ⑥ Time required for the kidney to reach CrCl>10 mL/min greater than 1 week. ⑦ Failure of creatinine to decline in the first 48 h in the absence of rejection.

iii. **Urine enzymes and biopsy**: ① Urine IL-18 in first 24 h>500 pg/mg. ②Urine NGAL on Day 0 >1000 ng/mg and IL-18 on Day 0 > 500 pg/mg. ③Pre-transplant soluble IL-6R of 35 000 pg/mL. ④ Pathologic findings that support acute renal tubular necrosis.

4. No more graft function (NGF): Postoperative failure of graft function that requires dialysis.
5. Hyper delayed graft function (HDGF): In rare cases, the anuria stage persists longer than one month, even several months after renal transplantation, followed by gradual renal function recovery, a phenomenon we called HDGF. In 2000, we performed a second renal transplantation in a female patient. In this patient, the anuria stage lasted 109 days postoperatively, and urine output increased gradually, with serum creatinine decrease to normal on day 155 postoperatively. Ten years of follow-up indicated the graft function to be normal.

3. Risk factors for DGF

DGF is a complex pathologic process usually involved donor- and recipient-related factors. Donor-related factors include age, cause of death, and transplantation and cold ischemia time of graft. Recipient-related factors include rejection, anti-HLA antibody level, and times of renal transplantation, cytomegalovirus infection, obesity, body size difference with the donor, pre-transplant dialysis type, and ethnicity.

1. Donor-related factors Due to an organ shortage, organs from donors of advanced age or organs with other confounding diseases are also used as sources for organ transplantation. The quality of renal graft is crucial. Renal graft function is closely associated with the donor's age, cause of death and primary disease. Renal graft of poor quality may not survive for long because of immune or non-immune damage to the graft.
   i. Brain death Animal study has demonstrated that changes in physiology, hemodynamics, endocrinology, and histomorphology as well as early inflammation damage peripheral organs following brain death. Cytokine storm after brain death may upregulate HLA expression in the graft and make the graft susceptible to attack by preexisting anti-HLA antibody. Rejection occurred earlier in renal grafts from rats after brain death than in the control group. The survival rate of renal grafts from non-kinship living donors is much higher than that of cadaveric renal grafts. Brain death influences the quality of donor organ, increasing the incidence of DGF.
   ii. Senile donors It has been clinically shown that senility of donors is a major risk factor for DGF, and it influences the long-term survival of grafts. The UN data demonstrate that senility of donor increases the incidence of DGF significantly. For instance, the incidence of DGF is 15% if the donors' age is 20 years, and is up to 40% if the donor's age is over 65 years. The cause for such difference may lie in the fact that the number of functioning nephrons decreases in healthy individuals with aging. In addition, renal grafts may be injured by ultrafiltration following transplantation.
   iii. Cause of death The cause of death is another major risk factor influencing the long-term survival of graft. According to the UNOS data, the incidence of DGF was 18%

if the donors died of traffic accident, was 30% if the donors died of cerebrovascular accident, and was 45% in 400 non-heart-beating donors (NHBDs) (possibly related to long periods of warm ischemia).

iv. Ischemia-reperfusion injury Cessation of blood flow leads to anaerobic metabolism and adenosine triphosphate depletion in the organ. The incidence of DGF is 12% if the period of cold ischemia of renal graft is less than 12h, and is up to 45% if the period of cold ischemia exceeds 48h. In addition, the incidence of DGF is less than 10% if the donor is young and the cold ischemia time is less than 12h, and is more than 20% if the donor is senile and the cold ischemia time is short. Given the cold ischemia time of 36-48h, the incidence of DGF is up to 50% if the donor is senile and, and is only 30% if the donor is young. Animal study has shown that the donor's age and cold ischemia time exert additive effect on chronic graft rejection.

2. Recipient-related factors
The incidence of DGF is relatively high given suboptimal HLA matching, high sensitization status and a second transplantation. The severity of immune injury depends mainly on the severity of early post-transplantation rejection. High sensitization status increases the risk of immune injury. DGF may mask rejection, but rejection may aggravate preexisting injury. It has been demonstrated that the incidence of DGF increases significantly in the presence of early graft rejection and DGF is a predictor for aggravation of rejection. Cytomegalovirus infection, obesity, type of pre-transplant dialysis, and ethnicity are all factors influencing the incidence of DGF. For instance, black recipients are more likely to develop DGF than other people. However, the mechanisms involved remain largely unknown.

3. Other factors
   i. Organ preservation: Continuous pulsatile perfusion or pulsatile perfusion plus simple cold preservation of grafts from NHBDs helps decrease the incidence of DGF and improve the long-term survival rate of graft. In NHBDs, comparison of bilateral kidneys subjected to pulsatile perfusion and simple cold preservation, respectively, showed that the incidence of DGF was 10% for grafts subjected to pulsatile perfusion, and was 30% for grafts subjected to simple cold preservation. Valero, et al analyzed in situ perfusion (ISP), total body cooling (TBC), and normothermic recirculation (NR) for grafts from NHBDs, and found that the incidence of DGF was significantly lower in grafts subjected to NR than in those subjected to ISP and TBC. The viability of grafts from NHBDs can be assessed by perfusion parameters, and be improved through infusing drugs. In 2009, Cyril Moers reported that Lifeport Transporter can significantly decrease the incidence and duration of DGF following renal transplantation, while significantly increasing the 1-years survival rate of graft. In addition, Lifeport Transporter provides useful information for professionals to make wise clinical decisions, and helps them choose renal grafts. Hence, Lifeport Transporter is an effective, economical device for renal graft preservation.

Shortening the ischemia time: Topical ischemia/reperfusion injury is the pathogenetic basis for DGF, and the severity of DGF depends on the duration of ischemia. The incidence of DGF is lower in China than in other countries. This is because the warm ischemia time (WIT) of cadaveric renal graft is usually maintained between 10 and 15min in the transplantation centers in China. The warm ischemia time should also be shortened during nephrectomy in living donors. It helps reduce the incidence of DGF to shorten the time for graft trimming and possible second warm ischemia of graft. The cold ischemia time (CIT) directly influences the incidence of DGF and graft survival. It was demonstrated that the risk of DGF increased by 23% every 6h.

Kidney preservatives: They are used to minimize topical ischemic injury. They comprise special components to relieve cellular swelling, maintain calcium homeostasis, reduce the production of oxyradicals and provide energy-rich substances. The UW preservative is superior to Euro-Collins solution in reducing the incidence of DGF. The research on preservatives is now focusing on additives to the standard formulas, e.g., Trimetazidine.

ii. Recipient management: Many patients have inadequate blood volume preoperatively, and the use of crystalline or colloid solutions under central venous pressure monitoring can reduce the incidence of DGF. The kidney is one of the organs that need plentiful blood supply, and the volume of blood supplied to the kidneys accounts for approximately 1/4 of cardiac output. The kidney is sensitive to ischemia, and the ischemia time is correlated to the severity of reperfusion-related injury. Appropriate blood pressure is a prerequisite for adequate graft perfusion. In particular, the blood pressure in the recipient prior to reperfusion determines the recovery of metabolism of graft after a series of ischemic events. A proper blood pressure ensures oxygenated blood perfusion and benefits graft functional recovery. The incidence of DGF is lower in patients receiving peritoneal dialysis prior to transplantation than those receiving hemodialysis. This may relate to decreased blood volume in patients receiving hemodialysis upon the procedure of transplantation. Therefore, sufficient fluid extension is beneficial for patients. Effective blood pressure must be maintained intra- and post-operatively, and blood pressure should better be kept 10-20mmHg (1mmHg=0.133kPa) above the basic blood pressure upon reperfusion and in the first three days postoperatively, thus ensuring effective graft perfusion. Stable blood pressure but poor graft vessel tension and anuria during operation may relate to arteriospasm that results from traction of the renal artery. Polyuria may be induce by postoperative administration of dopamine to dilate the renal artery and elevate systolic pressure.

iii. Vasodilators: During reperfusion, direct infusion of calcium channel blockers into the renal artery improves early renal function due to direct vasodilation and relief of lipid peroxide. A randomized trial has demonstrated that dilthiazem treatment of the donor or treatment of the recipient with other calcium channel blockers benefits early graft function. Atrial natriuretic peptide (ANP), a peptide hormone increasing glomerular filtration rate and urine output, improves renal function and histopathologic changes in animals with acute ischemic renal failure. After infusion of ANP increases serum creatinine clearance quickly and reduces the need for dialysis. In addition, ANP antagonizes vasoconstrictors following topical ischemic injury and promotes renal function recovery. Furosemide suppresses prostaglandin lyases and increases prostaglandin E, thus dilating renal vessels, decreasing renal vascular resistance, and increasing blood flow to the kidney, particularly to the tissues under renal cortex. Therefore, furosemide can relieve ischemic renal injury, promote renal function recovery, and decrease the incidence of DGF.

iv. HLA mismatching: Based on our data, HLA is no a risk factor for DGF, possibly because we controlled the number of HLA mismatches strictly. In addition, HLA matching directly influences the incidence of AR, and AR is one risk factor for

DGF. We also found that early urinary fistula and ureteral obstruction are not risk factors for DGF.

v. Type of dialysis: The type of pre-transplant dialysis may influence the incidence of DGF. A review of a number of cases showed that peritoneal dialysis is in favor of immediate recovery of renal function after renal transplantation, which was attributed to fluid load in the recipient. After analysis of multiple variables, e.g., DGF, ARF in patients who underwent preoperative hemodialysis (HD) or peritoneal dialysis (PD) and received the first cadaveric renal transplantation, it was found that there were 33 cases of DGF (27 cases of HD and 6 cases of PD, p=0.03, and there were 14 cases of ARF (14 cases of HD and 0 case of PD, p=0.01). The time for serum creatinine to decrease to 50% of the pre-transplant level correlates positively to the cold ischemia time and body weight increase in the recipient, and correlates negatively to the urine output in the first 24h, fluid load, and central venous pressure. PD is thought to decrease the incidence and severity of DGF after renal transplantation. Joseph, et al investigated acute rejection, DGF, graft survival, and patient survival in 325 patients who underwent preoperative HD and PD and the first cadaveric renal transplantation, and found 56 DGF cases in 183 PD patients and 58 DGF cases in 117 HD patients. The incidence of DGF was significantly higher in HD patients than in PD patients.

4. Mental disorders and interventions in DGF patients
With technical advance in renal transplantation, mental problems in patients with renal failure or undergoing renal transplantation have drawn more and more attention. These problems include personality change, emotional disorders, mental disorders, psychological rejection, and psychosocial dysfunction. Mental problems may directly influence graft function recovery, and even lead to graft nonfunction or serious adverse events, such as non-compliance to treatment or automutilation (suicide). Therefore, it is crucial to pay close attention to the patient's mental status before and after renal transplantation and manage mental disorders promptly.

Because of biological factors, e.g., renal failure and rejection, immunosuppressant-associated adverse reactions and psychosocial factors, patients may develop various mental disorders before and after renal transplantation, including anxiety, depression, psychotic symptoms, and psychological rejection. Anxiety/depression disorder is characterized by mental stress, excessive anxiety, worry, depression, self-abasement, self-blame, and decreased interest. Some patients may present with panic attack and social anxiety disorder, and serious patients may have suicidal idea and commit suicide. Psychotic symptoms include delusion, hallucination, lack of self-awareness due to mental and somatic disorders, and detachment of the real world. Patients with psychotic symptoms may suffer from secondary behavioral disorders. These symptoms persist for varying length of time. Psychological rejection occurs mainly after renal transplantation. The patients are unable to accept the grafts mentally, and they cannot cope with the mental stress associated with transplantation. They may refuse to take anti-rejection drugs or ask for removal of the grafts. These mental disorders may cause autonomic nerve dysfunction, immune dysfunction and behavioral disorders, e.g., somatic pain, insomnia, anorexia (or apastia), and non-compliance to treatment or automutilation (suicide).

Most patients expect much from renal transplantation, and they are likely to develop mental disorders in case of DGF. There are interacting biological and psychosocial factors that underlie mental disorders.

1. Biological factors:
    i. Acute renal failure
    Following renal transplantation, ATN leads to accumulation of toxic substances which damage nerve cells directly or indirectly and influence nerve cell functions. For instance, alteration in intracerebral monamine neurotransmitters may lead to anxiety, depression and psychotic symptoms.
    ii. Immunosuppressants
    Large doses of immunosuppressants may impair the immune system, and interfere with neuroendocrine function and neurotransmitters in the brain. Neuroendocrine and neurotransmitter dysfunction serve the principal biological mechanism for mental disorders in DGF patients.
    iii. Transplantation procedure
    Renal transplantation procedure per se is a traumatic stress, which can also cause mental disorders, particularly in patients with poor physical status. In addition, perioperative administration of medications, e.g., anesthetics, is one of the causes for mental disorders in DGF patients.
2. Psychosocial factors:
    i. Personality
    Positive and optimistic attitude, good cognition assessment system and coping capacity are crucial for mental health of patients undergoing renal transplantation. Personality traits such as anxiety, paranoid idea, and disadvantage-guided thought are the personality basis for mental disorders in DGF patients.
    ii. Stressful events
    In case of accumulation of adverse life events or major adverse life events, DGF patients may suffer from serious mental trauma and mental disorders.
    iii. Psychosocial supportive system
    The psychosocial supportive system for DGF patients involves social security system, family support and other interpersonal support. Social security system includes medical insurance and psychological support (e.g., unemployment). Family support mainly involves husband-wife and parent-child relationships and socioeconomic status of family. Other interpersonal support mainly includes career, friendship and special group relationships.

Proper assessment and effective management of DGF patients with mental disorders directly influence the efficacy of medical interventions and the life quality of patients.

3. Assessment of mental disorders:
    i. The patient is interviewed face-to-face by psychiatrist and psychologist to assess his/her mental status, personality traits and life events. Meanwhile, the need for medical management and the specific interventions, e.g., psychological intervention or medical treatment, are evaluated.
    ii. Mental status scale based measurements: including measurements of mental status, personality traits, life events and life quality.
4. Prevention of mental disorders:
    i. To establish an integrated social security supportive system, including medical insurance system and government funded special social security system.

   ii. To set up a team of psychiatrists or psychologists, who monitor the patients' mental status during the perioperative stage of renal transplantation, and diagnose and treat mental problems promptly.
   iii. To educate DGF patients, including introducing renal transplantation related issues and possible mental problems.
5. Treatment of mental disorders:
   i. Psychotherapy
   Individualized psychotherapy, primarily supportive psychotherapy, is considered. Cognitive and behavioral therapy may also be utilized. In addition, volunteers who ever suffered from DGF and now have their renal function recovered normal are invited to communicate with the patients, which is the most effective modality.
   ii. Drug treatment
   In DGF patients with serious mental disorders, antipsychotic drugs, e.g., Olanzapine, may be prescribed. The dose must be increased gradually. In case of serious emotional disorder, e.g., anxiety-depression, particularly, high risk of suicide, antidepressant drugs should be administered immediately. SSRI and SSNI drugs may be prescribed. For patients with serious anxiety, benzodiazepines may be used. Electroshock should be considered with caution.

4. Prevention and management of DGF

DGF leads to adverse outcomes, including prolonged hospital stay, need for postoperative hemodialysis, significant increase in medical care costs, decrease in the 1-year survival rate of graft, increase in the rejection incidence, and decrease in the long-term graft survival and the short-term and long-term survival rate of patients. Various medical modalities may decrease the incidence of DGF:

1. To choose young donors and ensure good match of the graft with the recipient.
2. To reduce warm and cold ischemia time.
3. To assess the graft quality and utilize optimal renal grafts.
4. To preserve renal grafts by pulsatile mechanical perfusion.
5. To administer small doses of calcineurin inhibitors (CNIs), biological immunosuppressants and calcium channel blockers. Calcium channel blockers may regulate the immune system and reduce acute rejection. In addition, they prevent the toxic and adverse effects of CNIs and decrease blood pressure.
6. To maintain a proper level of mean arterial pressure in the recipient prior to graft reperfusion.

5. Summary

DGF is an early complication after transplantation caused jointly by immunologic and non-immunologic factors. Various novel immunosuppressants can effectively control or relieve immunologic graft injury, thus improving the short-term and long-term survival rate of grafts. However, the mechanism of pre-transplant injury to the renal graft remains largely unclear. The risk factors for DGF include the warm ischemia time, cold ischemia time, intraoperative and early postoperative hypotension, ATN, nephrotoxicity of CNIs and AR.

Further study should be carried out with large sample sizes to investigate the correlation of times of transplantation, number of HLA mismatch, early postoperative urinary fistula, ureteral obstruction, and preoperative blood transfusion with DGF. Renal graft protection has seldom been investigated. Further efforts should be made to prevent non-immunologic injury to the renal graft, so as to increase the quality of renal graft and the short-term and long-term survival rate of renal grafts.

6. References

L Polyak MM, Arrington BO. Stubenbord WT, et al. The influence of pulsatile preservation on renal transplantation in the 1990s. Transplantation. 2000, 69: 249.

Lane NJ, Thorniley MS, Manek S, et al. Effect of mannitol and polyethylene glycol on the action of frusemide during renal storage and transplantation. Transplantation, 1996, 62: 575. 2008. 07No.

Gonwa TA, Hricik DE, Brinker K, et al. Improved renal function in sirolimus—treated renal transplant patients after-early cyclosporine elimination. Transplantation, 2002, 74: 1560.

McTaggart RA, Gotflieb D, Brooks J, et al. Sirolimus prolongs recovery from delayed graft function after cadaveric renal transplantation. Am J Transplant, 2003, 3: 416.

Stallone G, Di Paolo S, Schena A, et al. Addition of sirolimus to cyclosporine delays the recovery from delayed graft function but does not affect 1-year graft function. J Am Soe Nephrol, 2004, 15: 228.

Boom H, Mallat MJ, de Fijter JW, et al. Delayed graft function influences renal function, but not survival. Kidney lnt, 2000, 58: 859.

Bunnapradist S, Lochlainn EN, Takemoto SK. Antibody induction therapy and their associated outcomes in cadaveric kidney transplants. Am J Transplant, 2004, 4(Suppl. 8): 264.

McCormick BB. Pierrctos A, Fenteon S, et al. Review of clinical outcomes in nocturnal haemodialysis patients after renal transplantation[J]. Nephrol Transplant, 2004, 19(3): 714-719.

Jacobs SC, Cho E, Foster C, et al. Laparoscopic donor nephrectomy: the University of Maryland 6-year experience EJ]. J Urol, 2004, 171(1): 47-51.

Shosakes DA, Shahed AR, Kim S. Delayed graft function: Influence on outcome and strategies for prevention. Urol Clin Noah Am 2001, 28: 721—732.

Fischer J, Kirste G Keller H, et al. Does ATN influence renal transplant function negatively. Transplant Proc 1 988, 20: 908.

Hemandez A, Light JA, Barhyte D, et al. Ablating the ischemia reperfusion injury in non-heart-beating donor kidneys. Transplantation 1999, 67: 200-206.

Ojo AO, Wolfe RA, Held, et al. Delayed graft function: risk factors an d implications for renal allograft surviva1. Transplantation 1997, 63: 968-974.

Gaber LW, Gaber AO, Hathwaway DK, et al. Routine early biopsy of allograft with delayed graft function of histolopathology and transplant outcome. Clin Transplant 1 996, 1 0: 629-634.

Lemay S, Rabb H, Postler G, et al. Prominent and sustained upregulation of gpl30-signaling cytokines and chemokine MIP in murine renal ischemic reperfusion. Transplantalion 2000, 69(5): 957-963.

Canaud B. Leblane M. Leray Moragues H, et al. Slow continuous and daily ultrafiltration for refractory congestive heart failure. Nephrol Dial Transplant l998, 13(14): 51 – 55.

Avihingsanon Y, Ma N, PavlakisMet, et al. On the intraoperative molecular status of renal allografts after vascular reperfusion and clinical outcomes. J Am Soc Nephrol 2005; 16: 1542–1548

Boom H, Mallat MJ, de Fijter JW, et al. Calcium levels as a risk factor for delayed graft function. Transplantation 2004; 77: 868–873

Rodrigo E, Ruiz JC, Pinera C, et al. Creatinine reduction ratio on posttransplant day two as criterion in defining delayed graft function. Am J Transplant 2004; 4: 1163- 1169

Turkowski-Duhem A, Kamar N, Cointault O, et al. Predictive factors of postrenal transplant anemia. Transplant Proc 2005; 37: 1009–1011

Giral-Classe M, Hourmant M, Cantarovich D, et al. Delayed graft function of more than six days strongly decreases long-term survival of transplanted kidneys. Kidney Int 1998; 54: 972–978

Nickerson P, Jeffery J, Gough J, et al. Identification of clinical and histopathologic risk factors for diminished renal function 2 years posttransplant.J Am Soc Nephrol 1998; 9: 482–487

Gonwa TA, MaiML, Smith LB, et al. Immunosuppression for delayedor slow graft function in primary cadaveric renal transplantation: use of low dose tacrolimus therapy with post-operative administration of anti-CD25 monoclonal antibody. Clin Transplant 2002; 16: 144–149

Schmidt R, Kupin W, Dumler F, et al. Influence of the pretransplant hematocrit level on early graft function in primary cadaveric renal transplantation. Transplantation 1993; 55: 1034–1040

Shoskes DA, Hodge EE, Goormastic M, et al. HLA matching determines susceptibility to harmful effects of delayed graft function in renal transplant recipients. Transplant Proc 1995; 27: 1068- 1069

Mehta Tk. Quantitative detection of promoter hypermethylation as a biomarker of acute kidney injury during transplantation. Transplant Proc 2006; 38(10): 3420–6

Parikh CR, Jani A, Melnikov VY, et al. Urinary interleukin-18 is a marker of human acute tubular necrosis. Am J Kidney Dis 2004; 43: 405–414

Parikh CR, Jani A, Mishra J et al. Urine NGAL and IL-18 are predictive biomarkers for delayed graft function following kidney transplantation. Am J Transplant 2006; 6: 1639–1645

Sadeghi M, Daniel V, Naujokat C, et al. Association of high pretransplant sIL-6R plasma levels with acute tubular necrosis in kidney graft recipients. Transplantation 2006; 81: 1716–1724

Cyril M, Jacqueline M. Smits, et al. Machine Perfusion or Cold Storage in Deceased-Donor Kidney Transplantation.N Engl J Med 2009; 360:7-19

T. Tsunoda, R. Yamashita, Y. Kojima, S. Takahara. Risk Factors for Depression After Kidney Transplantation. Transplantation Proceedings, 2010, 42(5):1679-1681

A. Virzì, M.S. Signorelli, M. Veroux, G. Giammarresi, S. Maugeri, A. Nicoletti, P. Veroux. Depression and Quality of Life in Living Related Renal Transplantation. Transplantation Proceedings, 2007, 39(6): 1791-1793

8

New Onset Diabetes After Solid Organ Transplantation

Phuong-Thu T. Pham[1], Phuong-Mai T. Pham[2], Parikh S[1], Son V. Pham[3], Phuong-Anh T. Pham[4] and Phuong-Chi T. Pham[5]
[1]*Department of Medicine, Nephrology Division, Kidney Transplant Program, David Geffen School of Medicine at UCLA*
[2]*Department of Medicine, Greater Los Angeles VA Medical Center and David Geffen School of Medicine at UCLA*
[3]*Department of Medicine, Cardiology Division, Bay Pines VA Medical Center, Bay Pines, Florida*
[4]*Department of Medicine, Division of Cardiovascular Diseases, VA Medical Center, University of Tennessee Health Science Center, Memphis, TN*
[5]*Department of Medicine, Nephrology Division, UCLA-Olive View Medical Center and David Geffen School of Medicine*
United States of America

1. Introduction

New onset diabetes mellitus after transplantation (NODAT) is a serious and common complication following solid organ transplantation. NODAT has been reported to occur in 2% to 53% of all solid organ transplants. Kidney transplant recipients who develop NODAT have variably been reported to be at increased risk of fatal and nonfatal cardiovascular events and other adverse outcomes including infection, reduced patient survival, graft rejection, and accelerated graft loss compared with those who do not develop diabetes. Limited clinical studies in liver, heart and lung transplants similarly suggested that NODAT has an adverse impact on patient and graft outcomes. The following chapter presents an overview of the literature on the current diagnostic criteria for NODAT, its incidence after solid organ transplantation, suggested risk factors and potential pathogenic mechanisms. The impact of NODAT on patient and allograft outcomes and suggested guidelines for early identification and management of NODAT will also be discussed.

2. Definition and diagnosis of new onset diabetes after transplantation

Historically, post-transplant diabetes has been variably defined as having random glucose levels greater than 200 mg/dl fasting, glucose levels greater than 140 mg/dl, or the need for insulin or oral hypoglycemic agents in the post-transplant period. In 2003, the International Expert Panel consisting of experts from both the transplant and diabetes fields set forth the International Consensus Guidelines for the diagnosis and management of NODAT (Davidson et al., 2003; Wilkinson et al., 2005). It was recommended that the definition and diagnosis of NODAT should be based on the definition of diabetes mellitus and impaired glucose tolerance (IGT) described by the World Health Organization (WHO) (Montori et al., 2002; Wilkinson et al, 2005). The current WHO and American Diabetes Association (ADA) guidelines for the diagnosis of prediabetic states (IFG and IGT) and diabetes mellitus are provided in Table 1 (modified from Davidson et al., 2003).

Criteria for the diagnosis of diabetes mellitus

- Symptoms[1] of diabetes mellitus + casual[2] PG concentrations ≥ 200 mg/dL (11.1 mM)

or

- FPG ≥ 126 mg/dL (7.0 mM). Fasting is defined as no caloric intake for at least 8 hours

or

- 2-hr PG ≥ 200 mg/dL (11.1 mM) during an oral glucose tolerance test[3]

A confirmatory laboratory test based on measurements of venous PG must be done on another day in the absence of unequivocal hyperglycemia accompanied by acute metabolic decompensation.

Criteria for normal FPG and IFG or IGT

FPG

WHO criteria

FPG < 110 mg/dL (6.1 mM) = normal fasting glucose

FPG ≥ 110 mg/dl (6.1 mM) and < 126 mg/dl (7.0 mM) = IFG

2003 ADA updated consensus report

FPG < 100 mg/dL (5.6 mM) = normal fasting glucose

FPG ≥ 100 mg/dl (5.6 mM) and < 126 mg/dl (7.0 mM) = IFG

or

OGTT

2-hr PG < 140 mg/dl (7.8 mM) = normal glucose tolerance

2-hr PG ≥ 140 mg/dl (7.8 mM) and < 200 mg/dl (11.1 nM) = IGT

WHO: World Health Organization; PG: plasma glucose; FPG: fasting plasma glucose; IFG: impaired fasting glucose; IGT: impaired glucose tolerance; OGTT: oral glucose tolerance test

[1] Classic symptoms of diabetes include polyuria, polydipsia, and unexplained weight loss.

[2] Casual is defined as any time of day without regard to time since last meal.

[3] OGTT: the test should be performed as described by WHO, using a glucose load containing equivalent of 75 g anhydrous glucose dissolved in water.

Table 1. WHO and 2003 updated ADA criteria for the diagnosis of diabetes mellitus

3. Incidence

New onset diabetes mellitus after transplantation has been reported to occur in 4% to 25% of renal transplant recipients, 2.5% to 25% of liver transplant recipients, 4% to 40% of heart transplant recipients, and 30% to 35% of lung transplant recipients (Baid et al., 2001; Davidson et al., 2003; Knobler et al., 1998; Ye et al., 2010a). There has been scant literature on the incidence of diabetes mellitus after a successful pancreas transplant. In one-single center study persistent diabetes mellitus despite evidence of functioning pancreas allografts occurred in 19% of patients (22/144) at 39 months post-transplant (Dean et al., 2008).

The variation in the reported incidence may be due in part to the lack of a standard definition of the condition, the duration of follow-up, the presence of both modifiable and non-modifiable risks factors, and the type of organ transplants among others. In HCV-infected liver recipients, the prevalence of NODAT has been reported to range between 40% to 60% (Baid et al., 2001; Bigam et al., 2000; Knobler et al., 1998). While the prevalence of diabetes reported to the International Society of Heart Lung Transplant (ISHLT) are 19% at 1-year and 28% at 5 years for lung transplant recipients, and 15.4% at 1-year and 20% at 5-years for heart-lung transplant recipients (Trulock et al., 2007), a lower prevalence has been reported (Silverborn et al., 2005). In one single-center study consisting of 126 lung and heart-lung transplant recipients, diabetes has a reported prevalence of 6% at 1 year and 7% at 5 years. The lower prevalence of diabetes in this study was thought to be due in part to a lower frequency of cystic fibrosis patients (8.7% vs. 16.0% in the ISHLT database) and the exclusion of patients with pre-existing diabetes (Silverborn et al., 2005).

Similar to the nontransplant settings, the use of fasting plasma glucose (FPG) versus oral glucose tolerance test (OGTT) to define diabetes mellitus also changes the prevalence of NODAT. In a prospective study designed to evaluate the use of OGTT for risk-stratifying patients for NODAT, Sharif et al. demonstrated that among 122 renal transplant recipients without diabetes who had two FPG level measurements within the range of 100-125 mg/dl (5.6-6.9 mmol/l) for more than 6 months after transplantation, OGTTs revealed that 10% had overt diabetes mellitus, 9% had IGT alone, 18% had IFG alone (all defined by WHO criteria), and 14% had combined IFG and IGT (Sharif et al., 2006).

4. Risk factors for NODAT

Risk factors for the development of NODAT are categorized as non-modifiable and modifiable or potentially modifiable, the former category to facilitate the identification of high risk individuals, and the latter two categories to optimize the management of NODAT. Suggested risk factors for NODAT are summarized in Figure 1. It is noteworthy that most clinical studies evaluating the incidence and risk factors for NODAT have been performed in kidney and liver transplant recipients.

Limited studies in pancreas transplant recipients suggest that pre-transplant body mass index (BMI), high pretransplant insulin requirements and acute rejection episodes are risk factors for persistent post-transplant diabetes mellitus despite the presence of a functioning pancreas allograft (Dean et al., 2008).

Retrospective analysis of the UNOS/OPTN database demonstrated that the risk factors for NODAT after heart transplant are similar to those reported in kidney transplant recipients including older age, non-white race, higher BMI, recipient CMV positivity, tacrolimus (vs. cyclosporine) and steroid use (vs. no steroid) at discharge. Ischemic heart disease was also found to be associated with an increased incidence of NODAT (Ye et al., 2010b). In a single-center study consisting of 97 consecutive adult heart transplant recipients, a family history of diabetes and the need for insulin beyond the first 24 hours after transplantation were shown to be risk factors for the development NODAT (Depczynski et al., 2000).

4.1 Nonmodifiable risk factors

There has been ample literature suggesting that age, Hispanic and African American race and ethnicity are risks factors for NODAT (Cosio et al., 2001; Kasiske et al., 2003; P.T. Pham et al., 2007a, 2007b).

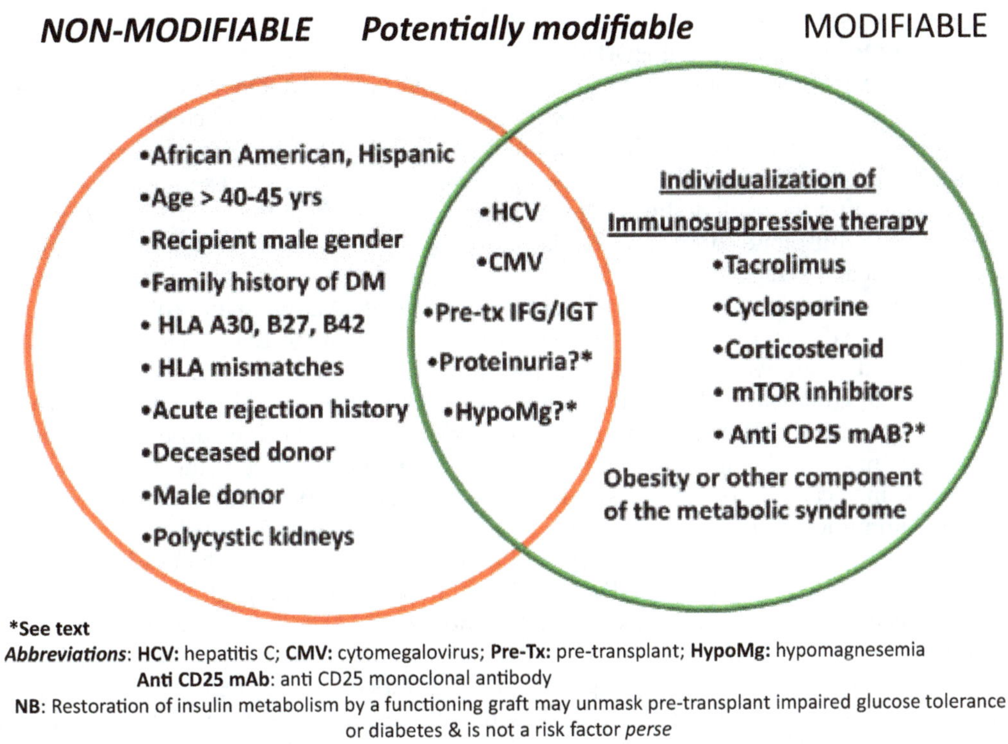

Fig. 1. Risk Factors for NODAT

Similar to type 2 diabetes in the general population, both genetic and environmental factors have been suggested to play a role in the development of NODAT. There is strong evidence suggesting that individuals with a family history of diabetes among first-degree relatives have an increased risk of developing NODAT with one study reporting a seven fold increase in the condition (Davidson et al., 2003). The increased prevalence of NODAT associated with a family history of diabetes has been documented across all types of solid organ transplantation. In a Spanish multicenter cross-sectional study consisting of 1410 recipients of kidney transplants, 489 liver transplants, 207 heart transplants, and 72 lung transplants, a positive family history of diabetes was associated with a 50% increased in the risk of developing NODAT (odds ratio of 1.51) (Martinez-Castelao et al., 2005).

Other non-modifiable risk factors include recipient male gender, the presence of certain HLA antigens such as HLA A 30, B27, B42, increasing HLA mismatches, DR mismatch, deceased donor kidneys, male donor, and acute rejection history (Depczynski et al., 2000). Adult polycystic kidney disease (ADPKD) has been suggested to confer an increased risk of developing NODAT in some studies but not in others (P.T. Pham et al., 2007b). The pathogenic mechanism of ADPKD-associated NODAT has not been studied. Of interest, ADPKD patients with normal native kidney function have been shown to have insulin resistance and compensatory hyperinsulinemia (Vareesangthip et al., 1997).

Although not a risk factor per se, increased insulin clearance after a successful kidney transplant can unmask pre-transplant impaired glucose tolerance or pre-existing diabetes mellitus that manifests clinically as NODAT.

4.2 Modifiable risk factors

4.2.1 Corticosteroid-associated NODAT

The now well-established contributory role of corticosteroid on NODAT was first described by Starlz in 1964 in renal transplant recipients. The diabetogenic effect of corticosteroids has been suggested to be dose-dependent. Single-center studies have demonstrated that oral prednisolone dose reduction to 5 mg daily significantly improves glucose tolerance during the first year after transplantation (Hjelmesaeth et al., 1997) while a 0.01 mg/kg/day increase in prednisolone dose is associated with a 5% risk of developing NODAT (Hjelmesaeth et al., 2001).

In a small study involving 57 stable renal transplant recipients, Midtvedt and colleagues found that prednisolone dose reduction from a mean of 16 mg daily (range 10 to 30) to 9 mg (range 5 to 12.5) resulted in an average increase in insulin sensitivity index of 24% (Midtvedt et al., 2004). However, complete withdrawal of 5 mg/day of prednisolone did not influence insulin sensitivity significantly. Whether complete withdrawal of chronic low dose corticosteroid therapy (prednisolone 5 mg daily) improves glucose metabolism remains to be studied. Nonetheless, in recent years several studies have suggested a potential beneficial effect of steroid-free immunosuppression on NODAT risk reduction (Luan et al., 2011).

In a retrospective analysis of the Organ Procurement Transplant Network/Scientific Registry of Transplant Recipient (OPTN/SRTR) database consisting of > 25,000 kidney transplant recipients engrafted between 1/2004 and 12/13/2006, Luan et al. demonstrated that steroid-free immunosuppression was associated with a significant reduction in the likelihood of developing NODAT compared with steroid-containing regimens (Luan et al., 2011). The cumulative incidence of NODAT within three years post-transplant were 12.3% in steroid-free vs. 17.7% in steroid-containing regimens, $p < 0.001$. Overall, steroid-containing regimens at the time of hospital discharge were associated with a 42% increased risk for NODAT. Notably, patients from programs that frequently adopted steroid-free regimens had reduced odds of NODAT compared with those from programs that commonly used steroid-contatining regimens.

The dose dependent diabetogenic effect of corticosteroid was also observed in recipients of nonrenal organ transplants. In a retrospective review involving 88 heart transplant recipients, Depczynski and colleagues found that patients who developed NODAT had received higher mean doses of prednisolone at 3 months compared with those who remained free of diabetes at a mean follow-up of 27 months (0.21 ± 0.03 vs. 0.19 ± 0.03 mg/kg/day, $p< 0.01$) (Depczynski et al., 2000).

4.2.2 Calcineurin inhibitor-associated NODAT: cyclosporine vs. tacrolimus

Although clinical trials comparing the incidence of NODAT in CSA- vs. Tac-treated patients have yielded mixed results, Tac has more consistently been shown to have a greater diabetogenic effect (Ekberg et al., 2007; P.T. Pham et al., 2007b; Woodward et al., 2003).

The DIRECT Study (Diabetes Incidence after Renal Transplantation: Neoral C2 monitoring versus Tacrolimus) was the first multi-center open label, randomized trial to assess glucose abnormalities in de novo kidney transplant patients who were randomized to cyclosporine microemulsion- (CsA-ME) or tacrolimus-based immunosuppression (Vincente et al., 2007). The incidence of NODAT or IFG (defined by WHO/ADA criteria) at 6-month post-transplant was significantly lower in CsA-ME- vs. tacrolimus- treated patients, (26% vs. 33.6%, p=0.046). Furthermore, a lower proportion of CsA-ME patients with NODAT required hypoglycemic medication or dual therapy with insulin and oral hypoglycemic agents compared with their tacrolimus-treated counterparts.

The greater diabetogenic effect of tacrolimus compared to CSA has been reported to occur across renal and nonrenal transplant groups. In a meta-analysis to evaluate the reported incidence of NODAT after solid organ transplantation, Heisel and colleagues found a higher incidence of insulin-dependent diabetes mellitus (IDDM) in Tac- vs. CSA-treated liver, heart, and lung transplant recipients (Heisel et al, 2004). In renal transplant recipients, IDDM occurred in 9.8% of Tac- vs. 2.7% of CSA-treated patients ($p<0.00001$). Similar trends were observed among recipients of non renal organ transplants (11.1% vs. 6.2%, respectively ($p<0.003$). Nonetheless, not all studies showed that Tac is more diabetogenic than cyclosporine (Meiser et al., 1998). It has been suggested that these study inconsistencies stemmed in part from the difference in the definitions of NODAT and the difference in calcineurin inhibitor dose and drug levels (Maes et al., 2001; Meiser et al., 1998). In a single-center study consisting of 139 renal transplant recipients without known pretransplant glucose abnormalities, Maes and colleagues have shown that high Tac trough levels, particularly levels greater than 15 ng/ml in the first month after transplant was a significant risk factor for persistent impaired fasting glucose or diabetes mellitus beyond the first year after transplantation (Maes et al., 2001). In a single-center study consisting of 45 OLT recipients treated with either CSA (n=9) or high- (n=15) vs. low- (n=13) dose Tac, the incidence of NODAT were 11%, 40% and 23%, respectively (Cai et al., 1998).

4.2.3 Interaction between tacrolimus and concomitant hepatitis C infection (HCV)

In a retrospective study of more than 400 kidney transplant recipients with no known pre-transplant diabetes, Bloom and colleagues have shown that among the HCV(+) cohort, NODAT occurred more often in the Tac- compared with the CSA-treated groups (57.8% vs. 7.7%, $p< 0.0001$) (Bloom et al., 2002). In contrast, among the HCV (-) cohort, the rates of NODAT were similar between the two calcineurin inhibitor (CNI) groups (Tac vs. CSA: 10% vs. 9.4%, respectively, $p= 0.521$). Whether concomitant exposure to tacrolimus and HCV plays a synergistic role in the development of NODAT remains speculative.

4.2.4 Effects of sirolimus on glucose metabolism

Early large randomized clinical trials suggested that sirolimus is devoid of diabetogenic effects either used alone or in combination therapy with CNI. However, the diabetogenicity of sirolimus has now been well-described. Teutenico et al. demonstrated that calcineurin inhibitors to sirolimus conversion therapy and tacrolimus withdrawal in a regimen consisting of tacrolimus and sirolimus were associated with a 30% increased incidence of impaired glucose tolerance (Teutenico et al., 2005). In one single-center study, tacrolimus and sirolimus combination therapy was found to be associated with a higher incidence of NODAT than tacrolimus alone immunosuppression (Sulanc et al., 2005). Subsequent large registry study also demonstrated an association between sirolimus and the development of NODAT. In an analysis of the USRDS database consisting of more than 20,000 primary kidney transplant recipients receiving sirolimus (Sir) or CNI (CsA or Tac) or both in various combination therapy with an antimetabolite (MMF or AZA), Johnston et al. demonstrated that patients treated with sirolimus in combination with a CNI (CsA or Tac) had the highest incidence of NODAT (Johnston et al., 2008). The authors further demonstrated that patients treated with (Sir + Tac) combination therapy had a hazard ratio of developing NODAT of 1.9 compared with those receiving (Tac + MMF/AZA), suggesting that sirolimus was associated with an increased risk for NODAT independent of any effect of tacrolimus.

4.2.5 Anti-CD25 monoclonal antibodies

In a single-center study consisting of 74 stable kidney transplant recipients with 3 month-follow-up, Bayes et al. demonstrated that basiliximab induction therapy is an independent risk factor for NODAT (OR: 3.28; p=0.041) (Bayes et al., 2007). Aasebo et al. similarly demonstrated that the use of basiliximab induction therapy significantly increased NODAT risk (n=264) (Aesebo et al., 2010). At 10 weeks post-transplant, NODAT, impaired glucose tolerance (IGT) or impaired fasting glucose (IFG) occurred in 51.5% in the basiliximab group compared with 36.9% in the group that did not receive basiliximab induction (p=0.017).

5. Potential pathogenic mechanisms of immunosuppressive drug--induced NODAT

5.1 Calcineurin inhibitors

Impaired insulin secretion has been suggested to contribute to the development of CNI-associated NODAT (Crutchlow & Bloom, 2007). Experimental studies have shown that CNIs impair the function of cultured β-cells by impairing insulin gene expression (Crutchlow et al., 2007; Van Hooff et al., 2004). In recipients of pancreas transplants, both calcineurin inhibitors CSA and Tac have been shown to cause reversible toxicity to islet cells. In a study of 26 pancreas allograft biopsies from 20 simultaneous kidney-pancreas transplant recipients, a significant correlation was seen between the presence of islet cell damage and serum levels of Tac and CSA, as well as with the Tac peak level (Drachenberg et al., 1999). Cytoplasmic swelling and vacuolization, and marked decrease or absence of dense-core secretory granules in β-cells were demonstrated on electron microscopy. The islet cell damage was more frequent and severe in the Tac- (10/13) compared to the CSA-treated groups (5/13). Serial biopsies from two patients with hyperglycemia and evidence of islet cell damage receiving Tac immunosuppression demonstrated reversibility of the damage upon discontinuation of tacrolimus.

5.2 Sirolimus (mTOR inhibitors)

Suggested pathogenic mechanisms of sirolimus-induced hyperglycemia include sirolimus-associated impaired insulin-mediated suppression of hepatic glucose production, ectopic triglyceride deposition leading to insulin resistance, and direct β cell toxicity (Crutchlow & Bloom, 2007). However, studies on the effects of sirolimus on insulin action and secretion have yielded variable and conflicting results. Currently existing literature suggests that the effects of sirolimus on glucose metabolism appear to be cell-species- and dose-dependent (Subramanian & Trence, 2007).

5.2.1 Anti-CD25 monoclonal antibodies

The pathogenic mechanisms of anti-CD25-induced NODAT have not been established. However, suppression of regulatory T-cells has been suggested to play a contributory role (Aasebo et al., 2010). Studies in diabetes-prone mice have shown that anti-IL2-antibody treatment trigger insulinitis and early onset diabetes through inhibition of Foxp3-expressing CD25+ CD4+ regulatory T-cells (Setoguchi et al., 2005).

Suggested pathogenic mechanisms of immunosuppressive drug-induced NODAT are summarized in table 2.

Immunosuppressive agent	Pathogenic mechanism(s)	Comments
Corticosteroids	•↓Peripheral insulin sensitivity • Inhibit pancreatic insulin production & secretion • ↑Hepatic gluconeogenesis • Promote protein degradation to free amino acids in muscle, lipolysis	•Dose-dependent •Impact of complete withdrawal of chronic low-dose steroids unclear •Potential ↓NODAT risk in steroid-free regimens
Cyclosporine	• ↓insulin secretion (CsA < Tac) • ↓insulin synthesis • ↓β-cell density	•Dose-dependent, •Diabetogenic effect ↑ with ↑ steroid dose*
Tacrolimus	• ↓insulin secretion (Tac > CsA) • ↓insulin synthesis	•Dose-dependent, •Diabetogenic effect ↑ with ↑ steroid dose*
Sirolimus	•↑Peripheral insulin resistance • Impair pancreatic β-cell response	↑Diabetogenicity when use with CNIs

Abbreviations: CNI: calcineurin inhibitors
* Demonstrated in some but not all studies

Table 2. Drug-Induced NODAT: potential pathogenic mechanism(s)

6. Obesity

Similar to the general population, obesity has been shown to be associated with the development of NODAT in most studies (Setoguchi et al., 2005). Analysis of the USRDS database revealed that obesity, defined as a BMI of $\geq$ 30 kg/m^2 is one of the strongest risk factors for NODAT (Relative risk of 1.73, $P < 0.0001$). Although some studies failed to demonstrate an association between obesity and the development of NODAT, obesity and its associated peripheral insulin resistance state is a known risk factor for type 2 diabetes. The mechanism whereby obesity induces insulin resistance is poorly understood. Nonetheless, the pattern of body fat distribution has been suggested to play a contributory role. Studies in healthy women showed that upper body or male-type obesity has a much greater association with insulin resistance and impaired glucose tolerance than lower body or female-type obesity (Kissebah et al., 1982). Similar studies in the transplant settings is lacking. It is speculated that intra-abdominal fat or waist-to-hip ratio may be more important risk factors for NODAT than total body weight or BMI (Davidson et al., 2003).

7. Hypertriglyceridemia / Hypertension

Early retrospective studies suggested that the greater the number of the metabolic syndrome components, the greater the risk for the development of NODAT (Eckel, 2007). In a recent retrospective analysis consisting of 640 nondiabetic renal transplant recipients Bayer et al. demonstrated that the prevalence of NODAT at 1-year increased with increasing number of metabolic syndrome score 0: 0%, 1: 24%, 2: 29%, 3: 31%, 4: 35%, 5: 74%, p=0.001) (Bayer et al., 2010). Multivariate analysis incorporating the individual metabolic syndrome components as covariates demonstrated that of all the pre-transplant metabolic syndrome components, only low-density lipoprotein was independently associated with the development of NODAT.

The precise role of the metabolic syndrome or metabolic syndrome component(s) in the development of NODAT remains to be defined. Nonetheless, the overlapping metabolic risk factors for type 2 diabetes and cardiovascular disease (e.g. obesity, hyperglycemia, dyslipidemia, hypertension) warrants early identification and aggressive management of individual risk factors

8. Proteinuria

Early report from single-center study suggested an association between proteinuria on day 5 after transplantation and the development of NODAT (Kuypers et al., 2008). However, these findings have been challenged because proteinuria on day 5 may just reflect the highly concentrated urine associated with hyperglycemia-induced osmotic diuresis from the early posttransplant use of high dose corticosteroid or residual native kidney proteinuria. Furthermore, it has been shown that immediate posttransplant proteinuria generally resolves several weeks after transplantation (Myslak et al., 2006). Nonetheless, in a subsequent single-center retrospective study designed to evaluate the impact of early proteinuria (3 and 6 months after transplantation) and urinary albumin excretion (UAE) on NODAT, Roland et al. demonstrated that low-grade (<1g/day) and very low-grade (< /0.3 g/day) proteinuria were independent risk factor for NODAT (p=0.0042 and p=.00025, respectively) (Roland et al., 2008). Furthermore, there was a dose-dependent relationship across UAE categories with NODAT. NODAT-free survival was greater in patients with normoalbuminuria than in those with microalbuminuria, and greater in those with microalbuminuria than in those with macroalbuminuria (p=0.0326). The authors also demonstrated that pulse pressure was an independent risk factor for NODAT, suggesting that early low-grade proteinuria and pulse pressure may be markers of the metabolic syndrome or vascular damage or both.

9. Hypomagnesemia

In the general population, not only has hypomagnesemia been shown to be associated with type 2 diabetes, but numerous studies have also reported an inverse relationship between glycemic control and serum Mg levels (P.C. Pham et al., 2007). Similar to the nontransplant settings, hypomagenesemia has also been shown to be an independent predictor of NODAT in recipients of renal and liver transplants. In a single-center retrospective analysis consisting of 254 renal transplant recipients Van Laecke et al. demonstrated that hypomagnesemia during the first-month posttransplantation was associated with the development of NODAT independent of the immunosuppressive regimen used (van Laecke et al., 2009). While the association between the use of CNIs was strongly related to hypomagnesemia, NODAT disappeared after adjustment for Mg levels suggesting that the diabetogenic effect of CNIs is at least in part related to hypomagnesemia. Conversely, the use of mTOR inhibitors appeared to be a risk factor for NODAT after adjustment for Mg levels. The same group of authors subsequently demonstrated that both pretransplant hypomagenesemia and hypomagnesemia in the first-month posttransplantation were independent predictors of NODAT in recipients of liver transplants (Van Laecke et al., 2010). Nonetheless, not all studies demonstrated that hypomagnesemia is a risk factor for NODAT. In one small single-center study consisting of 205 non-previously diabetic patients with > 1 year graft survival, neither the mean values of Mg nor the percentage of patients with hypomagnesemia differed between NODAT and non-NODAT patients (Santos et al., 2010).

Whether Mg supplementation and correction of Mg deficiency reduce the incidence of insulin resistance or NODAT remains to be studied.

10. Potentially modifiable risk factors

10.1 Impaired glucose tolerance before transplantation

Abnormal glucose metabolism has been reported to be a risk factor for the development of NODAT in some but not all studies. In a study consisting of 490 recipients of kidney transplants, Cosio et al. demonstrated that higher pretransplant glucose is a risk factor for NODAT at one year (Cosio et al., 2005). Using patients with pretransplant FPG levels between 90 and 100 as the reference group, patients with plasma glucose < 90 mg/dL have lower risk of NODAT (OR=.46, P=0.01). In contrast, the risk of NODAT increases as the pretransplant FPG levels increases (FPG =101-109, OR=1.5; and FPG = 110-125, OR=7.6, P < 0.0001). Among patients with IFG pretransplant, 70% had hyperglycemia at one year (IFG 43% and NODAT 27%). In one single-center study Eprinchard et al demonstrated that pretransplant IGT is a risk factor for NODAT with a relative risk of developing NODAT of 2.4 (Eprinchard et al., 2011).

10.2 HCV-associated NODAT

The association between HCV infection and impaired fasting glucose or the development of overt type 2 diabetes mellitus in the general population has long been suggested. Potential mechanisms of the diabetogenic effect of HCV infection include insulin resistance, decreased hepatic glucose uptake and glycogenesis, and direct cytopathic effect of the virus on pancreatic β cells (Bloom & Lake, 2006). Similar to the non-transplant settings, the link between hepatitis C and the development of NODAT has also been recognized in solid organ transplant recipients. The pathogenesis of HCV-associated NODAT, however, remains poorly understood. Clinical studies in recipients of orthotopic liver transplant (OLT) recipients have implicated insulin resistance associated with active HCV infection as a predominant pathogenic mechanism. Independent investigators have shown a temporal relationship between recurrent allograft hepatitis and increasing viral loads and the development of NODAT (Baid et al., 2001; Delgado-Borrego et al., 2004). Furthermore, patients who responded to antiviral therapy were observed to have improvement in glycemic control (Baid et al., 2001; Delgado-Borrego et al., 2004; Simo et al., 2006). In a small cohort of 17 non-diabetic HCV (+) and 33 non-diabetic HCV (-) OLT recipients, Baid and colleagues have shown that the presence of HCV infection was independently associated with a 62% increase in insulin resistance (P=0.0005) (Baid et al., 2001). It was suggested that the virus had a direct effect on insulin resistance as no difference in β cell function or hepatic insulin extraction between the HCV (+) and (-) groups was observed.

In a small study consisting of 16 renal transplant candidates with sustained virologic response to interferon treatment given in the pre-transplant period, none developed

NODAT at a mean follow-up of 22.5 months (range, 2 to 88 months) (Kamar et al., 2003). It is conceivable that successful pre-transplant treatment of hepatitis C could potentially reduce the incidence of NODAT after kidney transplantation.

10.3 Cytomegalovirus-associated NODAT

The link between cytomegalovirus (CMV) infection and the development of NODAT was first reported in 1985 in a renal transplant recipient (Lehr et al., 1985). Limited studies suggested that both asymptomatic CMV infection and CMV disease are independent risk factors for the development of NODAT. In a study consisting of 160 consecutive non-diabetic renal transplant recipients who were prospectively monitored for CMV infection during the first three months after transplantation, Hjelmesaeth and colleagues found that asymptomatic CMV infection was associated with a four-fold increased risk of new-onset diabetes (adjusted RR= 4.00; p=0.025) (Hjelmasaeth et al., 2004). Patients with active CMV infection had a significantly lower median insulin release compared to their CMV negative counterparts, suggesting that impaired pancreatic β cell insulin release may be involved in the pathogenic mechanism of CMV-associated NODAT. It is speculated that CMV-induced release of proinflammatory cytokines may lead to apoptosis and functional disturbances of pancreatic β-cells (Hjelmasaeth et al., 2005).

11. Impact of NODAT on patient and allograft outcomes

11.1 Kidney transplants

Clinical studies evaluating the impact of NODAT on patient and allograft outcomes after solid organ transplantation have yielded variable results. Nonetheless, there has been ample literature suggesting that kidney transplant recipients who developed NODAT are at two- to three- fold increased risk of fatal and nonfatal cardiovascular disease events as compared with nondiabetic patients (Ojo, 2006; Hjelmasaeth et al., 2006). The development of NODAT has also been shown to be associated with an adverse impact on patient survival and an increased risk of graft rejection and graft loss, as well as an increased incidence of infectious complications (Ojo, 2006). Data from the United Renal Data System consisting of over 11,000 Medicare beneficiaries who received primary kidney transplants between 1996 and 2000 demonstrated that compared to "no diabetes", NODAT was associated with a 63% increased risk of graft failure (p< 0.0001), a 46% increased risk of death-censored graft failure (p< 0.0001) and an 87% increased risk of mortality (p< 0.0001) (Kasiske et al., 2003).

In contrast to earlier reports, a retrospective analysis of the UNOS/OPTN database (involving patients transplanted between 2004-2007) failed to demonstrate the negative impact of NODAT on transplant survival or CV mortality during a median follow-up of 548 days. The study consisted of >37,000 renal transplant recipients with a functioning transplant for at least 1 year. Risk stratification according to diabetes status (pre-transplant diabetes, NODAT) and acute rejection (AR) at 1 year demonstrated that pre-transplant diabetes is the major predictor of all-cause and cardiovascular mortality whereas acute rejection during the first year is the major predictor of death-censored transplant failure. In contrast, NODAT alone was not associated significantly with any study outcomes (Kuo et al., 2010). Nonetheless, the study results were regarded as inconclusive due to the wide confidence intervals and the relatively short duration of follow-up. It is noteworthy that in a large registry study consisting of more than 27,000 primary kidney transplant recipients with graft survival of at least 1 year and with longer-term follow-up, Cole et al. demonstrated that patients with NODAT had decreased survival compared with those who developed neither NODAT nor acute rejection (HR 3.85; $p < 0.0001$) (Cole et al., 2008).

11.2 Non-renal solid organ transplants

Clinical studies evaluating the impact of NODAT on patient and allograft outcomes after non-renal solid organ transplantation have yielded variable results (Baid et al., 2001; John & Thuluvath, 2002; Valentine et al., 2001).

In a study consisting of 66 heart transplant recipients, post-transplant insulin resistance or post-transplant hyperglycemia (glucose levels > 8.9 mmol/L 2 hours after a standard oral glucose tolerance test) was found to be a predictive factor for transplant coronary artery stenosis ($p \leq 0.01$) and death ($p \leq 0.005$) during a 5-year post-tarnsplant follow-up period (Valentine et al., 2001). Patients with post-transplant hyperglycemia were also found to have a higher mean coronary artery intimal thickness than those without post-transplant hyperglycemia (0.35 ± 0.05 vs. $0.20 \pm .02$, respectively; $p \leq 0.05$).

In a single-center study consisting of 435 liver transplant recipients John et al. demonstrated that cardiovascular complications, major and minor infections, neurologic and neuropsychiatric complications were twice as common in patients who developed NODAT (n= 46) compared with their age- and sex-matched counterparts without pre- or post-transplant diabetes (n=92) (John & Thuluvath, 2002). However, there was no difference in patient survival between the two groups at 1-, 2- and 5-years follow-up. In contrast, Baid et al. demonstrated that NODAT was an independent risk factor for mortality after liver transplantation (HR 3.67, $p < 0.0001$) particularly in those with hepatitis C. The cumulative mortality in HCV (+) NODAT (+) vs. HCV (+) NODAT (-) patients was 56% vs. 14%, respectively ($p=0.001$) (Baid et al., 2001).

12. Detection and management of diabetes mellitus in recipients of solid organ transplants

12.1 Pre-transplant baseline evaluation

Suggested guidelines for pre-transplant baseline evaluation of potential transplant candidates is shown in Figure 2. Patients with evidence of IGT or abnormal OGTT before transplantation should be counseled on lifestyle modifications including weight control, diet, and exercise. The goals for the life-style modification involved achieving and maintaining a weight reduction of at least 7 percent of initial body weight through a healthy low-calorie, low-fat diet and at least 150 minutes of physical activity per week.

Pre-transplant treatment of HCV-infected renal transplant candidates should be considered. Selection of an immunosuppressive regimen should be tailored to each individual patient, weighing the risk of developing diabetes after transplantation against the risk of acute rejection.

12.2 Early detection of NODAT after transplantation

Studies investigating the best predictive tool for identifying patients at risk for developing NODAT early after transplantation are currently lacking. While fasting plasma glucose (FPG) is readily available in clinical practice it may be normal in kidney transplant recipients with abnormal glucose homeostasis. It has been suggested that transplant patients have an atypical form of insulin resistance and their plasma glucose often peeks before lunch. Hence the use of FPG alone may preclude the accurate diagnosis of NODAT. Kuypers et al. demonstrated that a normal (vs. diabetic) OGTT on day 5 was associated with a significantly reduced risk for NODAT (odds ratio 0.03, P=0.0002) (Kuypers et al., 2008). However, it is noteworthy that while acute rejection has been suggested to increase the risk for NODAT, it usually does not occur before day 5. Obtaining OGTT and FPG at day 5, therefore, may preclude the subset of patients with higher risk of developing NODAT. Hence, it has been suggested that performing OGTT at 10-12 weeks post-transplantation might be useful as an alternative or supplementary test to day 5 OGTT (P.T. Pham & P.C. Pham, 2008).

The routine recommendation of performing an OGTT early after transplantation awaits further studies. Suggested pre-transplant baseline evaluation and post-transplant screening for NODAT is shown in Figure 2.

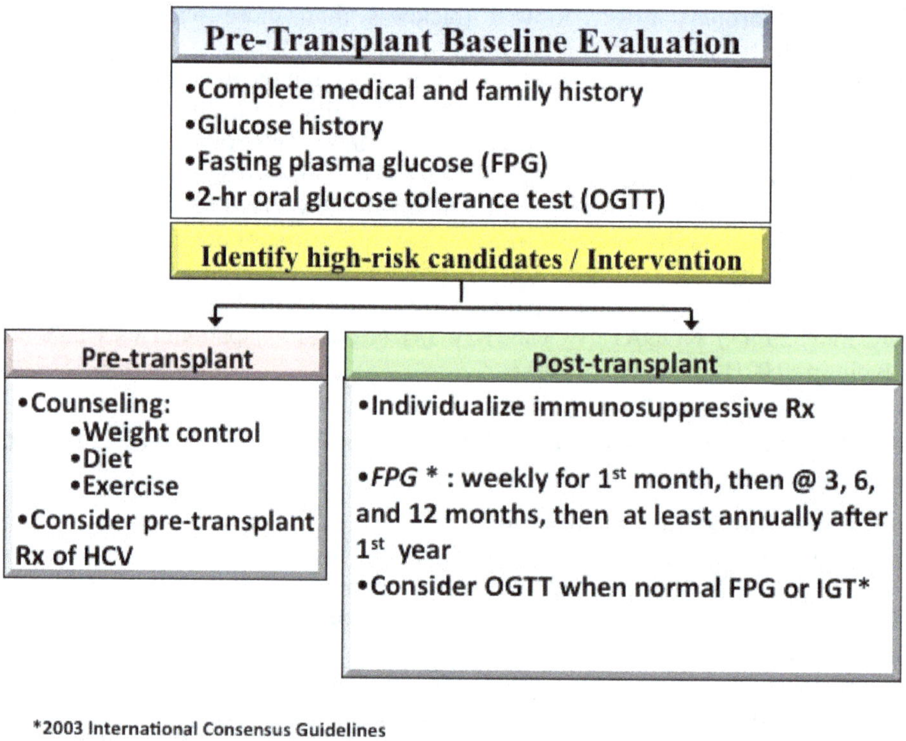

Fig. 2. Sugested guidelines for pre-transplant baseline evaluation and post-transplant screening for NODAT

12.3 Management of established NODAT

The management of NODAT should follow the conventional approach for patients with type 2 diabetes mellitus as recommended by many clinical guidelines established by well-recognized organizations including the American Diabetes Association (ADA).

Similar to the nontransplant settings, a target hemoglobin A1C level < 6.5%-7% is recommended. Fasting plasma glucose should be below 100 mg/dL (6.11 mmol/L), and a 2-hour postprandial plasma glucose should be below 140 mg/dL (7.77 mmol/L) (Mannon,

2008). Nonetheless, it should be noted that the Action to Control Cardiovascular Risk in Diabetes (ACCORD) trial was discontinued prematurely because of a satistically significant increase in all-cause mortality in the intensive- compared with the standard- glycemic treatment groups (Gerstein et al., 2008). At 1 year, stable median A_{1C} levels of 6.4% and 7.5% were achieved in the intensive-therapy and standard groups, respectively. The intensive-therapy group had a relative increase in mortality of 22% and an absolute increase of 1.0% during a follow-up period of 3.5 years. Death from cardiovascular causes were similar between the two treatment groups. It is also notable that hypoglycemia requiring assistance and weight gain of more than 10 kg were more frequent in the intensive-therapy group ($P < 0.001$). Long-term follow-up of the ACCORD study demonstrated that intensive therapy failed to reduce the risk of advanced measures of microvascular outcomes but delayed the onset of micro- and macro-albuminuria and some measures of ocular complications and peripheral neuropathy which persisted over the 5 year study period despite the transition from intensive to conventional treatment of glycemia after 3.7 years (Ismail-Beigi et al., 2010).

Study similar to that of the ACCORD study in recipients of solid organ transplantation is lacking. Nonetheless, the determination of hemoglobin A1C target levels for solid organ transplant recipients should be individualized based on hypoglycemia risks.

13. Modifiable risk factor management strategy

13.1 Dietary modification and physical activity

The Diabetes Prevention Program has demonstrated that a structured diet and physical activity program that achieves and maintains modest weight loss for overweight adults with IGT can significantly reduce the development of diabetes. Defining realistic goals such as a target weight loss of 5-10% of total body weight and patient- centered approach to education may be invaluable in achieving success. Suggested non-insulin management of NODAT is shown in table 3.

13.2 Modification of immunosuppression

Modification of immunosuppression should be considered in high-risk patients. Corticosteroid dose reduction has been shown to significantly improve glucose tolerance during the first year after transplantation (Kasiske et al., 2003). However, any dose reduction should be weighed against the risk of acute rejection. Steroid-sparing regimen or steroid avoidance protocol should be tailored to each individual patient. Tac to CSA conversion therapy in patients who fail to achieve target glycemic control or in those with difficult to control diabetes has yielded variable results. The use of CNI and mTOR inhibitor combination therapy should probably be avoided. Belatacept -- a selective T cell costimulation blocker, is a promising new immunosuppressant that has been suggested to have better cardiovascular and metabolic risk profiles compared with cyclosporine (lower blood pressure, better lipid profiles and lower NODAT incidence) (Vanrenterghem et al., 2011).

13.3 Renin-angiotensin inhibition

A meta-analysis of 10 randomized controlled trials to assess the effects of renin angiotensin inhibition [five with angiotensin-converting enzyme inhibitors (ACEIs) and five with

Agents	Action	Adverse effects / Comments
INSULIN SENSITIZERS (e.g. Metformin, Butoformin, Phenformin)	↓ hepatic glucose production, ↑ glucose uptake by skeletal muscle	• Diarrhea, dyspepsia, lactic acidosis w/ renal insufficiency • No weight gain, no hypoglycemia
INSULIN SECRETAGOGUES	↑ pancreatic insulin secretion	
Sulfonylureas (SUs) (e.g. Glipizide, Glyburide, Glimepiride)		***SUs***: weight gain, edema, hypoglycemia (esp. in renal insufficiency & elderly)
Meglitinides (e.g. Repaglinide, Nateglinide)		***Meglitinides***: weight gain, hypoglycemia (lower risk than SUs) Rapid onset & offset, hepatically excreted (use w/ renal insufficiency)
OTHERS W/ DIFFERENT ACTIONS		
Thiazolidinedione derivatives (TZD) [e.g. Pioglitazone, Rosiglitazone (the drug has been suspended in Europe since 2010, use with caution, see text)]	Bind to peroxisome proliferator-activated receptors (PPARs) & stimulate insulin sensitive genes	• Weight gain, peripheral edema (esp. w/ insulin), anemia, pulmonary edema, CHF, fractures • Slow onset of action, no hypoglycemia, no reliance on renal excretion, contraindicated in class III-IV CHF or hepatic impairment
Glucagon-like peptide-1 analogues (e.g. Exenatide, Liraglutide)	↑ pancreatic insulin secretion	Either favorable or neutral effect on weight gain (delays gastric emptying, ↑ satiety)
Dipeptidyl peptidase 4 inhibitors (e.g. Sitagliptin, Saxagliptin)	↑ Endogenous incretins	• Avoid vildagliptin in hepatic impairment & stage IV-V CKD, dose should be adjusted for renal insufficiency. • Watch for immunosuppresive drug interaction • Weight neutral, no hypoglycemia, ? β cell preservation

Table 3. Non-insulin drug therapy for NODAT

angiotensin receptor blockers (ARBs)] on the incidence of new cases of type 2 diabetes mellitus in patients with arterial hypertension and congestive heart failure demonstrated that renin-angiotensin inhibition with either ACEIs or ARBs consistently and significantly reduced the incidence of type 2 diabetes mellitus compared with placebo, or beta-blockers/diuretics or amlodipine (Scheen, 2004). This finding has not yet been validated in either transplant recipients or prospective trials in the general population (Bosch et al., 2006). Nonetheless, ACE-I and/or ARB are commonly used due to its well-established antiproteinuric, cardioprotective, and blood pressure lowering effect.

13.4 Pharmacological management

When lifestyle modification fails to achieve adequate glycemic control, medical intervention is recommended. Orally administered agents can be used either alone or in combination with other oral agents or insulin. The choice of pharmacologic therapy is based on the potential advantages and disadvantages associated with the different classes of oral agents. Table 3 summarizes the mechanisms of action and potential advantages and disadvantages of different classes of oral agents.

It is noteworthy that the results of the Dialysis Outcomes and Practice Patterns Study (DOPPS) demonstrated that in long-term hemodialysis patients rosiglitazone was associated with a significantly higher all-cause (hazard ration 1.59) and cardiovascular mortality and a 3.5 fold increase of hospitalizations due to myocardial infarction (Ramirez et al., 2009). In contrast to the DOPPS study results, in an analysis of the national cohort study consisting of more than 5,000 dialysis patients with type 2 diabetes Brunelli et al. observed a lower incidence of all-cause mortality in patients not on insulin vs. insulin requiring diabetic patients (Brunelli et al., 2009). Similar studies in the transplant settings are lacking. Nonetheless, great caution should be exercised when rosiglitazone is used in the setting of kidney transplantation because all kidney transplant recipients should be regarded as having at least stage II-IV chronic kidney disease. It should be noted that rosiglitazone has been suspended in Europe since 2010

Incretin-based therapy appears to provide an attractive treatment option for patients with NODAT owing to its favorable effect on weight reduction /weight neutrality. Data on its safety and efficacy in renal transplant recipients are currently lacking. A randomized, placebo-controlled, double-blind, prospective trial to evaluate the safety and efficacy of vildagliptin in patients with NODAT is currently underway (Haidinger et al., 2010). Caution should be exercised when these agents are used in the transplant setting, particularly with regards to drug to drug interactions. Vildagliptin should be avoided in patients with hepatic impairment and stage IV-V chronic kidney disease and the dose of sitagliptin should be adjusted for renal insufficiency.

Finally, drug to drug interactions should be carefully considered. Interested readers are referred to the following references (Cheng & Fantus, 2005; Hatorp et al., 2003; Niemi et al., 2000).

14. Summary

NODAT is a common complication after solid organ transplantation and has variably been reported to have an adverse impact on patient and allograft outcomes. Risk stratification and intervention to minimize risk should be an integral part in the management of the transplant recipients. Clinicians must be familiar with the patients' immune history prior to manipulating their immunosuppressive therapy.in an attempt to ameliorate NODAT risk. When lifestyle modification fails to achieve adequate glycemic control, medical intervention is often necessary.

The routine care of patients with NODAT should include an evaluation of hemoglobin A1C level every three months and regular screening for diabetic complications. It should be noted that hemoglobin A1C cannot be accurately interpreted within the first three months post transplantation due to various factors including possible blood transfusions in the early posttransplant period and the presence of anemia or impaired allograft function. Blood transfusions may render the test invalid until new hemoglobin is formed and the presence of anemia and kidney impairment can directly interfere with the A1C assay. An artifactual reduction in A1C level has been reported in islet cell transplant recipients taking dapsone for pneumocystis carinii (P. jiroveci) prophylaxis. The cause is yet unknown, but a reduction in red blood cell lifespan and/or hemolysis has been implicated (Froud et al., 2007).

Fasting lipid profile should be measured annually. In transplant recipients with multiple CVD risk factors, more frequent monitoring of lipid profile should be performed at the discretion of the clinicians. Statins or the HMG-CoA reductase inhibitors are the most widely used lipid lowering agents in both the nontransplant and transplant settings. Table 4 summarizes the suggested guidelines for the management of NODAT (P.T. Pham et al., 2007c; Qaseem et al., 2011).

Non-pharmacological

Dietary modification
Dietitian referral
Diabetic dyslipidemia: diet low in saturated fats and cholesterol & high in complex carbohydrates & fiber
AHA[1] guidelines: limiting cholesterol (< 200 mg/day for those with DM), < 7% calories from saturated fats, 2-3% calories from trans-fatty acids, < 2,400 mg sodium a day, > 25g/day of dietary fiber & 2 servings of fish a week

Lifestyle modification
Exercise
Weight reduction or avoidance of excessive weight gain
Smoking cessation

Modification of immunosuppressive medications[2]

Rapid steroid taper, steroid-sparing or steroid avoidance protocols
Tacrolimus to cyclosporine conversion therapy
Avoid CNI and mTOR inhibitors combination therapy

Pharmacological therapy

Acute, marked hyperglycemia (may require in-patient management)
Consider insulin drip when glucose > 400 mg/dL[3]
Chronic hyperglycemia: treat to target HbA1C < 6.5%[4]
Oral glucose-lowering agent monotherapy or combination therapy[5] and/or insulin therapy
Consider diabetologist referral if HbA1C remains > 9.0%

Monitoring of patients with NODAT

HbA1C every 3 months
Screening for microalbuminuria
Regular ophthalmologic exam
Regular foot care
Annual fasting lipid profile
Aggressive treatment of dyslipidemia nd hypertension

---

[1]AHA: American Heart Association
[2]Clinicians must be familiar with the patients'immune history prior to manipulating their immunosuppressive therapy
[3]The American College of Physicians expert panel recommends not using intensive insulin therapy to normalize blood glucose in general surgical and medical intensive care unit (SICU/MICU) patients with or without diabetes (reference 84). Studies in the transplant settings are lacking. The determination of target blood glucose for transplant recipients should be individualized at the discretion of the clinician.
[4]See text

Table 4. Management of NODAT

15. References

Aasebo, W., Midvedt, K., Valderhaugh, T.G., et al. (2010). Impaired gluose homeostasis in renal transplant recipients receiving basiliximab. *Nephrology Dialysis Transplantation*, Vol. 25, No. 4, (November 2010), pp. 1279-1286, ISSN 0931-0509

Baid, S., Cosimi, A.B., Farrell, et al. (2001). Posttransplant diabetes mellitus in liver transplant recipients: risk factors, temporal relationship with hepatitis C virus allograft hepatitis, and impact on mortality. *Transplantation*, Vol. 72, No. 6, (September 2010), pp. 1066-1072, ISSN 0041-1337

Bayer, N.D., Cochetti, P.T., Kumar, M.S.A., et al. (2010). Association of metabolic syndrome with development of New-Onset Diabetes after transplantation. *Transplantation*, Vol. 90, No. 8, (October 2010), pp. 861-866, ISSN 0041-1337

Bayes, B., Pastor, M.C., Lauzurica, R., et al. (2007). Do anti-CD25 monoclonal antibodies potentiate posttransplant diabetes mellitus? *Transplantation Proceedings*, Vol. 39, No. 7, (February 2007), pp. 2248-2250, ISSN 0041-1345

Bigam, D., Pennington, J., Carpentier, A., et al. (2000). Hepatitis-C related cirrhosis: a predictor of diabetes after liver transplantation. *Hepatology*, Vol. 32, No. 1, (July 2000), pp. 87-90, ISSN 1527-3350

Bloom, R.D., Rao, V., Weng, F., et al. (2002). Association of hepatitis C with posttransplant diabetes in renal transplant patients on tacrolimus. *Journal of American Society of Nephrology*, Vol. 13, No. 5, (May 2002), pp. 1374-1380, ISSN 1046-6673

Bloom, R.D., Lake, J.R. (2006). Emerging issues in hepatitis C virus-positive liver and kidney transplant recipients. *American Journal of Kidney Transplantation*, Vol. 6, No. 10, (October 2006), pp. 2232-2237, ISSN 1600-6135

Bosch, J., Yusuf, S., Gerstein, H.C., et al. (2006). Effect of ramipril on the incidence of diabetes. *New England Journal of Medicine*, Vol. 355, No. 15, (October 2006), pp. 1551-1562, ISSN 0028-4793

Brunelli, S.M., Thadhani, R., Ikizler, T.A., et al. (2009). Thiazolidinedione use is associated with better survival in hemodialysis patients with non-insulin dependent diabetes. *Kidney International*, Vol. 75, No. 9, (May 2009), pp. 961-968, ISSN 0085-2538

Cai, T.H., Esterl, R.M., Nichols, F., et al. (1998). Improved immunosuppression with combination tacrolimus (FK506) and mycophenolic acid in orthotopic liver transplantation. *Transplantation Proceedings*, Vol. 30, No. 4, (June 1998), pp. 1413-1414, ISSN 0041-1345

Cheng, A.Y.Y., Fantus, I.G. (2005). Oral antihyperglycemic therapy for type 2 diabetes mellitus. *Canadian Medical Association Journal*, Vol. 172, No. 2, (January 2005), pp. 213-226, ISSN 0820-3946

Cole, E.H., Johnston, O., Rose, C.L., et al. (2008). Impact of acute rejection and new-onset diabetes on long-term transplant graft and patient survival. *Clinical Journal of the American Society of Nephrology*, Vol. 3, No. 3, (May 2008), pp. 814-821, ISSN 1555-9041

Cosio, F.G., Pesavento, T.E., Osei, K., et al. (2001). Post-transplant diabetes mellitus: Increasing incidence in renal allograft recipients transplanted in recent years. *Kidney International*, Vol. 59, No. 2, (February 2001), pp. 732-737, ISSN 0085-2538

Cosio, F.G., Kudva, Y., van der Velde, M., Larson, T.S., et al. (2005). New onset hyperglycemia and diabetes mellitus are associated with increased cardiovascular risk after kidney transplantation. *Kidney International*, Vol. 67, No. 6, (June 2005), pp. 2415-2421, ISSN 0085-2538

Crutchlow, M.F., Bloom, R.D. Transplant-associated hyperglycemia: A new look at an old problem. (2007). *Clinical Journal of the American Society of Nephrology*, Vol. 2, No. 2, (March 2007), pp. 343-355, ISSN 1555-9041

Davidson, J., Wilkinson, A.H., Dantal, J., et al. (2003). New-onset diabetes after transplantation: 2003 International Consensus Guidelines. *Transplantation*, Vol. 75, No. 10, (May 2003), pp. SS3-SS24, ISSN 0041-1337

Dean, P.G., Kudva, Y.C., Larson, T.S., et al. (2008). Post transplantation diabetes after pancreas transplantation. *American Journal of Transplantation*, Vol. 8, No. 1, (January 2008), pp. 175-182, ISSN 1600-6135

Delgado-Borrego, A., Casson, D., Schoenfeld, D., et al. (2004). Hepatitis C virus is independently associated with increased insulin resistance after liver transplantation. *Transplantation*, Vol 77, No. 5, (March 2004), pp. 703-710, ISSN 0041-1337

Depczynski, B., Daly, B., Campbell, D., et al. (2000). Predicting the occurrence of diabetes mellitus in recipients of heart transplants. *Diabetic Medicine*, Vol. 17, No. 1, (January 2000), pp. 15-19, ISSN 1464-5491

Drachenberg, C.B., Klassen, D.K., Weir, M.R., et al. (1999). Islet cell damage associated with tacrolimus and cyclosporine: morphological features in pancreas allograft biopsies and clinical correlation. *Transplantation*, Vol. 68, No. 3, (August 1999), pp. 396-402, ISSN 0041-1337

Eckel, R.H. (2007). Mechanisms of the components of the metabolic syndrome that predispose to diabetes and atherosclerotic CVD. *Proceedings of the Nutrition Society*, Vol. 66, No. 1, (February 2007), pp. 82-95, ISSN 0029-6651

Eprinchard, C.S., Braun, P.P., Heibel, F., et al. (2011). Incidence and risk factors of glucose metabolism disorders in kidney transplant recipients: role of systematic screening by oral glucose tolerance test. *Transplantation*. Vol. 91, No. 7, (April 2011), ISSN 0041-1337

Ekberg, H., Tedesco-Silva, H., Demirbas, A., et al. (2007). Reduced exposure to calcineurin inhibitors in renal transplantation. *New England Journal of Medicine,* Vol. 357, (December 2007), pp. 2562-2575, ISSN 0028-4793

Froud, T., Faradji, R.N., Monroy, K., et al. (2007). Dapsone-induced artifactual A1C reduction in islet transplant recipients. *Transplantation*, Vol. 83, No. 6, (March 2007), pp. 824-825, ISSN 0041-1337

Gerstein, H.C., Miller, M.E., Byinhton, R.P., et al. (2008). Effects of intensive glucose lowering in type 2 diabetes. *New England Journal of Medicine*, Vol. 358, No. 24, (June 2008), pp. 2545-2559, ISSN 0028-4793

Haidinger, M., Werzowa, J., Voigt, H-C., et al. (2010). A randomized, placebo-controlled, double-blind, prospective trial to evaluate the effect of vildagliptin in new-onset diabetes mellitus after kidney transplantation. *Trials*, Vol. 11, No. 91, (October 2010), pp. 1-6, ISSN 1745-6215

Hatorp, V., Hansen, K.T., Thomsen, M.S. (2003). Influence of drugs interacting with CYP3A4 on the pharmacokinetics, pharmacodynamics and safety of the prandial glucose regulator repaglinide. *Journal of Clinical Pharmacology*, Vol. 43, No. 6, pp. 649-660, ISSN 0091-2700

Heisel, O., Heisel, R., Balshaw, R., et al. (2004). New onset diabetes mellitus in patients receiving calcineurin inhibitors: a systematic review and meta-analysis. *American Journal of Transplantation*, Vol. 4. No. 4, (April 2004), pp. 583-595, ISSN 1600-6135

Hjelmesaeth, J., Hartmann, A., Kofstad, J., et al. (1997). Glucose intolerance after renal transplantation depends upon prednisolone dose and recipient age. *Transplantation*, Vol. 64, No. 7, (October 1997), pp. 979-983, ISSN 0041-1337

Hjelmesaeth, J., Hartmann, A., Kofstad, J., et al. (2001). Tapering off prenisolone and cyclosporine the first year after renal transplantation: the effect on glucose tolerance. *Nephrology Dialysis Transplantation*, Vol. 16, No. 4, (April 2001), pp. 829-835, ISSN 0931-0509

Hjelmesaeth, J., Sagedal, S., Hartmannn, A. et al. (2004). Asymptomatic cytomegalovirus infection is associated with increased risk for new-onset diabetes and impaired insulin release after renal transplantation. *Diabetologia*, Vol. 47, No. 9, (September 2004), pp. 1550-1556, ISSN 0012-186X

Hjelmesaeth, J., Muller, F., Jenssen, T., et al. (2005). Is there a link between cytomegalovirus infection and new-onset posttransplant diabetes mellitus? Potential mechanisms of virus induced β-cell damage. *Nephrology Dialysis Transplantation*, Vol. 20, No. 11, (November 2005), pp. 2311-2315, ISSN 0931-0509

Hjelmesaeth, J., Hartmann, A., Leivestad, T. et al. (2006). The impact of early-diagnosed new-onset post-tarnsplantation diabetes mellitus on survival and major cardiac events. *Kidney International*, Vol. 69, No. 3, (February 2006), pp. 588-595, ISSN 0085-2538

Ismail-Beigi, F., Craven, T., Banerji, M.A., et al. Effect of intensive treatment of hyperglycemia on microvascular outcomes in type 2 diabetes: an analysis of the ACCORD randomized trial. *Lancet*, Vol. 376, No. 9739, (August 2010), pp. 419-430, ISSN 0140-6736

Kasiske, B.L., Snyder, J.J., Gilbertson, D., et al. (2003). Diabetes mellitus after kidney transplantation in the United States. *American Journal of Transplantation,* Vol. 3, No. 10, (October 2003), pp. 178-185, ISSN 1600-6135

Knobler, H., Stagnaro-Green, A., Wallenstein, S., et al. (1998). Higher incidence of diabetes in liver transplant recipients with hepatitis C. *Journal of Clinical Gastroenterology*, Vol. 26, No. 1 (January 1998), pp. 30-33, ISSN 0192-0790

Luan, F.L., Steffick, D.E., Ojo, A.O. (2011). New-Onset Diabetes Mellitus in kidney transplant recipients discharged on steroid-free immunosuppression. *Transplantation*, Vol. 91, No. 3, (February 2011), pp. 334-341, ISSN 0041-1337

John, P.R., Thuluvath, P.J. (2002). Outcomes of patients with new-onset diabetes mellitus after liver transplantation compared with those without diabetes mellitus. *Liver transplantation*, Vol. 8, No. 8, (August 2002), pp. 708-713, ISSN 1527-6465

Johnston, O., Rose, C.L., Webster, A.C., et al. (2008). Sirolimus is associated with New-Onset Diabetes in kidney transplant recipients. *Journal of American Society of Nephrology*, Vol. 19, No. 7, (July 2008), pp. 1411-1418, ISSN 1046-6673

Kamar, N., Toupance, O., Buchler, M., et al. (2003). Evidence that clearance of hepatitis C virus RNA after α-interferon therapy in dialysis patients is sustained after renal transplantation. *Journal of American Society of Nephrology*, Vol. 14, No. 8, (August 2003), pp. 2092-2098, ISSN 1046-6673

Kissebah, A.H., Vydelingum, N., Murray, R., et al. (1982). Relation of body fat distribution to metabolic complications of obesity. *Journal of Clinical Endocrinology and Metabolism*, Vol. 54, No. 2, (May 1982), pp. 254-260, ISSN 0021-972X

Kuo, H-T., Sampaio, M.S., Vincenti, F. ,et al. (2010). Associations of pretransplant diabetes mellitus, New-Onset Diabetes Mellitus after Transplant, and acute rejection with transplant outcomes: An analysis of the Organ Procurement and Transplant Network/United Network for Organ Sharing (OPTN/UNOS) database. *American Journal of Kidney Disease*, Vol. 56, No. 6, (December 2010), pp. 1127-1139, ISSN 0272-6386

Kuypers, D.R., Claes, K., Bammens, B., et al. (2008). Early clinical assessment of glucose metabolism in renal allograft recipients: Diagnosis and prediction of post-transplant diabetes mellitus. *Nephrology Dialysis Transplantation*, Vol. 23, No. 6, (June 2008), pp. 2033-2042, ISSN 0931-0509

Lehr, H., Jao, S., Waltzer, W.C., et al. (1985). Cytomegalovirus-induced diabetes mellitus in a renal transplant recipient. *Transplantation Proceedings*, Vol. 17, No. 5, (October 1985), pp. 2152-2154, ISSN 0041-1345

Maes, B.D., Kuypers, D., Messiaen, T., et al. (2001). Posttransplant diabetes mellitus in FK-506-treated renal transplant recipients: analysis of incidence and risk factors. *Transplantation*, Vol. 72, No. 10, (November 2001), pp. 1655-1661, ISSN 0041-1337

Mannon, R.B. (2008). Therapeutic management of posttransplant diabetes mellitus. *Transplantation Reviews*, Vol. 22, No. 2, (April 2008), pp. 116-124, ISSN 0955-470X

Martinez-Castelao, A., Hernandez, M.D., Pascual, J., et al. (2005). Detection and treatment of post kidney transplant hyperglycemia: A Spanish multicenter cross-sectional study. *Transplantation Proceedings*, Vol. 37, No. 9, (November 2005), pp. 3813-3816, ISSN 0041-1345

Meiser, B.M., Uberfuhr, P., Fuchs, A., et al. (1998). Single-center randomized trial comparing tacrolimus (FK506) and cyclosporine in the prevention of acute myocardial rejection. *The Journal of Heart and Lung Transplantation,* Vol. 17, No. 8(August 1998), pp. 782-788, ISSN 1053-2498

Midtvedt, K., Hjemesaeth, J., Hartmann, A., et al. (2004). Insulin resistance after renal transplantation: the effect of steroid dose reduction and withdrawal. *Journal of the American Society of Nephrology,* Vol. 15, No. 12, (December 2004), pp. 3233-3239, ISSN 1046-6673

Montori, V.M., Velosa, J.A., Basu, A. et al. (2002). Post transplantation diabetes: A systematic review of the literature. *Diabetes Care*, Vol. 25, No. 3, (March 2002), pp. 583-592, ISSN 0149-5992

Myslak, M., Amer, H., Morales, P. et al. (2006). Interpreting post-transplant proteinuria in patients with proteinuria pre-transplant. *American Journal of Transplantation*, Vol. 6, No. 7, (July 2006), pp. 1660-1665, ISSN 1600-6135

Niemi, M., Backman, J.T., Neuvonen, P.J., et al. (2000). Rifampin decreases the plasma concentrations and effects of repaglinide. *Clinical Pharmacology and Therapeutics*, Vol. 68, No. 5, (July 2000), pp. 495-500, ISSN 0009-9236

Ojo, A.O. (2006). Cardiovascular complications after renal transplantation and their prevention. *Transplantation*, Vol. 82, No. 5, (September 2006), pp. 603-611, ISSN 0041-1337

Pham, P.C., Pham, P.M., Pham, S.V. et al. (2007). Hypomagnesemia in patients with type 2 diabetes. *Clinical Journal of the American Society of Nephrology*, Vol. 2, No. 2, (March 2007), pp. 366-373, ISSN 1555-9041

Pham, P.T., Danovitch, G.M., Pham, P.C. (2007a). The medical management of the renal transplant recipient . In: *Comprehensive Clinical Nephrology, 3rd ed.*, R.J. Johnson & John Feehally, pp. 1085-1101, Mosby, ISBN 978-0-323-04602-2, Philadelphia, PA

Pham, P.T., Pham, P.C., Lipshutz, G., et al. (2007b). New onset diabetes mellitus after solid organ transplantation. *Endocrinology and Metabolism Clinics of North America,* Vol. 36, No. 4, (December 2007b), pp. 873-890, ISSN 0889-8529

Pham, P.T., Pham, P.C., Danovitch, G.M. (2007c). Posttransplant cardiovascular disease. *Seminars in Nephrology*, Vol. 27, No. 4, (July 2007c), pp. 430-444, ISSN 0270-9295

Pham, P.T., Pham, P.C. (2008). Assessing the risk of post-transplantation diabetes mellitus with an oral glucose tolerance test. *Nature Clinical Practice Nephrology*, Vol. 4, No. 11, (November 2008), pp. 600-601, ISSN 1759-5061

Qaseem, A., Humphrey, L., Chou, R., et al. (2011). Use of intensive therapy for the management of glycemic control in hospitalized patients: A clinical practice guideline from the American College of Physicians. *Annals of Internal Medicine*, Vol. 154, No. 4, (February 2011), pp. 260-267, ISSN 0003-4819

Ramirez, S.P., Albert, J.M., Blayney, M.J., et al. (2009). Rosiglitazone is associated with mortality in chronic hemodialysis patients. *Journal of the American Society of Nephrology*, Vol. 20, No. 5, (May 2009), pp. 1094-1101, ISSN 1046-6673

Roland, M., Gatault, P., Al-Naijjar, A., et al. (2008). Early pulse pressure and low-grade proteinuria as independent long-term risk factors for New-Onset Diabetes After kidney Transplantation. *American Journal of Transplantation*, Vol. 8, No. 8, (August 2008), pp. 1719-1728, ISSN 1600-6135

Santos, L., Rodrigo, E., Pinera, C., et al. (2010). Elevated serum Gamma-Glutaryltransferase and hypomagnesemia are not related with new-onset diabetes after transplantation. *Transplantation Proceedings*, Vol. 42, No. 8, (October 2010), pp. 2914-2916, ISSN 0041-1345

Scheen, A.J. Renin-angiotensin system inhibition prevents type 2 diabetes mellitus. Part 1. A meta-analysis of randomized clinical trials. *Diabetes and Metabolism*, Vol. 30, No. 6, (December 2004), pp. 487-496, ISSN 1262-3636

Setoguchi, R., Hori, S., Takahashi, T., et al. (2005). Hemoestatic maintenance of natural Fox3(+) CD25(+) CD4(+) regulatory T cells by interleukin (IL)-2 and induction of autoimmune disease by IL-2 neutralization. *The Journal of Experimental Medicine*, Vol. 201, pp. 723-735, ISSN 0022-1007

Sharif, A., Moore, R.H., Baboolal, K. (2006). The use of oral glucose tolerance tests to risk stratify for new-onset diabetes after transplantation: an underdiagnosed phenomenon. *Transplantation*, Vol. 82, No. 12, (December 2006), pp. 1667-1672, ISSN 0041-1337

Silverborn, M., Jeppsson, A., Martensson, G., & Nilsson, F. (2005). New-onset cardiovascular risk factors in lung transplant recipients. *The Journal of Heart and Lung Transplantation*, Vol. 24, No. 10, (October 2005), pp. 1536-1543, ISSN 1053-2498

Simo, R., Lecube, A., Genesca, J., et al. (2006). Sustained virological response correlates with reduction in the incidence of glucose abnormalities in patients with chronic hepatitis C virus infection. *Diabetes Care*, Vol. 29, No. 11, (November 2006), pp. 2462-2466, ISSN 0149-5992

Subramanian, S., Trence, D.L. (2007). Immunosuppression agents: effects on glucose and lipid metabolism. *Endocrinology and Metabolism Clinics of North America*, Vol. 36, No. 4, (December 2007), pp. 891-905, ISSN 0889-8529

Sulanc, E., Lane, J.T., Puumala, S.E., et al. (2005). New-onset diabetes after kidney transplantation: an application of 2003 International Guidelines. *Transplantation*, Vol. 80, No. 7, (October 2005), pp. 945-952, ISSN 0041-1337

Teutônico, A., Schena, P.F., Di Paolo, S. (2006). Glucose metabolism in renal transplant recipients: Effect of calcineurin inhibitor withdrawal and conversion to sirolimus. *Journal of American Society of Nephrology*, Vol. 16, No. 10, (October 2005), pp. 3128-3135, ISSN 1046-6673

Trulock, E.P., Christie, J.D., Edward, L.B., et al. (2007). Registry of the International society for heart and lung Transplantation: twenty-fourth official adult lung and heart-lung transplantation report. *The Journal of Heart and Lung Transplantation*, Vol. 26, No. 8, (August 2007), pp. 782-795, ISSN 1053-2498

Valentine, H., Rickenbacker, P., Kemna, M., et al. (2001). Metabolic abnormalities characteristics of dysmetabolic syndrome predict the development of transplant coronary artery disease: prospective study. *Circulation*, Vol. 103, pp. 2144-2152, ISSN 0009-7322

Van Hooff, J.P., Christiaans, M.H.L., van Duijhoven, E.M. (2004). Evaluating mechanisms of post-transplant diabetes mellitus. *Nephrology Dialysis Transplantation*, Vol. 19, Suppl. 6, (December 2004), pp. vi18-vi12, ISSN 0931-0509

Van Laecke, S., Van Biesen, W., Verbeke, F., et al. (2009). Posttransplantation hypomagnesemia and its realtion with immunosuppression as predictors of New-Onset Diabetes after Transplantation. *American Journal of Transplantation*, Vol. 9, No. 9, (September 2009), pp. 2140-2149, ISSN 1600-6135

Van Laecke, S., Desideri, F., Geerts, A., et al. (2010). Hypomagenesemia and the risk of New-Onset Diabetes after liver transplantation. *Liver Transplantation*, Vol. 16, No. 11, (November 2010), pp. 1278-1287, ISSN 1527-6465

Vanrenterghem, Y., Bresnahan, B., Campistol, J., et al. (2011). Belatacept-based regimens are associated with improved cardiovascular and metabolic risk factors compared with cyclosporine in kidney transplant recipients. (BENEFT- and BENEFITEXT Studies). *Transplantation*, (March 2011), [Epub ahead of print], ISSN 1534-0608

Vareesangthip, K., Tong, P., Wilkinson, R., et al. (1997). Insulin resistance in adult polycystic kidney disease. *Kidney International*, Vol. 52, No. 2, (August 1997), pp. 503-508, ISSN 0085-2538

Vincenti, F., Friman, S., Sceuermann, E., et al. (2007). Results of an International, randomized trial comparing glucose metabolism disorders and outcome with cyclosporine versus Tacrolimus. *American Journal of Transplantation*, Vol. 7, No. 6, (June 2007), pp. 1506-1514, ISSN 1600-6135

Wilkinson, A.H., Davidson, J., Dotta, F., et al. (2005). Guidelines for the treatment and management of new-onset diabetes after transplantation. *Clinical Transplantion*, Vol. 19, No. 3, (June 2005), pp. 291-298, ISSN 0902-0063

Woodward, R.S., Schnitzler, M.A., Baty, J., et al. (2003). Incidence and cost of new onset diabetes mellitus among U.S. wait-listed and transplanted renal allograft recipients.

American Journal of Transplantation, Vol. 3, No. 5, (May 2003), pp. 590-598, ISSN 1600-6135

Ye, X., Kuo, H-T., Sampaio, M.S., et al. (2010a). Risk factors for the development of new-onset diabetes mellitus after transplant in adult lung transplant recipients. *Clinical Transplantation,* (December 2010a), DOI:10.1111/j.1399-0012.2010.01383.x, ISSN 1399-0012

Ye, X., Kuo, H-T, Sampaio, M, et al. (2010b). Risk factors for development on New-Onset Diabetes Mellitus in adult heart transplant recipients. *Transplantation,* Vol. 89, No. 12, (June 2010b), ISSN 0041-1337

9

Donor Characteristics in 1,000 Consecutive Simultaneous Pancreas-Kidney Transplants

Hans W. Sollinger, Jon S. Odorico, Glen E. Leverson, Barbara J. Voss, and Anthony M. D'Alessandro
Department of Surgery, Division of Transplantation, University of Wisconsin, U.S.A.

1. Introduction

In 2003, Krieger et al. from our group published a manuscript which investigated the use of pancreas grafts for transplantation in different UNOS regions in the United States (1). It was reported that the utilization of pancreata showed a wide variation depending on the region. To approach some degree of standardization, we calculated the ratio of pancreata used for transplantation with the number of livers procured and transplanted. Using the data from our own institution, we had experienced that at least 70% of liver donors should provide acceptable pancreas grafts. The results of the study, however, demonstrated that in some regions, less than 20% of liver donors yielded pancreas grafts. Ensuing discussion revealed that the lack of established criteria to predict the outcome of pancreas transplantation based on available donor criteria was one of the reasons many centers, in particular less experienced programs, were hesitant to accept donors other than those expected to provide excellent pancreas grafts, and therefore, outcomes. Since then, few publications have addressed the correlation between available donor criteria and short- or long-term outcomes. One single center report analyzing outcomes in 61 simultaneous pancreas-kidney transplants (SPK) was published in 1995 by Douzdjian et al. (2), and a multi-center European report by Vinkers et al. (3) attempted to establish a donor quality score. During the preparation of this manuscript, the online version of a large-scale analysis using data from the Scientific Registry of Transplant Recipients (SRTR) in 9,401 transplants from 2000 to 2006 became available for review (4).

The purpose of this manuscript is to report the donor characteristics in 1,000 consecutively performed SPK transplants at a single center. Pancreas-kidney retrieval and donor management, as well as donor evaluation, were performed by the same organ procurement organization (UW OPO). Retrieval was performed by surgeons trained at our institution. Using only donor data easily available to OPO personnel and surgeons, we attempt here to provide straightforward guidelines regarding the acceptability of pancreas grafts. A unique feature of this study is the fact that long-term follow up is available up to 22 years.

2. Materials and methods

Between December 18, 1985 and December 3, 2007, 1,000 consecutive donor pancreatectomies were performed by the members of the University of Wisconsin transplant team and the University of Wisconsin OPO. In general, the retrieval team consisted of a transplant surgeon or a Board-certified/eligible surgeon, a transplant fellow and a procurement specialist. Over the 20-year interval, only a small number of surgeons and transplant specialists—all trained at our institution—were involved, keeping the surgical approach standardized. The principles of the donor operation have been previously described in detail (5). Our routine consisted of *in situ* flushing with UW solution (ViaSpan®, Bristol-Myers Squibb, Garden City, NY), after dissection of the pancreas and liver. A point was made not to exceed 2 liters of flush solution. The mesenteric vessels were always ligated. Donor demographics are shown in Table 1. Donor management was conducted by the intensive care staff of the referring hospital in consultation with OPO personnel. No OPO personnel was on site until the retrieval procedure. During organ retrieval, generous use of colloids was used to reduce pancreatic edema. All organs were stored in UW solution. Surgical implant technique, recipient management and immunosuppressive therapy have been previously described (6). It is of note that we never used any systemic anticoagulation in the recipients post-transplant.

Data for analysis was obtained from the UW OPO records and transferred into the UW Transplant database.

Histocompatibility testing was performed prior to all transplants, but no attempt was made to match donor and recipient as closely as possible. The only absolute requirement was a negative T-cell crossmatch using the NIH technique.

Statistical Analysis

For statistical analysis, continuous variables were summarized by reporting mean and standard deviation, and categorical variables were summarized by reporting percentages. Event rates were estimated using methods of Kaplan and Meier and compared between groups using a log rank test. $P<0.05$ was considered significant. All analyses were performed using SAS statistical software (SAS Institute, Inc., Cary, NC).

3. Results

For reporting purposes, the highest value among donor laboratory values was chosen for our calculations. BMI was determined by weight at the time of admission. Vasopressor use was defined as the use of any vasopressor at any time from the patient's admission to the time of the retrieval procedure. As expected, long-term outcomes for pancreas graft survival correlated with donor age (Figure 1). Donor age as previously reported by others appears to be a major risk factor. As previously reported by Fernandez, et al., young donors do extremely well despite higher technical difficulties (7). The youngest SPK donor in our experience was three years of age. These grafts should be placed into smaller recipients. BMI also had a significant correlation with inferior long-term outcomes (Figure 2). Obese donors, even in the younger age groups, have pancreata which are infiltrated by fatty tissue and respond poorly to preservation. In addition, fat necrosis after transplantation may lead to intra-abdominal fluid collections and subsequent abscess formation. Nevertheless, on occasion a donor with a high BMI may have a normal-appearing pancreas which can be safely used for transplantation.

Laboratory determinations such as amylase and lipase ($p>0.08$) have not shown any correlation with outcomes, as previously reported by Odorico et al. in a smaller cohort (8). In addition, maximum glucose levels have no predictive value. Glucose values often reflect the resuscitation effort and may be skewed by the co-administration of other drugs such as corticosteroids. In an unpublished study by our group, determination of HbA_1C in 100 consecutive donors did not elicit a single abnormal value which would allow the conclusion that medical history is sufficient to rule out diabetes or pre-diabetes. At the start of our program, we were hesitant to retrieve pancreata from donors with abdominal trauma and prior surgery, which frequently included splenectomy. With growing experience, we have learned to use these donors after careful inspection of the pancreas and duodenum. There is no difference in long-term outcomes ($p=0.6585$). Pancreatic grafts from young trauma victims are frequently very edematous, but return to normal texture after preservation in UW solution. Furthermore, the use of vasopressors is not associated with inferior long-term survival ($p=0.9196$).

4. Discussion

Data published by UNOS/SRTR reveal that the number of SPKs performed has not increased despite an increase in the number of potential pancreas donors by an average of 482 per year since 2003 (4). Most of these consented organs have not been recovered. The non-recovery rate among pancreata is at an all-time high of about 72% (4). Among the possible reasons are a) an older donor population; b) allocation criteria which lists kidney recipients and SPK recipients on the same list; and c) surgeons' fears of achieving inferior results, which in turn might result in termination of insurance coverage for the program. These fears are heightened by the fact that few objective criteria for donor selection exist. In 1998, Odorico et al. from our group analyzed donor factors affecting outcome after pancreas transplantation in 240 recipients (8). The relevant conclusions were that pancreata from donors >45 years of age are associated with a higher failure rate. This finding was consistent with the observations of Gruessner et al. reported in 1994 (9). Odorico et al. also conclude that serum amylase and glucose did not correlate with graft failure (8). Furthermore, in a small series of donation after cardiac death (DCD) donors, no difference in short-term outcomes was noted. Douzdjian et al. analyzed their single-center experience in 61 SPKs and found that duration of brain death before procurement, length of donor admission and donor age were the major factors associated with inferior outcomes (2). In accordance with our observations, serum glucose and serum amylase did not correlate with outcomes.

Recently, the online version of a manuscript by Axelrod et al. was available for review (10). SRTR data from over 9,401 pancreas donors were used to develop a Pancreas Donor Risk Index (PDRI). As pointed out by Krieger (1), the authors emphasize that pancreas utilization shows great regional variation in the United States and that donor selection is widely used as a key factor to successful pancreatic transplantation. The study is based on retrospective data from multiple centers using a variety of procurement techniques.

The uniqueness of this manuscript is that universal procurement and retrieval techniques were used and that the implant team primarily consisted only of a small group of uniformly trained surgeons. Our message is that the donor surgeon should not be discouraged from exploring a donor with high amylase, lipase and glucose levels. Also, the use of vasopressors should not be a reason to decline. Data by Bellingham et al. demonstrate that the same criteria apply in DCD pancreas donors (11).

Using these simplified criteria (age and BMI) for evaluating prospective pancreas donors, together with visual inspection of the graft, suitable pancreas grafts can be chosen to achieve excellent long-term functional outcomes (12). Adequately trained OPO personnel and procurement surgeons will be able to use these simple guidelines in order to maximize potential utilization of pancreas donors.

	Mean (range)
Age (years)	29 (3-60)
Weight (kg)	72 (15-156)
Amylase (U/L)	99 (2-2,002)
Glucose (mg/dL)	189 (6 – 824)
Pancreas cold storage time (hours)	15 (0-43)
	N (%)
Gender: Male Female	 604 (62.5%) 363 (37.5%)
Race: Caucasian African-American Asian Native American	 944 (97.5%) 16 (1.7%) 6 (6.2%) 1 (0.1%)

Table 1. Donor demographics

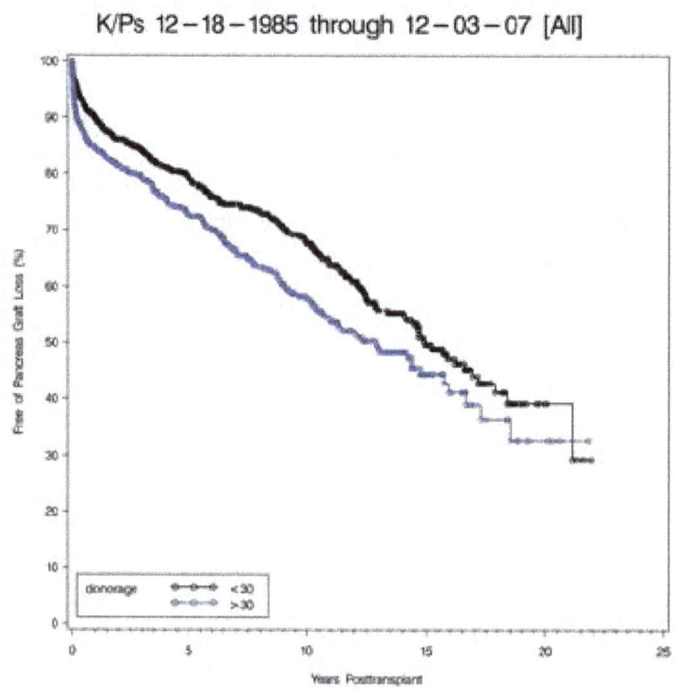

Fig. 1. Age and pancreas transplant outcome

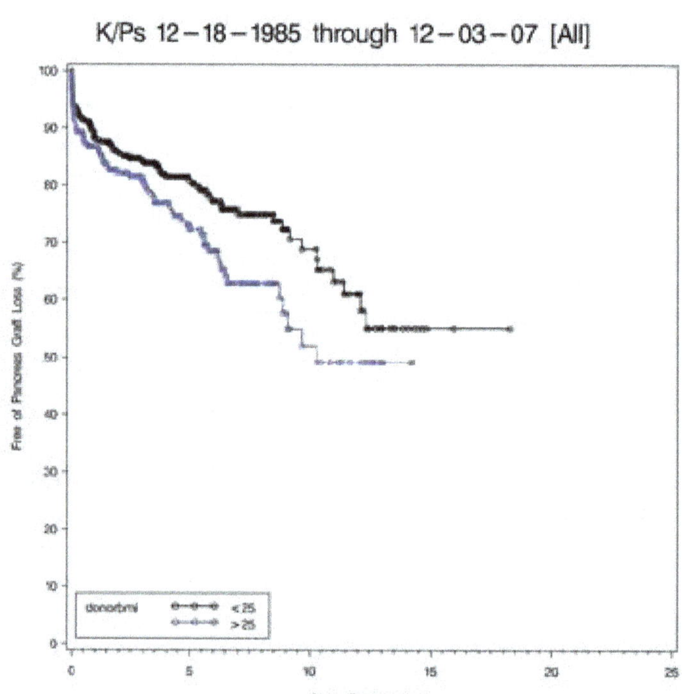

Fig. 2. BMI and pancreas transplant outcome

5. References

Krieger NR, Odorico JS, Heisey DM, et al. Underutilization of pancreas donors. Transplantation 2003;75:1271-6.

Douzdjian V, Gugliuzza KG, Fish JC. Multivariate analysis of donor and recipient risk factors for renal and pancreas allograft failure after pancreas-kidney transplantation. Transplant Proc 1995;27:3128-9.

Vinkers MT, Rahmel AO, Slot MC, Smits JM, Schareck WD. How to recognize a suitable pancreas donor: a Eurotransplant study of preprocurement factors. Transplant Proc 2008;40:1275-8.

Scientific Registry of Transplant Recipients [Internet]. www.ustransplant.org

Sollinger HW, Odorico JS, Knechtle SJ, D'Alessandro AM, Kalayoglu M, Pirsch JD. Experience with 500 simultaneous pancreas-kidney transplants. Ann Surg 1998;228:284-96

Sollinger HW, Odorico JS, Becker YT, D'Alessandro AM, Pirsch JD. One thousand consecutive simultaneous pancreas-kidney transplants at a single center with 22- year follow-up. Ann Surg 2009;250:618-30.

Fernandez LA, Turgeon NA, Odorico JS, et al. Superior long-term results of simultaneous pancreas-kidney transplantation from pediatric donors. Am J Transplant 2004;4:2093-101.

Odorico JS, Heisey DM, Voss BJ, et al. Donor factors affecting outcome after pancreas transplantation. Transplant Proc 1998;30:276-7.

Gruessner RW, Troppmann C, Barrou B, et al. Assessment of donor and recipient risk factors on pancreas transplant outcome. Transplant Proc 1994;26:437.

Axelrod DA, Sung RS, Meyer KH, Wolfe RA, Kaufman DB. Systematic Evaluation of Pancreas Allograft Quality, Outcomes and Geographic Variation in Utilization. Am J Transplant (in press).

Bellingham J, Goodman J, Leverson G, et al. Ten-year outcomes of simultaneous pancreas-kidney transplantation from donation after cardiac death. Am J Transplant 2008;8(suppl. 2):201 (published abstract).

Sollinger HW, Odorico JS, Becker YT, D'Alessandro AM, Pirsch JD. One thousand consecutive simultaneous pancreas-kidney transplants at a single center with 22- year follow-up. Ann Surg 2009;250:618-30.

10

Factors Related to Graft Outcome in Pediatric Renal Transplantation

Jean Herman and Rita Van Damme-Lombaerts
Department of Pediatric Transplantation
University Hospitals Leuven
Belgium

1. Introduction

Over the last decades, renal transplantation has evolved from an experimental procedure into the treatment of choice for children with end-stage renal disease. Differences in size and weight of the recipient, cause of renal failure, immune responsiveness, susceptibility to infection, pharmacokinetics of immunosuppressive drugs, and psychological aspects distinguish renal transplantation in children from adults. The longevity of an allograft is particularly important for the pediatric transplant recipient, because renal replacement therapy is necessarily a lifelong undertaking. The aim of the present study is to determine by means of a multivariable analysis the factors that significantly affect graft outcome in the paediatric transplant population. Knowledge of predictors of graft survival can be beneficial in planning the renal replacement therapy in children and improving transplantation results.

Registry studies, essentially from the North American Pediatric Renal Trials and Collaborative Studies (NAPRTCS) (Benfield et al., 1999; NAPRTCS, 2010) and from the United Network for Organ Sharing (UNOS) (Hwang et al., 2005), have been performed to analyse factors related to graft outcome in children. Registry studies have the advantage of being able to include large number of patients. However these studies usually involve heterogeneous populations with different pre-transplant selections, transplant procedures and post-transplant management. Therefore single center studies using a more homogeneous patient group and more uniform management protocols may be valuable in the analysis of transplant outcome. Nevertheless such single center studies using multivariable techniques to analyse transplant outcome are very scarce in paediatric renal transplantation (Vats et al., 2002).

We analysed all renal transplantations performed in children at our institution between 1980 and 2010 and included in our analysis various factors concerning recipient characteristics, donor characteristics, perioperative characteristics and post-transplant events.

2. Patients, materials and methods

2.1 Patients

The study population consisted of 151 kidney transplants performed between June 1980 and October 2010 in 135 children (81 boys and 54 girls) with mean age 10.7 years (± 4.9) at

transplantation. There were 132 first grafts, 15 second grafts, 3 third grafts and 1 fourth graft.
The original disease was congenital or hereditary in 74% and acquired in 26%. Thirteen children were transplanted preemptively. Kidney came from living related donors (LRD) in 33 cases (22%) and from deceased donors (DD) in 118 cases (78%). Four children underwent combined liver-kidney transplantation.
Immunosuppression consisted of an induction with antilymphocyte antibodies and a maintenance regimen with cyclosporine A (CsA) (since December 1984), azathioprine and prednisolone. Newer immunosuppressive agents were introduced more recently: tacrolimus in 1998, mycophenolate mofetyl in 1998, basiliximab and daclizumab in 1999.

2.2 Data source

Data were retrieved from the patients' medical files and from the archives and database of Eurotransplant. The follow-up period ended in February 2011.

2.3 Analytic variables and statistical analysis

The following variables were studied as potential factors affecting graft outcome:

- *Recipient characteristics*: age (years), gender, height (cm), weight (kg), body surface area (BSA, m^2), body mass index (BMI, kg/m^2), prior transplant, primary kidney disease, peak and current panel-reactive antibody percentage (PRA), ABO blood group, CMV serological status, number of prior blood transfusions (0-5 vs. >5), native nephrectomy, dialysis modality before transplantation, dialysis duration (years), time on the waiting list (years), hypertension (defined as the use of antihypertensive medications), year of transplantation.
- *Donor characteristics*: age, gender, height, weight, BSA, BMI, ABO group, CMV status, donor type (LRD vs. DD), cause of death for the deceased donors, serum creatinine level (mg/dl) at organ retrieval, diuresis (ml) during the last 24 hours and the last hour before organ retrieval.
- *Donor recipient relationships*: donor/recipient age ratio, height ratio, weight ratio, BSA ratio, BMI ratio, gender mismatch, human leukocyte antigen (HLA) mismatch, ABO mismatch (all grafts were ABO compatible but one), CMV mismatch (D+/R-, D-/R+, D+/R+, D-/R-).
- *Organ preservation and perioperative characteristics*: donor kidney preservation solution (Eurocollins (EC) vs. University of Wisconsin (UW) vs. histidine-tryptophan-ketoglutarate (HTK)), cold ischemia time (hours), warm ischemia time (minutes).
- *Immunosuppression*: induction therapy (polyclonal vs. monoclonal vs. none) and maintenance immunosuppression at time of discharge from the initial hospitalization including use of calcineurin inhibitors and type (CsA vs. tacrolimus), use of antimetabolites and type (azathioprine vs. mycophenolate mofetyl).
- *Post-transplant characteristics*: duration of initial transplant hospitalization (days), occurrence of delayed graft function (DGF) defined as the need for dialysis in the first week post-transplant, occurrence of acute rejection episodes, creatinine clearance (ml/min/1.73 m^2) at 1 year post-transplant (calculated using the Schwartz formula: creatinine clearance = 0.55*height (cm)/plasma creatinine (mg/dl)), hypertension (defined as the use of antihypertensive medications) and its severity as reflected by the

number of antihypertensive medications at 1 year post-transplant, proteinuria (>1 g/24 h) at 1 year post-transplant, hemoglobin (g/dl) at 1 year post-transplant.

Acute Rejection was defined as any rejection treatment. Acute rejection was suspected when the serum creatinine level increased to 20% above the baseline level and was biopsy proven in most cases.

Univariable analysis was performed on each of these variables using the Cox proportional hazards regression model. Variables with a p-value <0.10 in the univariable analysis were then entered into the multivariable analysis. Cox regression was applied with forward stepwise selection using likelihood-ratio tests. Variables were retained in the model at p<0.05. Acute rejection was considered as a time dependent covariate.

The hazard ratios (HR) for graft failure and corresponding 95% confidence intervals were estimated. Graft failure was defined as return to dialysis, re-transplantation or death with a functioning graft. Graft survival time was defined as the time between the date of transplantation and graft failure or the end of the study period.

Two models were constructed: one starting at the time of transplantation thus including all transplants (n=151) and one starting after the end of the first year post-transplant including transplants that functioned beyond the first year (n=140). Hypertension at 1 year, creatinine clearance at 1 year, proteinuria at 1 year (>1 g/24 h), hemoglobin at 1 year were included in the second model as additional potential predictors for graft survival after 1 year.

Patient and graft survivals were calculated with the Kaplan-Meier method.

Statistical analyses were performed using Statistica 8.1 (StatSoft Inc., Tulsa, OK., USA) and SPSS 18.0 (SPSS Inc., Chicago, IL., USA). Statistical significance was defined as p<0.05.

3. Results

3.1 Patient and graft survival

The actuarial patient survival was 97% at 1 year, 96% at 3 years, 94% at 5 years and 92% at 10 years (Figure 1). Nine patients died, three of them with a functioning graft. The cause of death was bacterial infection in four children, Pneumocystis carinii infection in one, malignant lymphoproliferative disorder in one, and a cardiovascular complication in three (two of whom died following cerebral haemorrhage and one following a myocardial infarction).

The overall actuarial graft survival was 94% at 1 year, 86% at 3 years, 80% at 5 years and 64% at 10 years (Figure 1). Mean follow-up time was 9.3 ± 6.5 years.

The actuarial graft survival at 1, 3, 5, 10 years was 94%, 90%, 83% and 68% respectively for recipients of living-related donor and 94%, 83%, 79% and 63% respectively for recipients of deceased donor (Log-Rank Test p=0.95). In children younger than 5 years the graft survival was 92% at 1 and 3 years, and 83% at 5 and 10 years; in this group the prevalence of LRD was rather high (11/24; 46%).

In total 68 grafts were lost during the study period, 9 of them during the first year post-transplant. The causes of graft loss are given in Table 1; chronic rejection being the leading cause. Non compliance was documented in 19% of the failure due to chronic rejection (9 cases). Recurrence of the initial disease was the second most frequent cause of graft failure.

The main characteristics of the study population are detailed in Table 2.

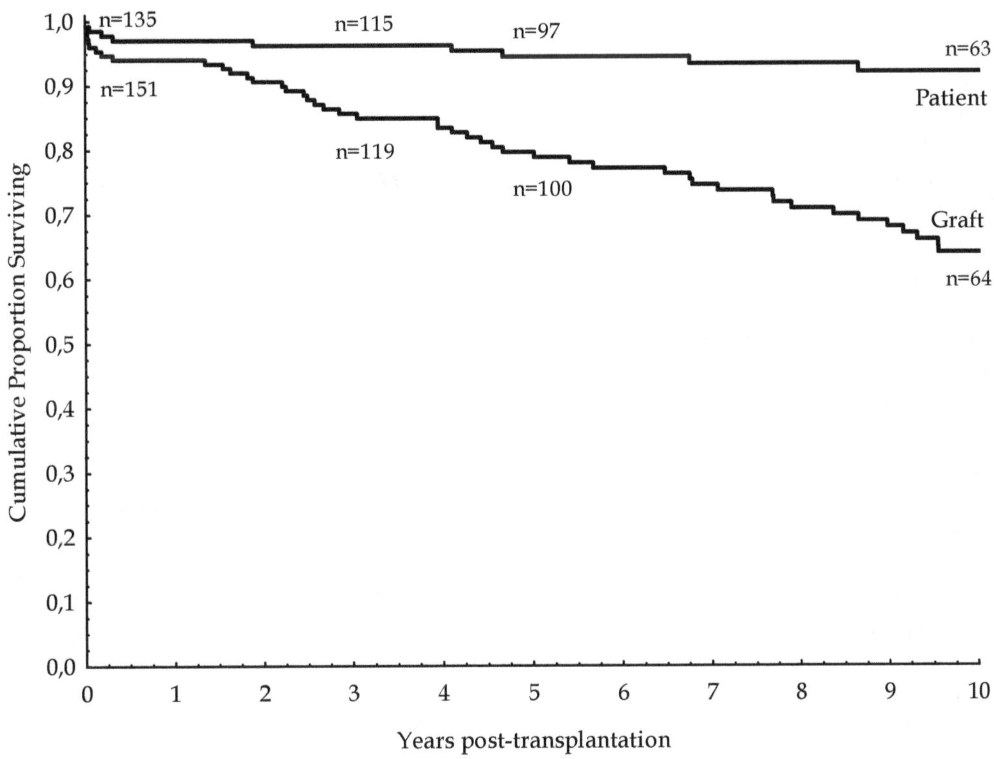

Fig. 1. Kaplan Meier plot of patient and graft survivals (n indicates the number of subjects at risk at 0, 3, 5 and 10 years).

	n	%
Chronic rejection	47	69.1
Recurrence of primary disease	8	11.8
Death with functioning graft	3	4.4
Malignancy	2	2.9
Infection	2	2.9
Technical failure	2	2.9
Primary non-function	2	2.9
Polyoma nephropathy	1	1.5
Thrombosis renal artery	1	1.5

Table 1. Causes of graft failure

	N*	Mean ± SD or n	Range or %
Recipient characteristics			
Age (year)		10.7 ± 4.7	1.3-21.9
0-4		24	15.9%
5-9		38	25.2%
≥10		56	59.0%
Gender M/F		91/60	59.6/40.4%
Weight (kg)		20.5 ± 14.5	8.4-76.4
Primary Tx/ReTx		132/19	87.4/12.6%
Primary kiney disease			
Congenital uro-nephropathy		72	47.7%
Hereditary nephropathy		40	26.5%
Acquired nephropathy		39	25.8%
Renal replacement therapy at Tx			
Hemodialysis		125	76.1%
Peritoneal dialysis		22	14.6%
Transplantation		1	0.7%
None		13	8.6%
Years of pre-transplant dialysis		1.93 ± 1.73	0-8.18
Years on waiting list	106	1.26 ± 1.12	0.04-6.25
>5 pre-transplant transfusions		62	41.1%
Current PRA>50%/Peak PRA>50%		16/33	10.6/21.9%
CMV serology: neg/pos/unknown		114/36/1	75.5/23.8/0.7%
On Antihypertensiva at time of Tx	149	81	54.4%
Donor characteristics			
Age (year)		23.8 ± 14.8	0.5-54.5
0-4		18	11.9%
5-19		48	31.8%
20-39		54	35.8%
40-55		31	20.5%
Gender M/F	150	86/64	57.3/43.7%
Weight (kg)	127	55.5 ± 23.5	7-101
Donor type			
DD/LRD		118/33	78.1/21.9%
Cause of donor death	117		
Trauma/CVA/others		71/24/22	60.7/20.5/18.8%
Donor /Recipient relationships			
Donor/Recipient Weight ratio	127	2.35 ± 1.78	0.29-8.47
Donor/Recipient BSA ratio	125	1.70 ± 0.88	0.21-4.51
Donor/Recipient BMI ratio	125	1.28 ± 0.28	0.53-2.15
CMV serology	134		
D-/R-		68	
D-/R+		23	
D+/R-		33	
D+/R+		10	

Table 2. Characteristics of the study population

	N*	Mean ± SD or n	Range or %
HLA Mismatch	150		
HLA-A		0.83 ± 0.60	
0/1/2		42/91/17	28.0/60.7/11.3%
HLA-B		1.03 ± 0.51	
0/1/2		17/111/22	11.3/74.0/14.7%
HLA-DR		0.77 ± 0.55	
0/1/2		44/97/9	29.3/64.7/6.0%
HLA-ABDR		2.62 ± 1.06	
0		7	4.7%
1		9	6.0%
2		46	30.7%
3		67	44.7%
4		15	10.0%
5		5	3.3%
6		1	0.7%
Perioperative characteristics			
Organ preservation solution	149		
Eurocollins/UW/HTK		48/64/37	32.2/43.0/24.8%
Cold ischemia time (hours) for DD	117	20.34 ± 7.70	8.40-50.47
>30 hr		10	9.3%
Warm ischemia time (min)	148	38.1 ±.11.8	15.0-95.0
>40 min		53	35.8%
Immunosuppression (IS)			
Induction	150		
Polyclonal (ALS/ATG)		92 (43/49)	61.3%
Monoclonal (anti-IL2r/OKT3)		52 (51/1)	34.7%
None		6	4%
Maintenance IS at discharge			
Cyclosporine A/Tacrolimus/No		104/31/16	68.9/20.5/10.6%
Azathioprine/MMF/No		104/45/2	68.9/29.8/1.3%
Post-transplant characteristics			
Tx hospitalization (days)		19.3 ± 12.9	7-113
Delayed graft function(DGF)		25	16.6%
Acute rejection			
Yes vs. No		69/82	45.7/54.3 %
Within the first year post Tx		58	38.4 %
Beyond the first year post Tx		23	15.7 %
Time first rejection episode (days)		46 (10-174)§	1-5474
Hemoglobin level at 1 yr (g/dl)	139	11.5 ± 1.4	6.4-14.0
Proteinuria (>1 g/24 h) at 1 yr	140	10	7.1%
Creatinine Clearance at 1 yr (ml/min/1.73 m^2)	140	72.1 ± 22.0	14.7-156.5

*N=number of transplants for whom data are available; if not specified n=151. §data given as median (interquartile range). CVA: cardiovascular accident; DD: deceased donor; DGF: delayed graft function ; LRD: Living related donor.

Table 2. Cont.

3.2 Univariable analysis of factors influencing graft outcome

Table 3 summarizes the predictors of graft outcome in univariable analysis ($p<0.10$).

Duration of pre-transplant dialysis, multiple blood transfusions pre-transplant (>5), warm ischemia time (superior to 40 min), cold ischemia time, delayed graft function (DGF) and acute rejection were found to significantly affect outcome adversely. Transplants that did not benefit from calcineurin inhibitors had a fourfold increased risk of graft failure ($p<0.0001$). In addition, over the time of our transplant program, there was a significant lower risk for graft failure with each subsequent year ($p=0.008$). As far as HLA matching is concerned, two mismatches on HLA-A tended to be detrimental ($p=0.064$).

Kidney function (creatinine clearance) at 1 year, proteinuria (>1 g/24 h) at 1 year and the level of hemoglobin at 1 year were found to be significant predictors of graft outcome for the transplants that functioned beyond the first year. Risk of graft loss increased with the presence of proteinuria and decreased with an increase in hemoglobin level and an increase in creatinine clearance.

Variables that were not retained as predictors ($p>0.10$) of graft outcome included among others: primary kidney disease, recipient and donor gender and age, recipient and donor anthropometric parameters (weight, height, BSA, BMI), age ratio and anthropometric parameters ratio between the donor and the recipient, peak and current PRA levels, recipient and donor blood group, donor type, organ preservation solution type, CMV matching status, repeat transplant, and hypertension at transplantation and at 1 year post-transplant.

	df	HR	95% CI	p Value
Time on dialysis (years)	1	1.17	1.02-1.34	0.030
>5 Transfusions pre-Tx	1	1.82	1.12-2.97	0.016
HLA-A mismatch (2 vs. 0-1)	1	1.96	0.96-3.98	0.064
Cold ischemia time (h) (DD)				
continue variable	1	1.03	1.002-1.065	0.034
>30 h vs. ≤ 30 h	1	2.63	1.31-5.26	0.006
Warm ischemia time (min)				
as continue variable	1	1.016	0.996-1.037	0.11
>40 min vs. ≤ 40 min	1	1.66	1.02-2.71	0.042
Year of transplantation	1	0.95	0.91-0.99	0.008
Absence of calcineurin inhibitors	1	4.31	2.44-7.63	<0.0001
Dialysis in the first week post-Tx (DGF)	2			0.001
Risk graft failure within first 3 months	1	16.89	3.41-83.80	0.001
Risk graft failure after first 3 months	1	1.05	0.54-2.04	0.88
Acute rejection	1	2.61	1.55-4.40	0.0003
Proteinuria (>1 g/24 h) at 1 year	1	4.13	2.01-8.48	0.0001
Hemoglobin at 1 year (g/dl)	1	0.67	0.54-0.82	0.0002
Creatinine clearance at 1 year (ml/min/1.73 m^2)	1	0.97	0.95-0.98	<0.0001

df: degrees of freedom; HR: hazard ratio; CI: confidence interval

Table 3. Predictors of graft outcome in univariable analysis ($p<0.10$)

3.3 Multivariable analysis of factors influencing graft outcome

3.3.1 Considering all transplants - graft survival from the time of transplantation

Multivariable Cox regression analysis showed that the significant factors contributing to graft failure were: absence of calcineurin inhibitors, two mismatches on HLA-A, occurrence of acute rejection and occurrence of DGF. The need for dialysis in the first week post-transplant was linked with a very high risk for graft failure within the first three months post-transplant; beyond this period it had no significant impact on graft outcome. The hazard ratios for graft failure and their confidence intervals are given in Table 4. The other factors that were found significant in univariable analysis (multiple pre-transplant transfusions, cold and warm ischemia times, year of transplantation, duration of pre-transplant dialysis) did not significantly affect outcome when subjected to a multivariable analysis.

	df	HR	95% CI	p Value
Absence of calcineurin inhibitors	1	3.98	2.15-7.36	<0.0001
2 HLA-A mismatches	1	2.77	1.31-5.84	0.008
DGF	2			0.002
Risk graft failure within first 3 months	1	3.21	2.62-66.50	0.002
Risk graft failure after first 3 months	1	1.31	0.66- 2.61	0.44
Acute rejection	1	2.10	1.25-3.52	0.005

Likelihood ratio Chi-square 46.208, df 5, p<0.0001 (n=150)

Table 4. Multivariable Cox regression analysis of graft survival from the time of transplantation: analysis of all grafts.

3.3.2 Considering transplants with ≥ 1 year survival - graft survival after 1 year

This analysis was done on the subset of transplants that were still functioning at 1 year. Nine grafts were lost in the first year. Multivariable Cox regression analysis showed that significant risk factors contributing to graft failure after 1 year were: absence of calcineurin inhibitors, two HLA-A mismatches, kidney function (creatinine clearance) at 1 year, proteinuria at 1 year (superior to 1 g/24 h) and hemoglobin level at 1 year.
The hazard ratios for graft failure and their confidence intervals are given in Table 5.

	df	HR	95% CI	p Value
Absence of calcineurin inhibitors	1	6.73	3.19-14.21	<0.0001
2 HLA-A mismatches	1	3.25	1.45-7.27	0.004
Creatinine clearance at 1 yr (ml/min/1.73 m^2)	1	0.97	0.96-0.99	0.002
Proteinuria (>1 g/24 h) at 1 yr	1	3.13	1.44-6.81	0.004
Hemoglobin level at 1 yr (g/dl)	1	0.76	0.61-0.94	0.011

Likelihood ratio Chi-square 52.383, df 5, p<0.0001 (n=139)

Table 5. Multivariable Cox regression analysis of graft survival after 1 year post-transplantation: analysis of grafts that survived beyond the first year.

4. Discussion

This single center study investigated factors that affect renal transplant outcome in children. Numerous factors concerning recipient characteristics, donor characteristics, perioperative characteristics and post-transplant events were included in the analysis.

Univariable analysis identified a number of factors associated with outcome. Multiple blood transfusions pre-transplant, duration of dialysis pre-transplant, prolonged cold and warm ischemia times, absence of calcineurin inhibitors, occurrence of acute rejection, occurrence of delayed graft function, absence of HLA-A matching, presence of marked proteinuria at 1 year post-transplant were associated with poor outcome. Risk of graft failure decreased with higher creatinine clearance at 1 year, higher level of hemoglobin at 1 year and later year of entry in the transplant program. Certainly in term of single variable determinants, these specific factors appear familiar to professionals in renal transplantation.

The following factors remained of significance after multivariable analysis: use of calcineurin inhibitors, absence of HLA-A matching, delayed graft function defined as the need for dialysis in the first week post-transplant, occurrence of acute rejection, proteinuria superior to 1 g/24 h at 1 year, hemoglobin level at 1 year and kidney function at 1 year.

Transplants that did not benefit from **calcineurin inhibitors** had a fourfold increased risk of graft failure. Most of these transplants (14 of 16) were performed in the period 1980-1984 before CsA was introduced. As the period 1980-1984 represents also the first years of our pediatric transplant program, the lack of center experience, the so called learning curve, may be partly a confounding factor. We found CsA to impact significantly and independently both on early and long term graft survival. This is similar to the findings of two single center pediatric studies (Chavers et al., 1994; Offner et al., 1999) reporting a beneficial effect of CsA up to 5 and 8 years post-transplant. The introduction of CsA in the mid-1980s for the prevention of acute rejection has been a major breakthrough in the transplantation field. However it has been reported to impact mostly on early graft survival by lowering acute rejection rates; its effect on long term outcome being much more controversial (Chapman & Nankivell, 2006; Pascual et al., 2002; Schurman & McEnery, 1997). One of the major concerns for long term outcome is the calcineurin inhibitor-induced chronic nephrotoxicity leading to progressive nephron loss and declining renal transplant function (Chapman & Nankivell, 2006; Nankivell et al., 2004). Hence with the broadening of the immunosuppressive drugs arsenal, calcineurin inhibitor minimization, calcineurin inhibitor withdrawal or avoidance strategies have been developed. Calcineurin inhibitor withdrawal and avoidance protocols have been associated with an amelioration of the renal function, however at the cost of a higher rejection rates (Guerra et al., 2007; Höcker & Tönshoff, 2011). The long-term safety and efficacy of calcineurin inhibitor withdrawal and avoidance strategies need to be further validated in controlled clinical trials. At present the safest therapeutic strategy for pediatric renal allograft with chronic calcineurin inhibitor induced nephrotoxicity appears to be a mycophenolate based regimen with low dose calcineurin inhibitor and corticosteroids (Höcker & Tönshoff, 2011).

Two **HLA-A** mismatches was in our population a strong predictive risk factor for graft failure. Matching for HLA-DR and HLA-B has generally received priority over matching for HLA-A in children as well as in adults. Multivariable analysis of the data from the large NAPRTCS registry showed that the absence of HLA-B match and the absence of HLA-DR match were significant risk factors for graft failure (NAPRTCS, 2010). Roberts and colleagues reported that matching at the HLA-DR locus has significant effect on the survival of renal grafts from DD whereas matching at the HLA-A and B loci has only small effect (Roberts et al., 2004). However, Zantvoort and colleagues from Eurotransplant (Zantvoort et al., 1996) found an independent HLA-A matching effect on long term survival of DD kidney grafts with an increasing effect over time (up to 6 years post-transplant). This was in contrast to the strong, short-lived, effects of HLA-DR and -B matching, which could only be detected up to 6 months and 2 years after transplantation, respectively. A clear additive beneficial effect of HLA-A matching was shown in the group without B and DR mismatches. They concluded that prospective matching for the HLA-A antigens remains important for renal allograft survival and our data are in agreement with this. Data from the Collaborative Transplant Study indicated that class II HLA-DR locus has a stronger impact than the class I HLA-A and HLA-B loci during the first post-transplant year but that during subsequent years the three loci have an equivalent and additive influence on graft survival: to obtain optimal long term survival all three loci must be considered in the donor-recipient matching procedure (Opelz et al., 1999). This has been our policy through the years of our program as reflected by the very low percentage of transplants with more than 3 HLA-A,-B,-DR mismatches (14%). Obtaining the best possible HLA match for children is also an important part of the Eurotransplant allocation process. In contrast, in the United States, matching for HLA-A and –B has been abandoned and only HLA-DR is considered during the kidney allocation process. Based on an retrospective analysis of the UNOS registry data from 1585 pediatric recipients of DD kidney between 1996-2004 showing no advantage for HLA-DR matching, it has been recommended that, in the modern era of immunosuppression, the HLA match should be entirely disregarded when allocating donor kidneys to pediatric recipients (Gritsch et al., 2008). This will allow shortening the waiting time on dialysis for children. This view has been challenged in a recent report by Opelz and Döhler who examined the outcomes of 9209 pediatric recipients of DD kidneys from the CTS registry (Opelz & Döhler, 2010). Comparing two decades (1988-1997 and 1998-2007), they showed that, although overall graft survival improved over time, HLA matching remained highly significant and similarly strong despite the introduction of newer and more potent immunosuppression. A hierarchical relationship was observed for the effect of increasing number of mismatches on graft survival in both periods. Interestingly, they found a strong association between two HLA-DR mismatches and non Hodgkin lymphoma, and recommended therefore to avoid transplants with 2 HLA-DR mismatches.

In our view, a well matched first kidney is especially important in children as they have a high likelihood of needing more than one transplant during their lifetime. A poor matched kidney is more likely to result in HLA allosensitization, resulting therefore in long waiting time for a second transplant when the first graft fails and compromising the chance of a successful retransplantation (Meier-Kriesche et al., 2009).

The need for dialysis in the first week after transplantation carried in our transplant population a very high risk of graft failure within the first months post-transplant but did not impact significantly on the long term outcome. Similar findings emerged out of the analysis of the NAPRTCS registry (Tejani et al., 1999). DGF was found to be a significant independent predictor of graft failure. However, when patients whose grafts had failed during the first year were censored, no differences in graft survival were noted between patients with and without DGF for either LRD or DD recipients. Similarly DGF was not an independent predictor of long term graft survival in a large single center analysis of pediatric renal recipients (Vats et al., 2002). Good long term graft survival has also been obtained with non-heart-beating donors despite a higher incidence of DGF (Koffman & Gambaro, 2003; Sanchez-Fructuoso et al., 2004; Summers et al., 2010). Others have reported a negative influence of DGF on long term graft outcome (Gjertson, 2000; Moreira et al., 2011). It remains however difficult to determine whether this negative impact of DGF is independent of two associated known risk factors for long-term outcome: acute rejection (AR) and degree of kidney function (Geddes et al., 2002; Troppmann et al., 1996). The combination of DGF and AR seems to be the most detrimental for graft survival (Matas et al., 2000; McLaren et al., 1999).

The **occurrence of acute rejection** was an independent predictor of graft survival when all transplants were included in the analysis. When only the grafts that functioned beyond the first year were considered, acute rejection disappeared from the significant factors in the multivariable analysis. The lack of significance can be due to the reduced power as acute rejection was introduced as a time dependent covariate and most of the events (acute rejection) occurred within the first year.

Acute rejection is an important predictor of chronic rejection which is the most common cause of graft loss. Single and multicenter studies in adult and children have shown an association between acute rejection and subsequent development of chronic rejection (Dart et al., 2010; Matas, 2000; Tejani & Sullivan, 2000). It is therefore expected that a reduction in the incidence of acute rejection - in our program the incidence of acute rejection in the period 2000-2010 has dropped to 7% - should result in the reduction of chronic rejection and thus in better long term graft survival. This is supported by a NAPRTCS study (Tejani et al., 2002). Moreover some studies clearly indicate that a rejection free milieu can truly provide improved long term survival. Vats et al. in one of the largest single center study to date on long term graft outcome in pediatric renal transplant patients found freedom from acute rejection in the first year post-transplant to be the strongest independent predictor of improved graft survival (Vats et al., 2002). In an analysis of the UNOS data on 93934 adult patients, Hariharan et al. reported an increase in graft half-life from 11.9 years for patients with an episode of clinical acute rejection during the first year post-transplant to 27.1 years for those who did not have such an episode (Hariharan et al., 2000). Meier-Kriesche group, on the contrary, reported that the significant reduction in the acute rejection rates observed in the modern era has resulted in a marked improvement of the short term graft survival but in negligible progress in longer term survival as the attrition rate beyond the first year show little improvements (Lamb et al., 2011; Meier-Kriesche et al., 2004).

We found **kidney function at 1 year** to be an independent predictor of long term graft survival indicating that preservation of renal function during the first year is important and that events occurring within the first year impacting on this function are of critical importance for long term survival. Several authors have reported that renal function after transplantation has a strong impact on long term graft survival. Hariharan et al. analysing factors influencing graft survival for 105742 adult renal transplants between 1988 and 1998 reported one year creatinine and delta creatinine 6 months-1 year values to be the best predictors of long term survival and that the recent improvement in graft half-lives are related to conservation of renal function within the first year post-transplant (Hariharan et al., 2002). As it is the case in our study, when renal function within the first year and clinical acute rejection were included in their model for long term graft failure it was the creatinine at 1 year that was significant and not clinical acute rejection. Thus in the setting of acute rejection it is the preservation of renal function that is more important for graft survival. Data from a multicenter study pointed the 1 year estimated glomerular filtration rate to be the most relevant predictor of long term graft function. The impact of DGF and acute rejection on the long term graft function appeared to be fully mediated by their influence on the 1 year GFR (Salvadori et al., 2006). Similar to us, three studies found allograft function at 1 year to be a significant and independent predictor of graft outcome in children (Filler et al., 2002; Mitsnefes et al., 2003; Muscheites et al., 2009). Kidney function at one year might be thus a useful surrogate end point for renal transplant clinical trials in children.

Anemia is a significant complication of renal failure being associated with numerous adverse outcomes, including compromised renal and cardiac function, cardiovascular disease, decreased exercise tolerance, cognitive impairment, poorer quality of life, increased risk for hospitalization and mortality (Koshy & Geary, 2008; Warady & Ho, 2003). Anemia is expected to resolve after transplantation. More and more data indicate on the contrary that anemia is a common phenomenon in pediatric kidney recipients with reported prevalence rates ranging from 25% to 80% depending on the definition of anemia used and the time post-transplantation (Al-Khoury et al., 2006; Mitsnefes et al., 2005; Yorgin et al., 2002). The prevalence of anemia at 1 year (defined as hemoglobin level <11 g/dl (Al-Khoury et al., 2006; Mitsnefes et al., 2005)) was 30% among our transplanted children. The pathogenesis of post-transplant anemia is multifactorial and include iron deficiency, bone marrow suppression effects of immunosuppressive medications and other therapeutic agents, chronic inflammatory conditions caused by infections, frequent blood draws, and deteriorating renal function (Al-Uzri et al., 2003). In our multivariable analysis, hemoglobin level at 1 year post-transplant was a significant predictor of long term graft outcome, a higher level of hemoglobin being associated with a lower risk of graft failure. When hemoglobin was dichotomized at 11 g/dl, the HR for anemia in the multivariable model was 1.93 (p=0.024; 95% CI 1.09-3.42) while the HRs of the other covariates (table 5) remained in the same order of magnitude (data not shown). It was significant in the presence of "kidney function" indicating that anemia is just not merely a surrogate marker of a declining function of the allograft. Anemia is an independent risk factor for progression of renal failure in pre-dialysis adults (Kovesdy et al., 2006) and treating anemia slows down the decline of kidney function in these patients (Gouva et al., 2004). Our findings are in line with several studies in the adult population showing post-transplant anemia to be associated with increased risk for subsequent graft loss (Chhabra et al., 2008; Imoagene-Oyedeji et al., 2006; Kamar & Rostaing, 2008; Molnar et al., 2007). In these studies, anemia was also associated with impaired patient survival and with a higher proportion of cardiovascular deaths. Whether this is also the case in children remains to be determined but a cross sectional study of pediatric kidney recipients pointing anemia to be predictive of left ventricular hypertrophy - an independent predictor of cardiovascular morbidity and mortality in adults - raises concern. Post-transplant anemia has also been reported to impact on the quality of life; anemic children presenting more physical discomfort (Riano-Galan et al., 2009). For all these reasons including our findings that anemia predicts poorer graft survival, anemia deserves to be recognized early after transplantation, properly investigated and corrected.

The presence of marked **proteinuria** at 1 year was in our study population a strong and independent predictor of impaired graft outcome. This is in good agreement with several studies in adults showing increasing levels of proteinuria at 1 year post-transplant to be associated with increasing risk of graft failure (Amer et al., 2007; Fernandez-Fresnedo et al., 2004; Roodnat et al., 2001). Persistent proteinuria is also associated in these studies with increased mortality. In our population, persistent proteinuria was attributed to biopsy proven chronic allograft nephropathy, recurrence of primary kidney disease (FSGS and dense deposit disease) and de novo glomerulonephritis; this is in line with reports in adult kidney recipients (Barama, 2008). The underlying cause of proteinuria and not the proteinuria per se could thus be the factor contributing to transplant dysfunction and failure. However it is now recognized that proteinuria is not only a sensitive marker of renal disease but is directly damaging to the kidney by various mechanisms including direct mesangial toxicity, tubular overload, induction of a proinflammatory state and release of substances associated with the development of fibrogenesis and glomerulosclerosis (Baines & Brunskill, 2008). Recent reports indicate that even early (1-3 months post-transplant) very low (<0.5 g/24 h) and low grade (<1 g/24 h) proteinuria - often referred as 'subclinical' or 'negligible' - is a potent predictor of graft loss in adult kidney recipients and that short term reduction in proteinuria is associated with improved long term graft survival (Halimi et al., 2005; Sancho Calabuig et al., 2009).

While ACE inhibitors have been shown to be effective and safe in proteinuric adult kidney recipients (Barama, 2008; Hiremath et al., 2007), there is a paucity of data in the pediatric transplant population. In one retrospective study, children treated with ACEI had slightly lower proteinuria than those who did not receive such treatment (Arbeiter et al., 2004). A recent uncontrolled small prospective study showed a reduction of proteinuria in nearly all children treated with ACEI (Seeman et al., 2010).

Several factors such as donor source, donor age, recipient age and hypertension were in contrast with the literature not found significant in our study.

Large registry and single centers studies show better graft survival for recipients of LRD as compared to recipient of DD kidney (Gjertson & Cecka, 2001; Magee et al., 2008; NAPRTCS, 2010). Data from the NAPRTCS indicate that the 1 year graft survival obtained with deceased donors has reached that of the living donors. In our population, graft survival is also equivalent with both donor sources at 1 year and thereafter superior for LRD. However, this difference is not statistically significant, possibly because of the small number of LRD recipients. Another explanation is that we achieved good survival rates with the DD recipients, due to our strict policy of donor selection, good HLA matching and short ischemia times.

There are a number of reports indicating poorer results with kidney from **young donors**, essentially due to an increase incidence of vascular thrombosis, primary non function and other technical causes (Cransberg et al., 2000; Postlethwaite et al., 2002; Seikaly et al., 2001). Earlier NAPRCTS reports of poor graft survival with young donors have led to a constant decrease of the use of these donors in pediatric recipients: donor younger than 10 years represented 38% of the DD for pediatric recipients in the 1988 cohort, 13% in the 2000 cohort, 8% in the 2005 cohort and less than 5% in the 2009 cohort (NAPRTCS, 2010). We have obtained good results with young deceased donors with short and long term survival comparable to older donor (Van Damme-Lombaerts et al., 2001). Data indicate also that pediatric donor organs perform better than adult donor organs in pediatric patients (Nashan, 2004; Pape et al., 2004) and it seems thus justify that pediatric donors should preferentially be allocated to pediatric recipients. This might be stimulated by a very recent analysis of the NAPRTCS registry showing comparable 3-year graft survival and comparable kidney function in recipient of young donors (Moudgil et al., 2011).

Young recipient age (<5 yr) has been traditionally associated with poorer short term graft survival due to a high incidence of vascular thrombosis, technical complications and acute rejection (Cransberg et al., 2000; Gagnadoux et al., 1993; Kari et al., 1999; Postlethwaite et al.,

2002). However, there are a few single center reports, including ours, indicating that excellent renal transplantation results can be obtained in this high risk group of patients with careful and meticulous surgical techniques, vigilant management of fluids administration, use of low molecular weight heparin in the early postoperative period and close monitoring of immunosuppression with early diagnosis and treatment of rejection (Gagnadoux et al., 1993; Ojogho et al., 2002; Vats et al., 2002). Furthermore, past the first post-transplant year, graft survival in these youngest children has been reported to be excellent: as good or even superior to older children and adults (Gjertson & Cecka, 2001; Ojogho et al., 2002; Vats et al., 2002).

In our study **hypertension** was not a significant predictor of graft failure. This may be due to the fact that we relied on the use of antihypertensive medications and their numbers as surrogates for defining hypertension and its severity. Studies using actual blood pressure measurements found early post-transplant hypertension to be a significant and independent predictor of early allograft function and long term graft outcome in pediatric renal transplant recipients (Mitsnefes et al., 2003; Mitsnefes et al., 2001).

5. Conclusion

Despite its limitation due to the small number of patients, our study shows that several factors influence the outcome of renal allograft in our pediatric population. The introduction of CsA had a very significant impact in improving graft survival. A good HLA match remains important and matching for HLA-A locus in children should not be neglected. Early recognition, investigation and treatment of post-transplant anemia and proteinuria may play an important role in ultimately improving outcomes.

Prevention and adequate management of DGF, prevention and effective treatment of acute rejection episodes, therapeutic monitoring of calcineurin inhibitors to limit their nephrotoxicity, prevention of other injuries to the allograft by factors such as severe infection, hypertension, obstruction should contribute to the preservation of the renal function during the first year and lead to improved long term outcome.

6. Acknowledgment

We are very grateful to Dr. Steffen Fieuws from the Department of Biostatistics for his help with statistical analysis.

7. References

Al-Khoury, S., Shah, N., Afzali, B., Covic, A., Taylor, J. & Goldsmith, D. (2006). Post-transplantation anaemia in adult and paediatric renal allograft recipients-Guy's Hospital experience. *Nephrol Dial Transplant*, Vol. 21, No. 7, (July 2006), pp 1974-1980, ISSN 0931-0509

Al-Uzri, A., Yorgin, P. D. & Kling, P. J. (2003). Anemia in children after transplantation: etiology and the effect of immunosuppressive therapy on erythropoiesis. *Pediatric Transplantation*, Vol. 7, No. 4, (August 2003), pp 253-264, ISSN 1397-3142

Amer, H., Fidler, M. E., Myslak, M., Morales, P., Kremers, W. K., Larson, T. S., Stegall, M. D. & Cosio, F. G. (2007). Proteinuria After Kidney Transplantation, Relationship to

Allograft Histology and Survival. *American Journal of Transplantation*, Vol. 7, No. 12, (December 2007), pp 2748-2756, ISSN 1600-6143

Arbeiter, K., Pichler, A., Stemberger, R., Mueller, T., Ruffingshofer, D., Vargha, R., Balzar, E. & Aufricht, C. (2004). ACE inhibition in the treatment of children after renal transplantation. *Pediatric Nephrology*, Vol. 19, No. 2, (February 2004), pp 222-226, ISSN 0931-041X

Baines, R. J. & Brunskill, N. J. (2008). The molecular interactions between filtered proteins and proximal tubular cells in proteinuria. *Nephron Exp Nephrol*, Vol. 110, No. 2, (November 2008), pp e67-71, ISSN 1660-2129

Barama, A. A. (2008). Mechanisms and Management of Proteinuria in Kidney Transplant Patients. *Drugs*, Vol. 68, No. Suppl.1, pp 33-39, ISSN 0012-6667

Benfield, M. R., McDonald, R., Sullivan, E. K., Stablein, D. M.& Tejani, A. (1999). The 1997 Annual Renal Transplantation in Children Report of the North American Pediatric Renal Transplant Cooperative Study (NAPRTCS). *Pediatric Transplantation*, Vol. 3, No. 2, (May 1999), pp 152-67, ISSN 1397-3142

Chapman, J. R. & Nankivell, B. J. (2006). Nephrotoxicity of ciclosporin A: short-term gain, long-term pain? *Nephrology Dialysis Transplantation*, Vol. 21, No. 8, (August 2006), pp 2060-2063, ISSN 0931-0509

Chavers, B. M., Kim, E. M., Matas, A. J., Gillingham, K. J., Najarian, J. S. & Mauer, S. M. (1994). Causes of kidney allograft loss in a large pediatric population at a single center. *Pediatric Nephrology*, Vol. 8, No. 1, (February 1994), pp 57-61, ISSN 0931-041X

Chhabra, D., Grafals, M., Skaro, A. I., Parker, M. & Gallon, L. (2008). Impact of Anemia after Renal Transplantation on Patient and Graft Survival and on Rate of Acute Rejection. *Clinical Journal of the American Society of Nephrology*, Vol. 3, No. 4, (July 2008), pp 1168-1174, ISSN 1555-9041

Cransberg, K., van Gool, J. D., Davin, JC., De Jong, M.C.J., Darby, M., Boendermaker, M. E., De Meester, J.M.J., Stijnen, T., Wolff, E. D. & Nauta, J. (2000). Pediatric renal transplantation in the Netherlands. *Pediatric Transplantation*, Vol. 4, No. 1, (February 2000), pp 72-81, ISSN 1397-3142

Dart, A. B., Schall, A., Gibson, I. W., Blydt-Hansen, T. D. & Birk, P. E. (2010). Patterns of Chronic Injury in Pediatric Renal Allografts. *Transplantation*, Vol. 89, No. 3, (February 2010), pp 334-340, ISSN 0041-1337

Fernandez-Fresnedo, G., Plaza, J. J., Sanchez-Plumed, J., Sanz-Guajardo, A., Palomar-Fontanet, R. & Arias, M. (2004). Proteinuria: a new marker of long-term graft and patient survival in kidney transplantation. *Nephrology Dialysis Transplantation*, Vol. 19, No. suppl 3, (June 2004), pp iii47-iii51, ISSN 0931-0509

Filler, G., Trompeter, R., Webb, N. J., Watson, A. R., Milford, D. V., Tyden, G., Grenda, R., Janda, J., Hughes, D., Offner, G. et al. (2002). One-year glomerular filtration rate predicts graft survival in pediatric renal recipients: a randomized trial of tacrolimus vs cyclosporine microemulsion. *Transplantation Proceedings*, Vol. 34, No. 5, (August 2002), pp 1935-1938, ISSN 0041-1345

Gagnadoux, M. F., Charbit, M., Beurton, D., Revillon, Y., Niaudet, P. & Broyer, M. (1993). Renal transplantation in children under five years of age. Experience at the Hopital des Enfants-Malades. *Annales de Pediatrie (Paris)*, Vol. 40, No. 2, (February 1993), pp 108-111, ISSN 0066-2097

Geddes, C. C., Woo, Y. M. & Jardine, A. G. (2002). The impact of delayed graft function on the long-term outcome of renal transplantation. *Journal of Nephrology*, Vol. 15, No. 1, (January-February 2002), pp 17-21, ISSN 1121-8428

Gjertson, D. W. (2000). Impact of delayed graft function and acute rejection on kidney graft survival. *Clinical Transplantation*, pp 467-480, ISSN 0902-0063

Gjertson, D. W. & Cecka, J. M. (2001). Determinants of long-term survival of pediatric kidney grafts reported to the United Network for Organ Sharing kidney transplant registry. *Pediatric Transplantation*, Vol. 5, No. 1, (February 2001), pp 5-15, ISSN 1397-3142

Gouva, C., Nikolopoulos, P., Ioannidis, J. P. & Siamopoulos, K. C. (2004). Treating anemia early in renal failure patients slows the decline of renal function: a randomized controlled trial. *Kidney International*, Vol. 66, No. 2, (August 2004), pp 753-760, ISSN 0085-2538

Gritsch, H. A., Veale, J. L., Leichtman, A. B., Guidinger, M. K., Magee, J. C., McDonald, R. A., Harmon, W. E., Delmonico, F. L., Ettenger, R. B. & Cecka, J. M. (2008). Should Pediatric Patients Wait for HLA-DR-Matched Renal Transplants? *American Journal of Transplantation*, Vol. 8, No. 10, (October 2008), pp 2056-2061, ISSN 1600-6143,

Guerra, G., Srinivas, T. R. & Meier-Kriesche, H.-U. (2007). Calcineurin inhibitor-free immunosuppression in kidney transplantation. *Transplant International*, Vol. 20, No. 10, (October 2007), pp 813-827, ISSN 0934-0874,

Halimi, J.-M., Laouad, I., Buchler, M., Al-Najjar, A., Chatelet, V., Houssaini, T. S., Nivet, H. & Lebranchu, Y. (2005). Early Low-Grade Proteinuria: Causes, Short-Term Evolution and Long-Term Consequences in Renal Transplantation. *American Journal of Transplantation*, Vol. 5, No. 9, (September 2005), pp 2281-2288, ISSN 1600-6143

Hariharan, S., Johnson, C. P., Bresnahan, B. A., Taranto, S. E., McIntosh, M. J. & Stablein, D. (2000). Improved graft survival after renal transplantation in the United States, 1988 to 1996. *New England Journal of Medicine*, Vol. 342, No. 9, (March 2000), pp 605-612, ISSN 1533-4406

Hariharan, S., McBride, M. A., Cherikh, W. S., Tolleris, C. B., Bresnahan, B. A. & Johnson, C. P. (2002). Post-transplant renal function in the first year predicts long-term kidney transplant survival. *Kidney International*, Vol. 62, No. 1, (July 2002), pp 311-318, ISSN 0085-2538

Hiremath, S., Fergusson, D., Doucette, S., Mulay, A. V. & Knoll, G. A. (2007). Renin angiotensin system blockade in kidney transplantation: a systematic review of the evidence. *American Journal of Transplantation*, Vol. 7, No. 10, (October 2007), pp 2350-2360, ISSN 1600-6135

Höcker, B. & Tönshoff, B. (2011). Calcineurin inhibitor-free immunosuppression in pediatric renal transplantation: a viable option? *Paediatr Drugs*, Vol. 13, No. 1, (February 2011), pp 49-69, ISSN 1174-5878

Hwang, A. H., Cho, Y. W., Cicciarelli, J., Mentser, M., Iwaki, Y. & Hardy, B. E. (2005). Risk Factors for Short- and Long-term Survival of Primary Cadaveric Renal Allografts in Pediatric Recipients: A UNOS Analysis. *Transplantation*, Vol. 80, No. 4, (August 2005), pp 466-470, ISSN 0041-1337

Imoagene-Oyedeji, A. E., Rosas, S. E., Doyle, A. M., Goral, S. & Bloom, R. D. (2006). Posttransplantation Anemia at 12 Months in Kidney Recipients Treated with Mycophenolate Mofetil: Risk Factors and Implications for Mortality. *Journal of the*

American Society of Nephrology, Vol. 17, No. 11, (November 2006), pp 3240-3247, ISSN 1046-6673

Kamar, N. & Rostaing, L. (2008). Negative impact of one-year anemia on long-term patient and graft survival in kidney transplant patients receiving calcineurin inhibitors and mycophenolate mofetil. *Transplantation*, Vol. 85, No. 8, (April 2008), pp 1120-1124, ISSN 0041-1337

Kari, J. A., Romagnoli, J., Duffy, P., Fernando, O. N., Rees, L. & Trompeter, R. S. (1999). Renal transplantation in children under 5 years of age. *Pediatric Nephrology*, Vol. 13, No. 9, (November 1999), pp 730-736, ISSN 0931-041X

Koffman, G. & Gambaro, G. (2003). Renal transplantation from non-heart- beating donors: a review of the European experience. *Journal of Nephrology*, Vol. 16, No. 3, (May-June 2003), pp 334-341, ISSN 1121-8428

Koshy, S. & Geary, D. (2008). Anemia in children with chronic kidney disease. *Pediatric Nephrology*, Vol. 23, No. 2, (February 2008), pp 209-219, ISSN 0931-041X

Kovesdy, C. P., Trivedi, B. K., Kalantar-Zadeh, K. & Anderson, J. E. (2006). Association of anemia with outcomes in men with moderate and severe chronic kidney disease. *Kidney International*, Vol. 69, No. 3, (February 2006), pp 560-564, ISSN 0085-2538

Lamb, K. E., Lodhi, S. & Meier-Kriesche, H. U. (2011). Long-Term Renal Allograft Survival in the United States: A Critical Reappraisal. *American Journal of Transplantation*, Vol. 11, No. 3, (March 2011), pp 450-462, ISSN 1600-6143

Magee, J. C., Krishnan, S. M., Benfield, M. R., Hsu, D. T. & Shneider, B. L. (2008). Pediatric Transplantation in the United States, 1997–2006. *American Journal of Transplantation*, Vol. 8, No. 4p2, (August 2008), pp 935-945, ISSN 1600-6143

Matas, A. J. (2000). Impact of acute rejection on development of chronic rejection in pediatric renal transplant recipients. *Pediatric Transplantation*, Vol. 4, No. 2, (May 2000), pp 92-99, ISSN 1397-3142

Matas, A. J., Gillingham, K. J., Humar, A., Dunn, D. L., Sutherland, D. E. & Najarian, J. S. (2000). Immunologic and nonimmunologic factors: different risks for cadaver and living donor transplantation. *Transplantation*, Vol. 69, No. 1, (January 2000), pp 54-58, ISSN 0041-1337

McLaren, A. J., Jassem, W., Gray, D. W., Fuggle, S. V., Welsh, K. I. & Morris, P. J. (1999). Delayed graft function: risk factors and the relative effects of early function and acute rejection on long-term survival in cadaveric renal transplantation. *Clinical Transplantation*, Vol. 13, No. 3, (June 1999), pp 266-272, ISSN 0902-0063

Meier-Kriesche, H.-U., Scornik, J. C., Susskind, B., Rehman, S. & Schold, J. D. (2009). A Lifetime Versus a Graft Life Approach Redefines the Importance of HLA Matching in Kidney Transplant Patients. *Transplantation*, Vol. 88, No. 1, (July 2009), pp 23-29, ISSN 0041-1337

Meier-Kriesche, H. U., Schold, J. D., Srinivas, T. R. & Kaplan, B. (2004). Lack of improvement in renal allograft survival despite a marked decrease in acute rejection rates over the most recent era. *American Journal of Transplantation*, Vol. 4, No. 3, (March 2004), pp 378-383, ISSN 1600-6143

Mitsnefes, M. M., Khoury, P. R. & McEnery, P. T. (2003). Early posttransplantation hypertension and poor long-term renal allograft survival in pediatric patients. The *Journal of Pediatrics*, Vol. 143, No. 1, (July 2003), pp 98-103, ISSN 0022-3476

Mitsnefes, M. M., Omoloja, A. & McEnery, P. T. (2001). Short-term pediatric renal transplant survival: blood pressure and allograft function. *Pediatric Transplantation*, Vol. 5, No. 3, (June 2001), pp 160-165, ISSN 1397-3142

Mitsnefes, M. M., Subat-Dezulovic, M., Khoury, P. R., Goebel, J. & Strife, C. F. (2005). Increasing incidence of post-kidney transplant anemia in children. *American Journal of Transplantation*, Vol. 5, No. 7, (July 2005), pp 1713-1718, ISSN 1600-6135

Molnar, M. Z., Czira, M., Ambrus, C., Szeifert, L., Szentkiralyi, A., Beko, G., Rosivall, L., Remport, A., Novak, M. & Mucsi, I. (2007). Anemia Is Associated with Mortality in Kidney-Transplanted Patients—A Prospective Cohort Study. *American Journal of Transplantation*, Vol. 7, No. 4, (April 2007), pp 818-824, ISSN 1600-6143

Moreira, P., SÃ¡, H., Figueiredo, A. & Mota, A. (2011). Delayed Renal Graft Function: Risk Factors and Impact on the Outcome of Transplantation. *Transplantation Proceedings*, Vol. 43, No. 1, (January 2011), pp 100-105, ISSN 0041-1345

Moudgil, A., Martz, K., Stablein, D. M. & Puliyanda, D. P. (2011). Good outcome of kidney transplants in recipients of young donors: a NAPRTCS data analysis. *Pediatric Transplantation*, Vol. 15, No. 2, (March 2011), pp 167-171, ISSN1397-3142

Muscheites, J., Wigger, M., Drueckler, E., Klaassen, I., John, U., Wygoda, S., Fischer, D.-C., Kundt, G., Misselwitz, J., Müller-Wiefel, D.-E. et al. (2009). Estimated one-yr glomerular filtration rate is an excellent predictor of long-term graft survival in pediatric first kidney transplants. *Pediatric Transplantation*, Vol. 13, (May 2009), pp 365-370, ISSN 1397-3142

Nankivell, B. J., Borrows, R. J., Fung, C. L.-S., O'Connell, P. J., Chapman, J. R. & Allen, R. D. M. (2004). Calcineurin Inhibitor Nephrotoxicity: Longitudinal Assessment by Protocol Histology. *Transplantation*, Vol. 78, No. 4, (August 2004), pp 557-565, ISSN 0041-1337

NAPRTCS. (2010). NAPRTCS 2010 Annual Transplant Report ,14.04.2011, Available from https://web.emmes.com/study/ped/annlrept/2010_Report.pdf.

Nashan, B. (2004). Renal allograft allocation for children: are we penalizing children to not penalize adults? *Transplantation*, Vol. 77, No. 8, (April 2004), pp 1145-1146, ISSN 0041-1337

Offner, G., Latta, K., Hoyer, P. F., Baum, H. J., Ehrich, J. H., Pichlmayr, R. & Brodehl, J. (1999). Kidney transplanted children come of age. *Kidney International*, Vol. 55, No. 4, (April 2004), pp 1509-1517, ISSN 0085-2538

Ojogho, O., Sahney, S., Cutler, D., Abdelhalim, F., Hasan, M., Baron, P. & Concepcion, W. (2002). Superior long-term results of renal transplantation in children under 5 years of age. *Am Surg*, Vol. 68, No. 12, (December 2002), pp 1115-1119, ISSN 0002-9610

Opelz, G. & Döhler, B. (2010). Pediatric Kidney Transplantation: Analysis of Donor Age, HLA Match, and Posttransplant Non-Hodgkin Lymphoma: A Collaborative Transplant Study Report. *Transplantation*, Vol. 90, No. 3, (August 2010), pp 292-297, ISSN 0041-1337

Opelz, G., Wujciak, T., Dohler, B., Scherer, S. & Mytilineos, J. (1999). HLA compatibility and organ transplant survival. Collaborative Transplant Study. *Rev Immunogenet*, Vol. 1, No. 3, pp 334-342, ISSN 1398-1714

Pape, L., Offner, G., Ehrich, J. H., de Boer, J. & Persijn, G. G. (2004). Renal allograft function in matched pediatric and adult recipient pairs of the same donor. *Transplantation*, Vol. 77, No. 8, (April 2004), pp 1191-1194, ISSN 0041-1337

Pascual, M., Theruvath, T., Kawai, T., Tolkoff-Rubin, N. &Cosimi, A. B. (2002). Strategies to Improve Long-Term Outcomes after Renal Transplantation. *New England Journal of Medicine*, Vol. 346, No. 8, (February 2002), pp 580-590, ISSN 1533-4406

Postlethwaite, R. J., Johnson, R. J., Armstrong, S., Belger, M. A., Fuggle, S. V., Martin, S., Middleton, D., Ray, T. C., Rigden, S. P., Verrier-Jones, K. et al. (2002). The outcome of pediatric cadaveric renal transplantation in the UK and Eire. *Pediatric Transplantation*, Vol. 6, No. 5, (October 2001), pp 367-77, ISSN 1397-3142

Riano-Galan, I., Malaga, S., Rajmil, L., Ariceta, G., Navarro, M., Loris, C. & Vallo, A. (2009). Quality of life of adolescents with end-stage renal disease and kidney transplant. *Pediatric Nephrology*, Vol. 24, No. 8, (August 2009), pp 1561-1568, ISSN 0931-041X

Roberts, J. P., Wolfe, R. A., Bragg-Gresham, J. L., Rush, S. H., Wynn, J. J., Distant, D. A., Ashby, V. B., Held, P. J. & Port, F. K. (2004). Effect of changing the priority for HLA matching on the rates and outcomes of kidney transplantation in minority groups. *New England Journal of Medicine*, Vol. 350, No. 6, (February 2004), pp 545-551, ISSN 1533-4406,

Roodnat, J. I., Mulder, P. G., Rischen-Vos, J., van Riemsdijk, I. C., van Gelder, T., Zietse, R., JN, I. J. &Weimar, W. (2001). Proteinuria after renal transplantation affects not only graft survival but also patient survival. *Transplantation*, Vol. 72, No. 3, (August 2001), pp 438-444, ISSN 0041-1337

Salvadori, M., Rosati, A., Bock, A., Chapman, J., Dussol, B., Fritsche, L., Kliem, V., Lebranchu, Y., Oppenheimer, F., Pohanka, E. et al. (2006). Estimated One-Year Glomerular Filtration Rate is the Best Predictor of Long-term Graft Function Following Renal Transplant. *Transplantation*, Vol. 81, No. 2, (January 2006), pp 202-206, ISSN 0041-1337

Sanchez-Fructuoso, A., Prats Sanchez, D., Marques Vidas, M., Lopez De Novales, E. & Barrientos Guzman, A. (2004). Non-heart beating donors. *Nephrol Dial Transplant*, Vol. 19, Suppl. 3, (June 2004), pp iii26-31, ISSN 0931-0509

Sancho Calabuig, A., Pallardó Mateu, L. M., Avila Bernabeu, A. I., Gavela Martínez, E., Beltrán Catalán, S. & Crespo Albiach, J. F. (2009). Very Low-Grade Proteinuria at 3 Months Posttransplantation Is an Earlier Marker of Graft Survival. *Transplantation Proceedings*, Vol. 41, No. 6, (August 2009), pp 2122-2125, ISSN 0041-1345

Schurman, S. J. & McEnery, P. T. (1997). Factors influencing short-term and long-term pediatric renal transplant survival. *J Pediatr*, Vol. 130, No. 3, (March 1997), pp 455-462, ISSN 0022-3476

Seeman, T., Dušek, J., Vondrák, K. & Janda, J. (2010). Ramipril in the treatment of proteinuria in children after renal transplantation. *Pediatric Transplantation*, Vol. 14, No. 2, (August 2009), pp 283-287, ISSN 1397-3142

Seikaly, M., Ho, P. L., Emmett, L. & Tejani, A. (2001). The 12th Annual Report of the North American Pediatric Renal Transplant Cooperative Study: renal transplantation from 1987 through 1998. *Pediatric Transplantation*, Vol. 5, No. 3, (June 2001), pp 215-231, ISSN 1397-3142

Summers, D. M., Johnson, R. J., Allen, J., Fuggle, S. V., Collett, D., Watson, C. J. & Bradley, J. A. (2010). Analysis of factors that affect outcome after transplantation of kidneys donated after cardiac death in the UK: a cohort study. *The Lancet*, Vol. 376, No. 9749, (October 2010), pp 1303-1311, ISSN 0140-6736

Tejani, A., Ho, P. L., Emmett, L. & Stablein, D. M. (2002). Reduction in acute rejections decreases chronic rejection graft failure in children: a report of the North American Pediatric Renal Transplant Cooperative Study (NAPRTCS). *American Journal of Transplantation*, Vol. 2, No. 2, (February 2002), pp 142-147, ISSN 0041-1337

Tejani, A. & Sullivan, E. K. (2000). The impact of acute rejection on chronic rejection: a report of the North American Pediatric Renal Transplant Cooperative Study. *Pediatric Transplantation*, Vol. 4, No. 2, (May 2000), pp 107-111, ISSN 0041-1337

Tejani, A. H., Sullivan, E. K., Alexander, S. R., Fine, R. N., Harmon, W. E. & Kohaut, E. C. (1999). Predictive factors for delayed graft function (DGF) and its impact on renal graft survival in children: a report of the North American Pediatric Renal Transplant Cooperative Study (NAPRTCS). *Pediatric Transplantation*, Vol. 3, No. 4, (November 1999), pp 293-300, ISSN 1397-3142

Troppmann, C., Gillingham, K. J., Gruessner, R. W., Dunn, D. L., Payne, W. D., Najarian, J. S. & Matas, A. J. (1996). Delayed graft function in the absence of rejection has no long-term impact. A study of cadaver kidney recipients with good graft function at 1 year after transplantation. *Transplantation*, Vol. 61, No. 9, (May 1996), pp 1331-1337, ISSN 0041-1337

Van Damme-Lombaerts, R., Herman, J., Coosemans, W. & Pirenne, J. (2001). Pediatric renal transplantation: a single Belgian center experience over 20 years. *Pediatric Transplantation*, Vol. 5, No. 6, (December 2001), pp 447-451, ISSN 1397-3142

Vats, A., Gillingham, K., Matas, A. & Chavers, B. (2002). Improved late graft survival and half-lives in pediatric kidney transplantation: a single center experience. *American Journal of Transplantation*, Vol. 2, No. 10, (November 2002), pp 939-945, ISSN 1600-6143

Warady, B. & Ho, M. (2003). Morbidity and mortality in children with anemia at initiation of dialysis. *Pediatric Nephrology*, Vol. 18, No. 10, (October 2003), pp 1055-1062, ISSN 0931-041X

Yorgin, P. D., Belson, A., Sanchez, J., Al Uzri, A. Y., Sarwal, M., Bloch, D. A., Oehlert, J., Salvatierra, O. & Alexander, S. R. (2002). Unexpectedly high prevalence of posttransplant anemia in pediatric and young adult renal transplant recipients. *Am J Kidney Dis*, Vol. 40, No. 6, (December 2002), pp 1306-1318, ISSN 0272-6386

Zantvoort, F. A., D'Amaro, J., Persijn, G. G., Cohen, B., Schreuder, G. M., Van Rood, J. J. & Thorogood, J. (1996). The impact of HLA-A matching on long-term survival of renal allografts. *Transplantation*, Vol. 61, No. 5, (March 1996), pp 841-844, ISSN 0041-1337

11

Sexual and Reproductive Function in Chronic Kidney Disease and Effects of Kidney Transplantation

Mahboob Lessan-Pezeshki[1] and Shirin Ghazizadeh[2]
[1]*Nephrology Research Center, Imam Khomeini Hospital,*
Tehran University of Medical Sciences,
[2]*Obstetrics and Gynecology Department,*
Tehran University of Medical Sciences,
Iran

1. Introduction

Chronic renal failure has been known to be associated with impotence and loss of libido in men and for many women, infertility and menstrual irregularities. There have been ongoing improvements in survival and quality of life after renal transplantation. These have been accompanied by an improvement in reproductive function and reversal of the relative infertility that occurs despite maintenance hemodialysis. One of the most impressive aspects of successful renal transplantation in the young person is the ability of the male patient to father a child and the female patient to give birth to a healthy baby.

Pregnancy does not appear to have any adverse effect on the long-term survival of renal allografts. Because the outcome of pregnancy in transplantation are so different than those in chronic dialysis, it is advisable to treat end-stage renal disease patients with transplantation and wait until renal function has been stable before undertaking a planned pregnancy. Women are usually advised to wait at least 1 year after living-related kidney Transplantation, and 2 years after cadaveric kidney transplantation; however, waits of 5 years or more have been associated with impaired renal function post-partum.

All women of child-bearing age should be counseled about the possibility and risks of pregnancy after kidney transplantation. Types of immunosuppressive regimens and assessment of graft function should be considered during preconception counseling. Contraceptive counseling should be provided before transplantation surgery, because ovulatory cycles may begin within 1 to 2 months after transplantation in women with grafts that are functioning well. It is strongly advised that every sexually active transplant recipient attend a family-planning counseling session, ideally before transplantation is performed. Breastfeeding is discouraged for patients taking any immunosuppressive drugs.

In this chapter we will first have a short review on reproductive physiology in male and female and irregularities caused by end stage renal disease and then we will review the experience of women undergoing child birth after transplantation, with a focus on outcomes and suggested management strategies including contraception counseling.

2. Male reproduction

2.1 Physiology of reproduction in men

The male reproductive tract consists of the testis, epididymis, vas deference, prostate, seminal vesicles, ejaculatory duct, bulbouretral glands, and urethra. The testes contain two cell types: the Sertoli cells, which line the seminiferous tubules (the site of spermatogenesis), and the Leydig cells (the site of androgen synthesis). In the male, the pituitary gland secretes luteinizing hormone (LH) and follicle-stimulating hormone (FSH), which act on the testes. LH stimulates the synthesis and secretion of testosterone by the Leydig cells, and FSH stimulates the sertoli cells to secrete inhibin. FSH and testosterone act on the seminiferous tubules to stimulate spermatogenesis. In human it takes about 75 days for spermatogonia to develop into mature sperm cells (Berek 2002).

During ejaculation, mature spermatozoa are released from the vas deferens along with fluid from the prostate, seminal vesicle, and the bulbourethral glands. The semen released is a gelatinous mixture of spermatozoa and seminal plasma; however it thins out 20 -30 minutes after ejaculation by a process called liquefaction (Berek 2002).

Both LH and FSH play roles in normal spermatogenesis. Thus, spermatogenesis does not occur spontaneously in men who have hypogonadotropic hypogonadism of prepubertal onset. Spermatogenesis can be initiated in these men by the administration of human chorionic gonadotropin (hCG), which has potent LH effects, and an FSH preparation, such as human menopausal gonadotropin (hMG) (Finkel 1985).

2.2 Male reproduction in end stage renal disease

For many male patients with renal failure, impotence and loss of libido have been seen frequently; these problems may improve but rarely normalize with the institution of maintenance dialysis, commonly resulting in a decreased quality of life (Holdsworth 1978; Diemont 2000; Rosas 2003). By comparison, a well-functioning renal transplant is much more likely to restore sexual activity; however, some features of reproductive function may remain impaired.

The uremic milieu plays an important role in the genesis of sexual dysfunction in end stage renal disease. Psychologic and physical stresses that may contribute to disturbances in sexual function are also commonly present in patients with chronic renal failure (Holdsworth 1978; Steele 1996; Toorians, Janssen et al. 1997).

2.2.1 Gonadal function

Advanced chronic kidney disease is associated with impaired spermatogenesis and testicular damage (Holdsworth 1977; Holdsworth 1978). Semen analysis typically shows a decreased volume of ejaculate, oligo- or complete azoospermia, and a low percentage of motile sperm. Testicular histology shows reduced spermatogenic activity varying from decreased numbers of mature spermatocytes to complete aplasia of germinal elements. Other findings include damage to the seminiferous tubules, atrophy of Sertoli cells, and interstitial fibrosis and calcifications.

The factors responsible for testicular damage in uremia are not well understood. It is possible that plasticizers in dialysis tubing, such as phthalate, may play a role in patients undergoing maintenance hemodialysis.

Uremia also impairs gonadal steroidogenesis. The serum total and free testosterone concentrations are typically reduced, although the binding capacity and concentration of sex hormone-binding globulin are normal (Lim 1976; Levitan 1984; de Vries 1984). Another manifestation of diminished testosterone secretory capacity is the subnormal and delayed testosterone response to the administration of human chorionic gonadotropin (HCG), a compound with luteinizing hormone-like actions (Stewart-Bentley 1974). By comparison, although the total plasma estrogen concentration is frequently elevated, the serum estradiol concentration is typically normal (Lim 1978).

2.2.2 Pituitary function

The serum concentration of luteinizing hormone (LH) is elevated in uremic men (Lim 1978); this is due to diminished testosterone feedback.

Follicle stimulating hormone (FSH) secretion is also elevated, although to a more variable degree (Holdsworth 1978; de Vries 1984). Elevated FSH levels are probably the result of decreased testosterone and inhibin, a Sertoli cell product. The plasma FSH concentration tends to be highest in those uremic patients with the most severe damage to seminiferous tubules and presumably the lowest levels of inhibin. It has been suggested that increased FSH levels may portend a poor prognosis for recovery of spermatogenic function after renal transplantation. The gonadotropin reserve is generally intact, since the plasma level of both gonadotropins increased appropriately following administration of gonadotropin-releasing hormone (GnRH) (LeRoith 1980). The appropriate increase in FSH and LH in response to the administration of clomiphene (a nonsteroidal antiestrogen that stimulates gonadotropin secretion by blockade of estrogen mediated negative feedback on the hypothalamus) (Lim 1978), also indicates a normal gonadotropin reserve.

2.2.3 Hyperprolactinemia

The basal levels of serum prolactin are elevated in the majority of uremic patients, and the response to thyrotropin-releasing hormone (TRH) is reduced and delayed (Hagen C 1976). The mechanisms for the hyperprolactinemia in chronic renal failure are not well defined. Increased autonomous production rate of prolactin is a major mechanism for the hyperprolactinemia but decreased metabolic clearance rate may also play a role (Cowden 1981). The demonstration of resistance to stimulation or suppression of prolactin in CRF is consistent with increased autonomous production (Pece 1979). The state of secondary hyperparathyroidism of CRF may contribute to the increased production rate of prolactin, because PTH stimulates prolactin secretion (Issac 1978). The treatment of CRF patients with erythropoietin was associated with a decreased in serum prolactin levels and improvement in sexual dysfunction (Schaefer, Stanhope et al. 1989), but did not normalize rate of the response to TRH (Ramirez 1976). These observations suggest that either anemia and/or deficiency of erythropoietin per se participate in the genesis of the hyperprolactinemia of CRF.

2.2.4 Gynecomastia

Variable degrees of gynecomastia are often encountered in the male uremic patient treated with maintenance hemodialysis (Lim 1978). Gynecomastia usually develops during initial months of dialysis and regresses as dialysis continues. It may be transient or may last for periods of several months. The etiology may be related to the improvement in the nutritional status of uremic patient with dialysis theray and, as such, is similar to the mechanism of refeeding gynecomastia. It must be emphasized that in almost all cases of

Gynecomastia, there is an alteration either in the ratio between the serum level of androgen and estrogen, in favor of the latter, or in the ratio between the action of androgen and estrogen at the tissue level (Sawin 1973). Indeed, in patients with advanced CRF and those treated with hemodialysis, the ratio between the serum levels of free testosterone and estradiol is reduced because of a decreased in testosterone levels.

2.3 Erectile dysfunction in end stage renal disease:

Erectile dysfunction is defined as the inability to achieve and maintain an erection sufficient to permit satisfactory sexual intercourse. It may result from psychologic, neurologic, hormonal, arterial or cavernosal impairment or from a combination of these factors. Most of the studies in sexual dysfunctions in CRF patients have focused on impotence. Erectile dysfunction is common in patients with CRF and is observed in excess of 50% of these patients (Procci 1981). These data are based on results obtained from interviews with or by the completion of questionnaires by the patients and/or their spouses. Several factors appear to participate in the genesis of impotence in CRF patients. These include abnormalities in the neurohormonal control system of erection hormones of the hypothalamic-pituitary-gonadal axis , secondary hyperparathyroidism and, dysfunction of the corporal smooth muscle of the penis or in their response to relaxing stimuli and/or derangements in the arterial supply or the venous drainage of the penis (Schrier RW 2001). Patients with a history of abnormal erectile function prior to the onset of renal disease may have a secondary cause, such as a neuropathy or peripheral vascular disease.

The presence of a neurogenic bladder suggests an underlying neuropathy, while findings of peripheral vascular disease point toward inadequate penile blood flow. The lack of secondary sexual characteristics combined with small soft testicles suggests hypogonadism. The ingestion of a number of medications, such as beta blockers and tricyclic antidepressants, may be a cause of erectile dysfunction.

Among those without an obvious cause of impotence after an initial evaluation, consideration should be given to a psychologic difficulty, such as stress or depression. The values of Nocturnal Penile Tumescence (NPT) among a large population of uremic patients are significantly lower than normal. The administration of a nocturnal penile tumescence test may help distinguish between an organic and a psychologic disorder; the absence of an erection during sleep suggests underlying organic dysfunction. A positive test, however, does not exclude a physical cause.

2.3.1 Management

The first step in the treatment of uremic men with sexual dysfunction is increasing the delivered dose of dialysis, discontinuing medications with side effects of impotence and correcting the anemia of chronic renal disease. As an example, the administration of recombinant human erythropoietin to raise the hematocrit to 33 to 36 percent may enhance sexual function (Delano 1989).

Sildenafil has been effectively used in the treatment of erectile dysfunction in both hemodialysis and peritoneal dialysis patients and is often used for psychologic, vascular, or neurogenic causes (Ifudu 1998; Palmer 1999; Turk 2001; Seibel 2002; Rosas 2003; Grossman 2004). Concurrent use of sildenafil and nitrates in any form, regularly or intermittently, is contraindicated.

Since the elevation of serum levels of prolactin plays a role in the impotence of male uremic patient, correction of hyperprolactinemia by bromocriptin is also associated with improvement of sexual dysfunction.

Cabergoline, which causes nausea much less often than does bromocriptine and is at least as effective in treating hyperprolactinemia, should be tried first (Biller BM; Molitch ME; Vance ML; Cannistraro KB; Davis KR; Simons JA; Schoenfelder JR; Klibanski A 1996). The administration of testosterone to uremic men usually fails to restore libido or potency, despite normalized serum testosterone.

A vacuum tumescence device may be effective in restoring potency in uremic impotent males unresponsive to medical therapy. Administration of zinc is also a reasonable therapeutic option in uremic men.

2.4 Renal transplantation

Kidney transplantation is the best and most effective option that can be offered to patients with severe renal damage to restore their health and the possibility of recovering their sexual and reproductive functions.

After successful transplantation, about two thirds of male patients observe improved libido and a return of sexual function to predialysis levels. Fertility as assessed by sperm counts, improves in half patients. The sex hormone profile tends to normalize; plasma testosterone and follicle stimulating hormone levels increase; and luteinizing hormone levels which may be high in dialysis patients, decrease to normal or low levels (Danovitch GM 2005).

The factors that might cause certain difficulties for the recovery of sexual and reproductive functions in this type of patients include prolonged use of peritoneal dialysis, high follicle stimulating hormone (FSH) serum levels before the transplant, and a deficient function of the graft (De Celis and Pedron-Nuevo 1999).

A certain improvement has been reported as to semen quality in the three main parameters (number, morphology, and motility of the spermatozoa) in patients after kidney transplantation (De Celis and Pedron-Nuevo 1999).

Several studies conducted to evaluate the effects of immunosuppressive regimens suggest that some of these agents are potentially gonadotoxic since they affect testicular function and decrease fertility. This is mainly due to an indirect effect on the hypothalamus-pituitary-gonadal axis, or directly suppressant on the germinal epithelium of the testis, where the spermatogenetic process is primarily affected because of an interruption of the cycle needed for the development of an adequate amount of normal spermatozoa.

This would result in oligo/asthenozoospermia, teratozoospermia, or azoospermia. Cyclosporine (CSA) is an important therapeutic agent and a common component in multiple immunosuppressive regimens used in recipients of kidney transplants and for a growing number of autoimmune disorders. Some studies imply that CSA is a potentially gonadotoxic drug, producing adverse effects on the reproductive capability in experimental models as well as in humans. In certain animal species, such as the Sprague-Dawley strain rats, Seethalakshmi et al. showed that the administration of CSA induces a deficient intratesticular synthesis of androgens and a reduction in spermatogenesis, although this reduction was reversible after exogenous gonadotrophins were administered (Seethalakshmi 1990). On the other hand, it has also been possible to observe the adverse effect of CSA by means of testicular biopsies performed in dogs (Seethalakshmi 1988) and rats (Seethalakshmi 1990) treated with CSA for short periods, where marked abnormalities in spermatogenesis were seen. Cyclosporine (CSA) may impair testosterone biosynthesis through direct damage to leydig cells and germinal cells, an indirect impairment of the hypothalamic-pituitary-gonadal axis has also been suggested.

Computer-aided sperm analysis (CASA) in infertile renal transplant recipients showed that both sperm concentration and straight line velocity (VSL) were inversely correlated to the cyclosporine whole blood trough levels. Stabilization of the cyclosporine whole blood trough level within the target therapeutic level could improve the fertility potential in kidney transplant recipients. Duration of hemodialysis before transplantation is also important in this regard. The time spent on hemodialysis is inversely correlated with the percentage of motile spermatozoa and the amplitude of lateral head displacement (ALH) (Eid, Abdel-Hamid et al. 1996).

Azathioprine (AZA), another drug that is frequently combined with CSA, is considered to be genotoxic (Olshan 1994). However, very few studies have analyzed the effects of AZA on the reproductive function of humans. Several studies suggest that prednisone might not be involved in sperm cell damage.

Kaczmarek and coworkers found that heart transplant recipients treated with sirolimus had significantly lower free testosterone levels and significant higher levels of gonadotropic hormones luteinizing hormone and follicle-stimulating hormone compared with calcineurin inhibitor-based immunosuppression group (Kaczmarek 2004). Patients treated with sirolimus throughout the post-transplant period have a significantly reduced total sperm count compared to patients who did not receive sirolimus and a decreased proportion of motile spermatozoa. Moreover, the fathered pregnancy rate was lower in patients receiving sirolimus-based regimens (Zuber, Anglicheau et al. 2008).

There is also concern about infertility associated with Ganciclovir which is used for treatment of cytomegalovirus (CMV) infection in transplant patients (Nevins and Dunn 1992). There is no increased incidence of neonatal malformations in pregnancies fathered by transplant recipients (Danovitch GM 2005).

2.4.1 Sexual functions in renal transplant patients

Renal transplant recipients have all suffered from uremia. They have frequently spent a significant amount of time on dialysis and often have other comorbidities including hypertension and diabetes. Although a successful transplant may improve erectile function and return of libido, in many cases some degree of sexual dysfunction may persist. On the contrary a recent study showed that, erectile function worsens after RT in patients<45 yr (Mirone, Longo et al. 2009).

Hypertension is common among transplant patients; CSA can exacerbate preexisting high blood pressure and also induce hypertension in patients, who had normal blood pressure prior to the kidney transplant.

Antihypertensive medications have negative effects on male sexual functions, such as libido and erection (Matthew RW 2005). Those medications which are implicated in erectile dysfunction include beta blockers (propranolol, labetalol), Alpha blockers (prazosin), sympatholytics (clonidine), vasodilators (hydralazine), and diuretics (thiazides, spironolactone).

Other drugs which may also play a role in erectile dysfunction in transplant patients are: HMG- CoA reductase inhibitors (lovastatin, simvastatin), antidepressant (serotonin reuptake inhibitors, tricyclics, monoamine oxidase inhibitors) and H2 antagonists (cimetidine, ranitidine, famotidine).

Ketoconazole which is used in some transplant centers in order to increase cyclosporine level and reducing the cost of calcineurin inhibitors can cause erectile dysfunction because of its antiandrogenic action.

Additional factors such as smoking and alcohol intake may account for failure of male sexual function to improve after transplantation.

Cigarette smoking may induce vasoconstriction and penile venous leakage because of its contractile effect on the cavernous smooth muscle (Juenemann 1987). Alcohol in small amounts improves erection and increases libido because of its vasodilatory effect and the suppression of anxiety; however, large amounts can cause central sedation, decreased libido, and transient erectile dysfunction. Chronic alcoholism may cause hypogonadism and polyneuropathy, which may affect penile nerve function (Miller 1988).

Autonomic neuropathy may impair erectile function, and interruption of both hypogastric arteries may occasionally impair vascular supply.

2.4.2 Management of erectile dysfunction in transplant patients

Male patients should be asked about their sexual function and referred for urologic evaluation when necessary. Historically, androgens were touted as enhancing male sexual function. Today, more effective treatments are available, and testosterone therapy should be discouraged in men in whom erectile dysfunction is not associated with hypogonadism (Lue T F 2000). Sildenafil is a selective inhibitor of phosphodiesterase type 5, which inactivates cyclic GMP. Since its release in March 1998, it has become the drug of choice for most men with erectile dysfunction. When sexual stimulation releases nitric oxide into the penile smooth muscle, inhibition of phosphodiesterase type 5 by sildenafil causes a marked elevation of cyclic GMP concentrations in the glans penis, corpus cavernosum, and corpus spongiosum, resulting in increased smooth-muscle relaxation and better erection. Sildenafil has no effect on the penis in the absence of sexual stimulation, when the concentrations of nitric oxide and cyclic GMP are low (Lue T F 2000). Sildenafil has little effect on libido. Among more than 3700 men with 1631 patient years of exposure to sildenafil, most adverse events were mild to moderate and self-limited in duration (Esteban de la Rosa, Bravo Soto et al. 2003). Among men taking 25 to 100 mg of sildenafil, 16 percent reported headache, 10 percent flushing, 7 percent dyspepsia, 4 percent nasal congestion, and 3 percent abnormal vision (described as a mild and transient color tinge or increased sensitivity to light). These rates were twice as high among men taking 100 mg of sildenafil as among men who were taking lower doses. The visual effect is probably related to inhibition of phosphodiesterase type 6 in the retina. No chronic visual impairment has been reported, and the incidence of visual side effects was similar in diabetic and nondiabetic men (Price 1998). Nevertheless, because of the short duration of the clinical trials and the difficulty in detecting subtle retinal changes, the long-term safety of sildenafil treatment is still unknown. In men with retinal diseases, an ophthalmologic consultation may be warranted before sildenafil treatment is initiated. Adverse cardiovascular events (nasal congestion, headache, and flushing) were mild and transient in the majority of men. The rate of serious cardiovascular events (angina and coronary-artery disorder) is low. Sexual activity was thought to be a likely contributor to myocardial infarction in only 0.9 percent of 858 men in one study (Muller, Munder et al. 2009). Thus, the absolute increase in risk caused by sexual activity is low (one chance in a million for a healthy man). According to data from the National Center for Health Statistics and the Framingham Heart Study, the rate of death from myocardial infarction or stroke for men in the age range in which erectile dysfunction is common is approximately 170 per million men per week. Therefore, it appears that sildenafil therapy is safe for most men. Nevertheless, given that most of the men who died had underlying cardiovascular disease; cardiovascular status should be carefully assessed before treatment. The combination of nitrates and sildenafil has resulted in severe hypotension and 16 deaths in the United States. Therefore, nitrate therapy is an absolute contraindication to sildenafil therapy (Lue T F 2000).

Sildenafil is absorbed well during fasting, and the plasma concentrations are maximal within 30 to 120 minutes (mean, 60). It is eliminated predominantly by hepatic metabolism, and the terminal half-life is about four hours. The recommended starting dose is 50 mg taken one hour before sexual activity. The maximal recommended frequency is once per day. On the basis of effectiveness and side effects, the dose may be increased to 100 mg or decreased to 25 mg (Lue T F 2000). There is no specific contraindication to use of sildenafil (Viagra) in transplant patients so long as standard precautions are taken regarding concomitant coronary artery disease.

Oral vardenafil (Phosphodiesterase-5 Enzyme Inhibitor) therapy has a high efficacy and a low incidence of adverse events for kidney transplant recipients with ED (Yang, Ju et al. 2008). Vardenafil enhances the effect of NO by inhibiting phosphodiesterase type 5 (PDE-5), which is responsible for degradation of cGMP in the corpus cavernosum; when sexual stimulation causes local release of NO, inhibition of PDE-5 by vardenafil causes increased levels of cGMP in the corpus cavernosum, resulting in smooth muscle relaxation and inflow of blood to the corpus cavernosum. so it can prolong erectile duration of ED patients (Wang and Huang 2009); at recommended doses, it has no effect in the absence of sexual stimulation.

Transurethral administration of alprostadil (synthetic form of prostaglandin E_1) or intracavernous injection resulting in an erection sufficient for intercourse has been used successfully. The most effective intracavernous therapy used is a three-drug mixture containing papaverine, phentolamine, and alprostadil (trimix). The usual dose of trimix solution ranges from 0.1 to 0.5 ml. The rate of response to this solution is as high as 90 percent (Bennett 1991). In case of drug treatment failure, penile prosthesis can be considered even in transplanted patients (Lasaponara, Pasquale et al. 2009; Phe, Roupret et al. 2009).

3. Female reproduction

3.1 Menstrual cycle

The menstrual cycle is a hormonally controlled process of events occurring through the hypothalamic-pituitary-ovarian axis and reflected by the histological changes in the endometrium.

The normal menstrual cycle is a tightly coordinated cycle of stimulatory and inhibitory effects that results in the release of a single mature oocyte from a pool of hundreds of thousands of primordial oocytes.

The menstrual cycle lasts 25 to 30 days in most women. It is divided into two successive phases: the follicular phase and the luteal phase. By convention, the day of menstruation is designated as day 1 of the menstrual cycle. The luteal phase is remarkably constant in length and lasts 13 to 15 days, but length of the follicular phase is variable. The average duration of flow is 4 to 6 days but can be as few as 2 days and as many as 7 days. A flow of longer than 7 days deserves evaluation (Higham 1990).The average blood loss during one menses is about 30 mL. A flow of 80 mL or more can lead to anemia and should be evaluated (Cohen and Galbraith 2001). However, it is not necessary to measure menstrual flow; a patient's perception of abnormal menses deserves evaluation and treatment.

By definition menorrhagia is excessive and prolonged uterine bleeding at regular intervals; metrorrhagia is irregular, intermenstrual bleeding. Menometrorrhagia is heavy, prolonged, irregular bleeding at frequent, irregular intervals. Polymenorrhea is frequent, regular episodes of uterine bleeding at intervals of less than 21 days. Oligomenorrhea is irregular bleeding occurring at prolonged intervals of more than 35 days. Amenorrhea is absence of uterine bleeding (Sciarra J 2001).

There is relatively little cycle variability among women between the ages of 20 and 40 years. In comparison, there is significantly more cycle variability for the first 5 to 7 years after menarche and for the last 10 years before cessation of menses (Treloar 1967).

3.2 Menstrual cycle irregularities in end stage renal disease

Menstrual problem is common among women with renal insufficiency. It is partly because of abnormal bleeding time due to platelet dysfunction and also because of failure to ovulate or sustain adequate corpus luteum function.

Amenorrhea is common by the time the patient reaches end-stage renal disease. The menstrual cycle typically remains irregular with scanty flow after the initiation of maintenance dialysis, although normal menses are restored in some women(Holley 1997) In others, menorrhagia develops, sometimes leading to significant blood loss and increased transfusion requirements.

Oligo/ anovulation is the major factor for these menstrual cycle abnormalities in uremic women. Uremia is associated with hypothalamic-pituitary-gonadal dysfunction.

Leptin is one of the responsible factors involving in this cycle abnormality. In general, serum leptin levels are significantly elevated in patients with renal failure, particularly when compared to age and body mass index (BMI)-matched controls (Wolf 2002). Leptin appears to be one of several factors that influence the maturation of the gonadotropin-releasing hormone (GnRH) pulse generator.

Hyperprolactinemia is common in women with chronic renal failure due to increased secretion and decreased metabolic clearance of this hormone (Sievertsen 1980). The elevated prolactin levels may impair hypothalamic-pituitary function and contribute to sexual dysfunction and galactorrhea in these patients. Although kidney transplantation greatly improves menstrual pattern, but irregular bleeding is still a major problem among women with a transplanted kidney. In a study on 114 women with a transplanted kidney we found normal menstruation in 49%, oligo/ hypomenorrhea or amenorrhea in 31.3% and hypermenorrhea in 19.8% (Lessan-Pezeshki, Ghazizadeh et al. 2004).

In order to reduce the chance of endometrial hyperplasia that results from chronic stimulation of the endometrium with estradiol, medroxyprogesterone acetate (Provera), 10 mg/day orally for 5 days is prescribed. Patients with adequate endogenous estrogens will bleed within 3 to 5 days after medication, indicating adequate endogenous estrogen stimulation of the endometrium. Patients with relatively low levels of endogenous estrogens may have a limited response to the progesterone challenge.

3.3 Sexual dysfunction in uremic women

Sexual desire or drive is defined as the frequency or intensity with which a person desires to participate in sexual activity. Both organic and psychological variables contribute to this interest. Hormones can act on sexual behavior indirectly by influencing general mood. They can influence sexual interest levels by their peripheral action, such as by increasing genital vasocongestion and sexual sensation or by enhancing the sexual attractiveness of the female by means of smell. Women receiving chronic dialysis tend to experience decreased libido and reduced ability to reach orgasm.

Uremic patient's sexual difficulties are often worsened by hemodialysis, with a lowered frequency of intercourse, reduced sexual desire, and an increased incidence of sexual failure (Thurm JA 1976). Initial treatment goals for uremic women with sexual dysfunction include increasing the adequacy of dialysis, and correcting the anemia of chronic renal failure.

Amenorrheic dialysis patients may have low estradiol levels; this may lead to vaginal atrophy and dryness, thereby resulting in discomfort during intercourse. Such patients may benefit from local estrogen therapy or vaginal lubricants. Successful transplantation is clearly the most effective means to restore normal sexual desire in women with chronic renal failure (Diemont 2000). Sexual desire increases significantly after successful transplantation in most patients, however improvement in frequency of sexual activity and overall sexual satisfaction is not as high as sexual desire.

Low dose testosterone may be effective but, due to potential toxicity, is rarely used. The administration of bromocriptine may help restore sexual function in those with hyperprolactinemia.

3.4 Pregnancy in end stage renal disease

Fertility is reduced in the presence of end-stage renal disease. Conception is rare for women on dialysis, and occurs at a rate of one in every 200 patients (Rizzoni, Ehrich et al. 1992). Pregnancy is often diagnosed late because of menstrual irregularities; thus, early spontaneous abortion may be overlooked. The diagnosis of pregnancy may be difficult in women with end-stage renal disease; particularly because serum levels of beta-human chorionic gonadotropin (beta-hCG) may be increased in the absence of pregnancy. The main risks for a fetus include death, prematurity, and growth retardation. A review by Hou of 37 pregnancies associated with chronic renal dialysis found that 75% to 80% resulted in spontaneous abortion, stillbirth, or neonatal death. (Hou S 1987) Placental abnormalities included abruption, infarction, and microscopic areas of necrosis. No developmental abnormalities were reported, and the incidence of congenital abnormalities appeared to be no greater than for normal pregnancies.

Hypertension is a major problem and may prove very difficult to control. Forty-nine percent of the patients reviewed by Hou became hypertensive during pregnancy. The infants of hepatitis carriers should receive hepatitis B immune globulin and vaccine in the first 72 hours to avoid becoming carriers.

Since 1976, chronic ambulatory peritoneal dialysis (CAPD) has been increasingly used to manage end-stage renal failure. It has several theoretical advantages over hemodialysis for the management of pregnant patients (Mahanty, Cherikh et al. 2001). A more constant intrauterine environment without rapid shifts in fluid, solutes, and electrolytes may benefit a fetus, Redrow compared eight pregnancies managed with peritoneal dialysis with seven managed with hemodialysis (Redrow 1988). Hypotensive episodes appear to be less frequent, hematocrits higher, and control of insulin and glucose levels more exact in the group on peritoneal dialysis. Further experience is needed to determine if this is the preferred mode of dialysis in pregnancy. If peritoneal dialysis is used, the exchange volumes should be decreased (eg, to 1.5 liters) and the frequency should be increased (Jungers and Chauveau 1997).

3.4.1 Management

An increased dose of dialysis appears to be beneficial, with reports of Kt/V values of 6 to 8, on hemodialysis 5-6 days per week (Henrich WL 2004), with the BUN being maintained at under 50 mg/dL or even under 45 mg/dL. Ameliorating the uremic milieu can avoid polyhydramnios, help control hypertension, and improve maternal nutrition. Increased doses of erythropoietin are required to maintain hemoglobin levels in an acceptable range (10 to 11 g/dl) and transfusions are sometimes required (Chao 2002). Protein intake should be 1 g/kg per day plus an additional 20 g/day for fetal growth. Diet should be supplemented with water soluble vitamins and zinc. Metabolic acidosis and hypocalcemia should be corrected. Careful uterine and fetal monitoring during hemodialysis, such as assessment of the fetal heart rate (particularly during the last portion of a session), combined with measures aimed at preventing dialysis-induced hypotension should be performed. In many cases, patients are hospitalized around week 20 of gestation for management of blood pressure, dialysis fluid balance, nutrition and anemia.

If peritoneal dialysis is used, the exchange volumes should be decreased (eg, to 1.5 liters) and the frequency should be increased.

3.5 Pregnancy in renal transplantation

Fertility is usually restored in women with renal transplants and pregnancy is common, occurring in 12% of women at childbearing age in one series (Sturgiss and Davison 1995). Pregnancy success rate exceeds 90% after the first trimester. The recovery of fertility is less common in women who undergo transplantation close to the end of their childbearing years (Hou S 1987). The first reported successful pregnancy occurred in a recipient of a kidney transplant from an identical twin sister performed in 1958 (Murray 1963). Since then, there have been hundreds of successful pregnancies reported in renal transplant recipients (Davison JM 1987). During the last decade there has been a steady increase in the number of pregnancies following renal transplantation (Sgro, Barozzino et al. 2002).

Pregnancy in transplant recipients provides an opportunity to investigate biological processes that may have an impact on graft outcome as well as pregnancy outcome. For example, immunologic adjustments are believed to be involved in implantation as well as a successful acceptance of the allogenic fetus by their mother (Matthew RW 2005).

3.5.1 Effect of pregnancy on graft function

Although pregnancy can cause an increase in the glomerular filtration rate, which could theoretically lead to hyperfiltration and resultant glomerulosclerosis, the hyperfiltration of pregnancy is flow related, with no concomitant increase in intraglomerular pressure (Denton and Baylis 2007).

In cyclosporine treated patients, graft dysfunction after pregnancy was seen in patients with higher mean serum creatinine levels and lower mean cyclosporine doses prior to conception (ArmentiVT, Radomski JS et al. 2000). Overall, in the majority of recipients studied, pregnancy does not appear to cause excessive or irreversible problems with graft function if the function of transplant organ is stable prior to pregnancy (Armenti, Constantinescu et al. 2008).

The long-term effect of pregnancy on renal function is less clear. Two small studies in which matched nonpregnant controls were used found conflicting results: no deleterious effect in one with 15 year follow-up; and an increase in the plasma creatinine concentration of 0.5 to

0.7 mg/dL at 3 to 12 months in the other (Salmela, Kyllonen et al. 1993; Sturgiss and Davison 1995). The latter report also suggested that a second pregnancy might carry a greater risk, as renal function deteriorated in three of seven women (Salmela, Kyllonen et al. 1993).

The incidence of acute rejection is not greater than expected for non-pregnant transplant patients. The incidence of acute rejection during pregnancy and three months after delivery varies between 9 and 14.5% in the published series. Rejection is sometimes difficult to diagnose and an ultrasound-guided biopsy may be helpful to diagnose acute pyelonephritis, recurrent glomerulonephritis, and severe pre-eclampsia. Renal biopsy should be performed before starting anti-rejection therapy, and high steroid doses are the first line of treatment. It has been suggested that acute rejection during the puerperium may be due to a return to a normal immune status or to a rebound effect from the altered gestational immune responsiveness. Therefore, immunosuppression should be re-adjusted immediately after delivery.

3.6 Immunosuppressive drugs in pregnancy

Immunosuppression in pregnancy is a concern from the perspective of both maternal and fetal safety issues. Blood volume and volume of distribution increase during pregnancy thus blood levels of immunosuppressive drugs are often lower, though there is no evidence that effective immunosuppression is inadequate if prepregnancy doses are used. We currently have limited information regarding the toxicities and teratogenic potentials of these agents, although our knowledge has recently increased as more women maintained on immunosuppressive therapy for solid organ transplants have opted to become pregnant.

3.6.1 Glucocorticoids

The most commonly used glucocorticoids are the short acting agents; prednisone, prednisolone and methyl prednisolone. Radiolabaled prednisone and prednisolone can cross the placenta, but maternal / cord blood ratios are approximately 10:1 (Beitins 1972). In utero exposure to high-dose steroid and immunosuppressive agents does not seem to be associated with an increased incidence of congenital anomalies in the offspring of pregnant women with a renal transplant. Adrenal insufficiency and thymic hypoplasia have occasionally been described in the infants of transplant recipients, but these problems are unlikely if the dose of prednisone has been decreased to 15 mg . Cases of cleft palate, mental retardation, have also been described in humans after in utero corticosteroid exposure. Glucocorticoid therapy during pregnancy can result in premature rupture of the membranes (PROM) and intrauterine growth restriction. The increased risk of PROM with prednisone therapy likely reflects the inhibitory effects of glucocorticoids on fetal membrane extracellular matrix synthesis. Alternatively, PROM may be the result of prednisone's stimulatory effects on fetal membrane, placental, and decidual corticotropin releasing hormone. Furthermore, pregnancy-induced hypertension, gestational diabetes, and osteoporosis can be exacerbated.

Doses of prednisone greater than 20 mg/d have been associated with serious maternal infection, however treatment of rejection with steroids, if necessary, should not be avoided during pregnancy (Lessan-Pezeshki M 2002).

Current data suggest that steroids and immunosuppressive agents in the doses used to prevent graft rejection in transplant recipients are well tolerated by the fetus. Long-term

studies are required to determine whether there may be other effects, particularly an increase in the incidence of malignancies or abnormalities in the subsequent generation.
FDA rates the risk of prednisone use in pregnancy as C which implies that "Risks can not be ruled out".

3.6.2 Azathioprine

Azathioprine is an antimetabolite, an imidazole derivative of 6- mercaptopurine . It is commonly used during pregnancy in transplant recipients. Radioactive labeling studies in humans have shown that 64 - 93 percent of azathioprine administered to mothers appears in fetal blood as inactive metabolites (Sarikoski 1973). Azathioprine can cause transient gaps or breaks in lymphocyte chromosomes. Germ cells and other tissues have not been studied. In the adult, azathioprine is metabolized to 6- mercaptopurine. The immature fetal liver lacks the enzyme inosinate pyrophosphorylase, needed for conversion, and the fetus is relatively protected from the effects of the drug (Lessan-Pezeshki M 2002). The desired drug dose of azathioprin is 2 mg/kg/day or less. In high doses (6 mg/kg), azathioprine is teratogenic in animals. In human studies low birth weights, prematurity, jaundice, respiratory distress syndrome and aspiration have been reported in kidney transplant recipients. Azathioprine has been associated with a dose related myelosuppression in the fetus, but leukopenia is not usually a problem in the neonate if the maternal white blood count is maintained at greater than 7500 /mm3 (Armenti, Constantinescu et al. 2008).
FDA rated azathioprine use during pregnancy as D which implies that "positive evidence of risk exists but potential benefit may outweigh the risk"

3.6.3 Cyclosporine

Cyclosporine is a small cyclic polypeptide of fungal origin that inhibits calcineurin. There is little or no transplacental passage of cyclosporine in rodents (Safwenberg, Backman-Bave et al. 1977). In comparison, there are conflicting reports on the transfer of cyclosporine across the human placenta. Studies in pregnant rats have generally shown no effect of cyclosporine on organogenesis, although some renal proximal tubular cell damage can occur (Bailie, Elder et al. 2007). Human data showed that administration of cyclosporine was associated with low birth weights and a higher incidence of maternal diabetes, hypertension and renal allograft dysfunction. Cyclosporine metabolism appears to be increased during pregnancy and higher doses may be required to maintain plasma levels in the therapeutic range (Murirhead 1992). In women several years post-transplant with stable renal function, the pre-pregnancy dose can be continued. Some of the pregnancies in cyclosporine- treated women were complicated by preeclampsia. Cyclosporine increases production of thromboxane and endothelin, which have both been implicated in the pathogenesis of preeclampsia. Because of this, some physicians have suggested that the dose be limited to 2 to 4 mg/kg per day (Lindheimer Md and 1992).
Although the safety of cyclosporine is not well established in pregnancy, but it does not appear to be a major teratogen, as suggested by the results of a meta-analysis of 15 studies (Bar Oz 2001).
FDA rates the risk of cyclosporine use in pregnancy as C.

3.6.4 Tacrolimus

Tacrolimus is another calcineurin inhibitor. Experience with tacrolimus in pregnancy is limited. Among 100 pregnancies in 84 women treated with tacrolimus, of whom 27 percent were renal transplant recipients, 68 progressed to a live birth, with 60 percent of deliveries being premature (Kaniz and 2000). It has been associated with neonatal hyperkalemia. As with cyclosporine, patients taking tacrolimus require frequent monitoring of renal function and drug levels. During pregnancy, the hepatic cytochrome p450 enzymes may be inhibited, which can lead to increased serum level of tacrolimus. The dose may therefore have to be significantly reduced to prevent toxicity (sometimes as much as 60 %) (Lessan-Pezeshki M 2002).

FDA rates the risk of tacrolimus use in pregnancy as C.

3.6.5 Mycophenolate Mofetil (MMF)

MMF is a selective antimetabolite which impairs lymphocyte function by blocking purine biosynthesis via inhibition of the enzyme inosine monophosphate dehydrogenase. Mycophenolate was developed as a replacement for azathioprine for maintenance immunosuppression. It is not nephrotoxic, and has less bone marrow toxicity than azathioprine.

MMF has been reported to cause head and eye malformations in the offspring of rat. Reported experience in human pregnancy with MMF is limited. There have been birth defects in few cases, but current data are insufficient to determine incidence of specific malformation. Among the 14 MMF-exposed offspring that has been reported, the underlying maternal conditions were kidney transplantation (N=7), lupus nephritis (N=4), liver transplantation, heart transplantation, and recurrent erythema multiforme. All were exposed in early pregnancy. The most distinctive malformation was moderate-to-severe microtia or anotia in 12, with external auditory canal atresia in 9. Other common craniofacial malformations and minor anomalies included orofacial clefts, hypertelorism, coloboma, and micrognathia. Six had cardiovascular malformations, of which three were either conotruncal or aortic arch defects (Anderka, Lin et al. 2009).

The manufacturer of MMF recommends that women of child-bearing age should have a negative pregnancy test prior to the initiation of therapy. We currently recommend that allograft recipients who wish to conceive should change from MMF to azathioprine, if there are no contraindications to the switch. MMF should be stopped 6 weeks prior to conception.

FDA rates the risk of MMF use in pregnancy as D.

3.6.6 Sirolimus

Sirolimus is a macrolide antibiotic compound that is structurally related to tacrolimus. Following entry into the cytoplasm, sirolimus binds to the FK binding protein and presumably modulates the activity of the mammalian target of rapamycin (mTOR). The mTOR inhibits interleukin-2 mediated signal transduction, resulting in cell cycle arrest in the G1-S phase (Danovitch GM 2005). It causes delayed ossification in animal reproductive studies, and its use is contraindicated in human until more data are available. Its use should also be discontinued at least 6 weeks prior to attempted conception.

In general, we recommend that women post-transplant who wish to conceive be switched prior to conception from sirolimus to cyclosporine. Upon delivery, it is recommended to switch the mother back to her basal immunosuppression in view of the potential benefits of the newer agents to prevent late acute rejection and chronic allograft nephropathy.

FDA rates the risk of sirolimus use in pregnancy as C.

3.6.7 OKT3 and polyclonal antibodies

OKT3 is a mouse antibody licensed for antirejection therapy, being directed against the CD3 antigen that is closely associated with the T cell receptor. It crosses the placenta. The National Transplantation Pregnancy Registry (NTPR) has reported the treatment of five women with OKT3 during pregnancy, with four surviving infants (Eisenberg 1997). The effect of polyclonal antibodies on the developing fetus is not known, but the IgG component would be expected to cross the placenta.

3.6.8 Intravenous Immune Globulins (IVIG)

Pooled human gamma-globulin preparations which were initially developed for the treatment of humoral immune deficiency disorders, proving to be invaluable in certain defined situations in clinical transplantation when used alone or in combination with plasmapheresis, such as antibody mediated rejection (Danovitch GM 2005). IgG is selectively transported across the placenta and the amount transferred increases with gestational age and dose. No cases of human deficiency virus (HIV) transmission have been reported with the use of IVIG, but adverse effects include thrombosis, alopecia, liver function disturbances, transient neutropenia, chills, nausea, flushing, tightness of chest and anaphylactic reaction in those with IgA antibodies.

There is little information regarding the teratogenicity of IVIG in animals. One report showed that IVIG was well tolerated in pregnant mice with induced antiphospholipid antibody syndrome (Bakimer 1993). In humans, IVIG appears to cross the placenta after 32 weeks of gestation, even after modification that alters the Fc binding sites (Hockel 1986). There have been no reports of fetal malformations in humans. However, IVIG is not completely benign, since hemolytic disease of the newborn and transmission of hepatitis C has been reported in selected cases.

3.6.9 Leflunomide

Leflunomide is an antimetabolite with both immunosuppressive and antiviral activities. It has been used successfully in the treatment of polyoma virus nephropathy (Danovitch GM 2005). It has marked teratogenic properties.

FDA rates its use during pregnancy as X. This medication should not be used during pregnancy or breast feeding.

3.7 Management of pregnancy in kidney transplant patient's guidelines:

All women of childbearing age should be counseled concerning the possibility and risks of pregnancy after kidney transplantation. Women who are not rubella immune should receive the rubella vaccine before transplantation, because live virus vaccines are contraindicated post transplantation (Hou S and 1999). Women are usually advised to wait at least one year after living related donor transplantation and two years after cadaveric renal transplantation (Lessan-Pezeshki M 2002). However, waiting 5 or more years may result in impaired renal function post partum that fails to recover, because of gradually deteriorating renal function secondary to chronic allograft nephropathy.

Criteria that should be ideally met before conception are shown in table 1.

Criteria
At least 1 year post transplantation
Stable renal function with creatinine< 1.5 mg/dl
No recent episodes of acute rejection
BP $\leq$ 140/90 mmHg on medications
Proteinuria <500 mg/ day
Prednisone $\leq$ 15 mg/day
Azathioprine $\leq$ 2 mg /kg/day
Cyclosporine 2- 4 mg/ kg/ day
Normal allograft ultrasound

Table 1. Criteria for transplant recipients contemplating pregnancy

3.7.1 Management of preeclampsia and chronic hypertension

Preeclampsia is the most common complication, affecting 30% of pregnancies in renal transplant recipients, especially those with pre-transplant hypertension. Women with mild to moderate hypertension should be watched closely, warned about signs of early superimposed preeclampsia.

In transplant recipients, changes in urinary protein excretion, plasma uric acid, platelet count, or liver function tests seem to be less useful as markers of preeclampsia than in the normal population. Blood pressure, renal function, proteinuria and weight should be monitored every 2-4 weeks, with more attention during the third trimester. Anti-hypertensive agents should be changed to those tolerated during pregnancy.

3.7.2 Antihypertensive drugs used in pregnancy

Safety and efficacy of Alpha Methyldopa are supported in several randomized trials and in 7.5 years follow up study of children born to treated mothers.

Beta Blockers; especially Atenolol and Metoprolol, appear to be safe and efficacious in late pregnancy; but fetal growth retardation has been noted when treatment was started in early or midgestation (Lindheimer MD.Davison JM 2001).

Hydralazine is safe and used frequently as adjunctive therapy with α methyldopa and β blockers.

Calcium Channel Blockers such as Nifedipine, Nicardipine and Verapamile have been used in severe hypertension. They do not appear to be associated with any increase in congenital anomalies when used in the first trimester.

Calcium channel blockers may potentiate the hypotensive effects and neuromuscular blockade of magnesium and the interaction should be kept in mind when the drugs are used in women with a possibility of developing preeclampsia (Dynder 1988).

Labetalol appears to be as effective as methyldopa, but there is little follow up information on children born to mothers treated with this drug.

The second and third trimester exposure to ACE inhibitors and AT1 antagonists may be associated with serious adverse fetal effects. Most of these problems have been disturbances of fetal and neonatal renal function, such as oligohydramnios, neonatal anuria, renal failure and death (Pryde 1993). The fetal outcome is generally good in women who present in early pregnancy while taking an ACE inhibitor if the drug is stopped.

Continued administration of an ACE inhibitor during pregnancy is contraindicated (Shotan 1994).

The use of thiazide diuretics has been approved in women with chronic hypertension if prescribed before gestation; however, the recommendation is against their use in preeclamptic women, who often manifest decreased intravascular volumes and poor placental perfusion.

3.7.3 Management of infection

Pregnancy is associated with suppression of the adaptive immune system. There is evidence that pregnant women in general are more susceptible to infection. Infection also is an important consideration in any patient receiving immunosuppressive drugs, including transplant patients.

3.7.3.1 Bacterial

Urinary tract infections are the most common bacterial infections and occur in up to 40% of pregnant transplant recipients, and are particularly common in patients who develop end-stage renal disease due to pyelonephritis. These women should have monthly screening urine cultures (Armenti, Constantinescu et al. 2008), if asymptomatic bacteriuria is present; the patient should be treated for 2 weeks and may be treated with suppressive doses of antibiotics for the rest of the pregnancy (Lessan-Pezeshki M 2002). If there is a need for invasive procedures such as fetal monitoring with scalp electrodes or intrauterine pressure monitoring, prophylactic antibiotics are recommended. Aseptic technique should be used for even minor surgery and steroid therapy augmented.

3.7.3.2 Viral

Cytomegalovirus (CMV) remains the most frequent cause of viral infection post transplantation, however if the patient waits the recommended time after transplantation to become pregnant, she has passed the peak time of risk for CMV infection.

Infection in the fetus can be diagnosed by culturing the amniotic fluid. Titers of anti-CMV IgG and IgM during pregnancy are recommended, Ganciclovir has caused birth defects in animals when administered at twice human dose (Hou S and 1999). Herpes Simplex Virus (HSV) infection before 20 weeks gestation is associated with an increased rate of abortion. A positive HSV cervical culture at term is an indication for cesarean section. This can minimize the risk for neonatal herpes. Acyclovir can be safely used in pregnancy (Andrew 1992).

Continuous exposure to CsA in utero seems to impair T-, B- and NK-cell development and function in neonates. This effect is prolonged throughout the first year of life. In addition, low levels of serum immunoglobulins occur at the same time. This leads to suggest a delayed administration of classical vaccinations (after the first 6 months of life) in view of the potential risks of both sub-optimal immunologic responses, and adverse events after the administration of live, attenuated vaccines in infants born from young female organ transplant recipients (Schen 2002).

An infant born to an HBSAg – positive mother should be given hepatitis B immunoglobulin within 12 hours of birth and HBV vaccine at another site within 48 hours followed by a booster injection at 1 and 6 month.

The combination of immunoglobulin and vaccine offers protection for more than 90% of infants.

Vertical transmission is believed to be low (<7%) with hepatitis C unless the patient is also infected with the human immunodeficiency virus (Lessan-Pezeshki M 2002).

3.7.4 Labor and delivery

The incidence of pre-term delivery is 50%, because of presence of preeclampsia, renal function deterioration, fetal distress, premature rupture of membrane and premature labor. Intrauterine uterine growth retardation showing small-for-age babies is present in 20% of pregnancies. In general, successful fetal outcome is related to better renal function at conception. Despite immunosuppressive therapy there is no increase of fetal abnormalities.

A transplanted kidney rarely obstructs labor, vaginal delivery is recommended in most transplant recipient women. Cesarean section should be performed only for standard obstetric reasons. Delivery should occur in a specialized centre. Care must be taken to avoid fluid overload and infection. At the time of delivery, instrumentation should be minimized. Patients with renal insufficiency may be particularly at risk for water retention secondary to oxytocin (Lessan-Pezeshki M 2002).

In the perinatal period, the steroid dose should be augmented to cover the stress of labor and to prevent postpartum rejection. Hydrocortisone, 100 mg every 6 hours, should be given during labor and delivery. In the puerperium, renal function, proteinuria, blood pressure, cyclosporine/tacrolimus blood levels and fluid balance should be closely monitored.

3.7.5 Breastfeeding

Breastfeeding is discouraged for patients taking any immunosuppressive drugs. Cyclosporine measurement in maternal blood and breast milk revealed a mean breast milk/ maternal blood level ratio of 84% (Munoz-Flores- thiagarajan and 2001).

Azathioprine is also appears in breast milk, these levels can be toxic to a newborn, and nursing is not recommended. Similar recommendations exist for tacrolimus or any other immunosuppressive agents.

In summary, Because the outcome of pregnancy in transplantation are so different than those in chronic dialysis, it is advisable to treat end-stage renal disease patients with transplantation and wait until renal function has been stable for 1 to 2 years before undertaking a planned pregnancy. Such planned pregnancies offer the mother and fetus the best chance of favorable outcome. Before any woman with a renal transplant embarks on a pregnancy, she should be counseled by an obstetrician and transplant physician. Pregnancy appears to have no significant effect on graft function or survival; however, an important concern is that a mother may not survive to bring up the child that she bears. (Davison JM 1987)

3.8 Contraception for transplant patients:

Most female transplant recipients are unaware that transplantation has reversed the relative infertility associated with end-stage renal disease. The incidence of unwanted pregnancy among female kidney transplant recipients is significantly higher than general population. An unplanned pregnancy puts this special group at higher risk; either an induced abortion or continuing the pregnancy without a preconceptional evaluation could be harmful (Lessan-Pezeshki and 2004). Outcomes for unwanted pregnancies are inferior to outcomes for planned pregnancies, so it is strongly advised that every sexually active transplant recipient attend a family-planning counseling session. Contraceptive counseling should be provided before transplantation surgery, because ovulatory cycles may begin within 1 to 2 months after transplantation in women with grafts that are functioning well. Women who do not desire pregnancy should be protected by an effective method of contraception. Surgical contraception (sterilization) should be considered for those who have completed their family. Tubal ligation can be performed at the time of transplantation surgery. Vasectomy is also an effective form of permanent contraception with little morbidity. The risk for infection may be increased with the use of an intrauterine device in immuno-compromised patients, and their efficacy decrease because of anti-inflammatory effects of immunosuppressive agents (Zerner J, Doil KL et al. 1981). New devices containing levonorgestrel are more effective than previous copper containing devices, with fewer side effects (Fong and Singh 1999).

Depot medroxyprogesterone acetate injection at three months interval is another effective method of contraception for these patients but return of fertility after discontinuation is not fast and loss of bone mineral density is a concern with its long-term use.

Although low dose estrogen progesterone oral contraceptive preparations are not contraindicated for transplant patients, but they should be used with caution because they may cause or aggravate hypertension or precipitate thromboembolism, especially in the context of cyclosporine immunosuppression. Calcineurin inhibitors levels should also be monitored soon after the contraceptive is started. Because of unfounded fear of using contraceptive pills, a significant number of kidney transplant recipients use less effective methods such as coitus interruptus. In our study on unwanted pregnancy we found that 92% of women with unwanted pregnancies were using coitus interruptus as the only method of contraception (Ghazizadeh 2005). Progestin-only pill is an option for women who have contraindication to use estrogen but their failure rate is higher than combined oral contraceptive pills. Barrier contraceptives such as male condom are the safest modality but depend on user compliance for efficacy. It provides some protection against sexually transmitted diseases. Patients should know about emergency contraception in case of a broken condom. Two tablets of 0.75 mg of Levonorgestrel pills are administered within 72 hours of unprotected intercourse. Considering the above mentioned issues, unplanned pregnancy should be avoided by proper use of effective contraception.

4. Conclusion

Chronic kidney disease affects reproductive and sexual functions in both sexes. Although adequate dialysis will improve this dysfunction to some extent, but successful kidney transplantation has a better impact on fertility and reproductive functions.

Reproductive success is a common, expected outcome for male and female recipients of kidney transplant. One of the most impressive aspects of successful renal transplantation in the young person is the ability of the male patient to father a child and the female patient to give birth to a healthy baby. There are, however, important maternal and fetal complications that need to be considered to provide optimal care to the mother and her infant.

5. References

Delano, B. (1989). "Improvements in quality of life following treatment with r-HuEPO in anemic hemodialysis patients." Am J Kidney Dis(14): 14.

Diemont, W., Vruggink, PA, Meuleman, EJ, et al. (2000). "Sexual dysfunction after renal replacement therapy." Am J Kidney Dis 35: 845.

Finkel, D., Phillips, JL, Snyder, PJ. (1985). "Stimulation of spermatogenesis by gonadotropins in men with hypogonadotropic hypogonadism." N Engl J Med(313): 651.

Grossman, E., Swan, SK, Muirhead, GJ, et al. (2004). "The pharmacokinetics and hemodynamics of sildenafil citrate in male hemodialysis patients." Kidney Int(66): 367.

Hockel, M., Kaufmann, R, (1986). "Placental transfer of class G immunoglobulins treated with B-propiolactone (P-PL) for intravenous application a case report." J Perinat Med 14: 205.

Holdsworth, S., Atkins, RC, de Kretser, DM. (1977). "The pituitary-testicular axis in men with chronic renal failure." N Engl J Med (296): 1245.

Holdsworth, S., de Kretser, DM, Atkins, RC (1978). " A comparison of hemodialysis and transplantation in reversing the uremic disturbance of male reproductive function." Clin Nephrol(10): 146.

Holley, J., Schmidt, RJ, Bender, FH, et al. (1997). "Gynecologic and reproductive issues in women on dialysis." Am J Kidney Dis 29: 685.

Ifudu, O. (1998). "Care of patients undergoing hemodialysis." N Engl J Med(339): 1054.

Levitan, D., Moser, SA, Goldstein, DA, et al. . . (1984). "Disturbances in the hypothalamic-pituitary-gonadal axis in male patients with acute renal failure." Am J Nephrol (4): 99.

Lim, V., Fang, VS. (1976). "Restoration of plasma testosterone levels in uremic men with clomiphene citrate." J Clin Endocrinol Metab(43): 1370.

Rosas, S., Joffe, M, Franklin, E, et al. (2003). "Association of decreased quality of life and erectile dysfunction in hemodialysis patients." Kidney Int(64): 232.

Sawin, C., Longcope, C, Schmitt, GW, Ryan, RJ. (1973). "Blood levels of gonadotropins and gonadal hormones in gynecomastia associated with chronic hemodialysis. ." J Clin Endocrinol Metab 36: 988.

Sievertsen, G., Lim, VS, Nakawatase, C, Frohman, LA, (1980). "Metabolic clearance and secretion rates of human prolactin in normal subjects and patients with chronic renal failure. ." J Clin Endocrinol Metab 50: 846.

Turk, S., Karalezli, G, Tonbul, HZ, et al. (2001). "Erectile dysfunction and the effects of sildenafil treatment in patients on haemodialysis and continuous ambulatory peritoneal dialysis." Nephrol Dial Transplant(16): 1818.

Wolf, G., Chen, S, Han, DC, Ziyadeh, FN, (2002). "Leptin and renal disease." Am J Kidney Dis 39: 1.

Anderka, M. T., A. E. Lin, et al. (2009). "Reviewing the evidence for mycophenolate mofetil as a new teratogen: case report and review of the literature." Am J Med Genet A 149A(6): 1241-8.

Andrew, E., Yankaskas, BC, Cordero, JF, Schoeffler, K, Hampp, S: (1992). "Acylovir in pregnancy registry: six years experience." Obstet Gynecol(79): 7-13.

Armenti, V. T., S. Constantinescu, et al. (2008). "Pregnancy after transplantation." Transplant Rev (Orlando) 22(4): 223-40.

ArmentiVT, Radomski JS, et al. (2000). "Report from the National Transplantation Pregnancy Registry(NTPR) outcome of pregnancy after transplantation." Clin Transpl 123-34.

Bailie, G. R., S. J. Elder, et al. (2007). "Sexual dysfunction in dialysis patients treated with antihypertensive or antidepressive medications: results from the DOPPS." Nephrol Dial Transplant 22(4): 1163-70.

Bakimer, R., Guilburd, B, Zurgil, N, Schoenfeld, Y, (1993). "The effect of intravenous gamma globulin on the induction of experimental antiphospholipid syndrome. ." Clin Immunol Immunopathol 69: 97.

Bar Oz, B., Hackman, R, Einarson, T, Koren, G, (2001). " Pregnancy outcome after cyclosporine therapy during pregnancy: a meta-analysis." Transplantation 71(8): 1051-5.

Beitins, I., Bayard, F, Ances, IG, et al. (1972). "The transplacental passage of prednisone and prednisolone in pregnancy near term." J Pediatr (81): 936.

Bennett, A., Carpenter, AJ, Barada, JH, (1991). "An improved vasoactive drug combination for a pharmacological erection program. ." J Urol 146 1564-5.

Berek, J. S. (2002). Novak's Gynecology, Lippincott Williams & Wilkins.

Biller BM; Molitch ME; Vance ML; Cannistraro KB; Davis KR; Simons JA; Schoenfelder JR; Klibanski A (1996). "Treatment of prolactin-secreting macroadenomas with the once-weekly dopamine agonist cabergoline." J Clin Endocrinol Metab 81(6): 2338-43.

Chao, A., et al (2002). "Pregnancy in women who undergo longterm dialysis." Am J Obstet Gynecol 187: 152-156.

Cohen, D. and C. Galbraith (2001). "General health management and long-term care of the renal transplant recipient." Am J Kidney Dis 38(6 Suppl 6): S10-24.

Cowden, E., Ratcliff, WA, Ratcliff, JG, et al (1981). "Hypothalamic-Pituitary function in uremia." Acta Endocrinol 98: 488.

Danovitch GM (2005). Handbook of Kidney Transplantation, Lippincott Williams&Wilkins.

Davison JM (1987). "Renal transplantation and pregnancy. ." Am J Kidney Dis 9: 374.

De Celis, R. and N. Pedron-Nuevo (1999). "Male fertility of kidney transplant patients with one to ten years of evolution using a conventional immunosuppressive regimen." Arch Androl 42(1): 9-20.

de Vries, C., Gooren, LJG, Oe, PL. (1984). "Hemodialysis and testicular function." Int J Androl(7): 97.

Denton, K. and C. Baylis (2007). "Physiological and molecular mechanisms governing sexual dimorphism of kidney, cardiac, and vascular function." Am J Physiol Regul Integr Comp Physiol 292(2): R697-9.

Diemont, W., Vruggink, PA, Meuleman, EJ, et al. (2000). "Sexual dysfunction after renal replacement therapy." Am J Kidney Dis (35): 845.

Dynder, S., Cardwell, MS, (1988). "Neuromuscular blockade with magnesium sulfate and nifedipine." Am J Obstet Gynecol(161): 35-36.

Eid, M. M., I. A. Abdel-Hamid, et al. (1996). "Assessment of sperm motion characteristics in infertile renal transplant recipients using computerized analysis." Int J Androl 19(6): 338-44.

Eisenberg, J., Armenti, VT ,Mc Grovy, CH, et al (1997). "National transplantation pregnancy registry(NTPR) : Use of muromonab-CD3(OKT3) during pregnancy in female transplant recipients." Am Soc Transplant phys(20): 108.

Esteban de la Rosa, R. J., J. A. Bravo Soto, et al. (2003). "Influence of age, sex, and hepatitis C virus infection on peripheral blood lymphocyte subsets in stable kidney transplantation." Transplant Proc 35(8): 2905-7.

Fong, Y. F. and K. Singh (1999). "Effect of the levonorgestrel-releasing intrauterine system on uterine myomas in a renal transplant patient." Contraception 60(1): 51-3.

Ghazizadeh, S., Lessan-Pezeshki, M, Khatami, MR, Mahdavi, M, (2005). "Unwanted Pregnancy in Kidney Transplant Recipients in Iran." Transplantation Proceedings 37(7): 3085-3086.

Hagen C, O. K., McNeilly AS (1976). "Prolactin and the pituitary gonadal axisin male uremic patients on regular dialysis. ." Acta Endocrinol (Copenh)(82): 29.

Henrich WL (2004). Principles and Practice of Dialysis, Lippincott Williams&Wilkins.

Higham, J., O'Brien, PMS, Shaw, RM, (1990). "Assessment of menstrual blood loss using pictorial chart." Br J Obstet Gynaecol 97: 734.

Hou S (1987). " Pregnancy in women requiring dialysis for renal failure." Am J Kidney Dis 9 368.

Hou S and (1999). "Pregnancy in chronic renal insufficiency and end stage renal disease. ." Am J Kidney Dis (33): 235.

Issac, R., et al (1978). " Effect of parathyroid hormone on plasma prolactin men." (47): 18.

Juenemann, K.-P., Lue, TF, Luo, JA, Benowitz, NL, Abozeid, M, Tanagho, EA. (1987). "The effect of cigarette smoking on penile erection." J Urol 138 438-41.

Jungers, P. and D. Chauveau (1997). "Pregnancy in renal disease" Kidney Int 52: 871-885.

Kaczmarek, I., Groetzner, J, Adamidis, I, Landwehr, P, (2004). "Sirolimus impairs gonadal function in heart transplant recipients. ." Am J of Transplantation 4: 1084.

Kaniz, A., Harabacz, I, Cowirick, IS, et al. and (2000). "Review of the course and outcome of 100 pregnancies in 84 women treated with tacrolimus. ." Transplantation proceeding(70): 1718.

Lasaponara, F., G. Pasquale, et al. (2009). "[Penile prosthesis implantation in kidney-transplanted patients.]." Urologia 76(2): 95-97.

LeRoith, D., Danovitz, G, Trestian, S, Spitz, IM. (1980). "Dissociation of pituitary glycoprotein response to releasing hormones in chronic renal failure." Acta Endocrinol (Copenh)(93): 277.

Lessan-Pezeshki M (2002). "Pregnancy After Renal Transplantation, Points to Consider " Nephrol Dial Transplant 17: 703-707.

Lessan-Pezeshki, M., S. Ghazizadeh, et al. (2004). "Fertility and contraceptive issues after kidney transplantation in women." Transplant Proc 36(5): 1405-6.

Lessan-Pezeshki, M., Ghazizadeh, S, Khatami, M, R, Mahdavi, M, Razeghi, E, Seifi, S,Ahmadi, F, Maziar,S, and (2004). "Fertility and contraceptive issues after kidney transplantation in women " Transplantation proceeding (36): 1405-1406.

Lim, V., Kathpalia, SC, Henriques, C. (1978). "Endocrine abnormalities associated with chronic renal failure." Med Clin North Am 62:. 1341.

Lindheimer Md, K. A. and (1992). "Pregnancy in the renal transplant patients." Am J Kidney Dis (19): 173.

Lindheimer MD.Davison JM, K. A. (2001). "The kidney and hypertension in pregnancy: twenty exciting years." Semin Nephrol 21 (2): 173-189.

Lue T F (2000). "Erectile dysfunction." The New England Journal of Medicine 342(24): 1802, 12.

Mahanty, H. D., W. S. Cherikh, et al. (2001). "Influence of pretransplant pregnancy on survival of renal allografts from living donors." Transplantation 72(2): 228-32.

Matthew RW (2005). Medical Management of Kidney transplantation, Lippincott Williams & Wilkins.

Miller, N., Gold, MS. (1988). "The human sexual response and alcohol and drugs." J Subst Abuse Treat 5: 171-7.

Mirone, V., N. Longo, et al. (2009). "Renal transplantation does not improve erectile function in hemodialysed patients." Eur Urol 56(6): 1047-53.

Muller, I., M. Munder, et al. (2009). "Polymorphonuclear neutrophils and T lymphocytes: strange bedfellows or brothers in arms?" Trends Immunol 30(11): 522-30.

Munoz-Flores- thiagarajan, K., Easterling, T, Davis, C, Bond, EF. and (2001). " Breast-feeding by a cyclosporine- treated mother." Obstet Gynecol(97): 816 -8.

Murirhead, N., Sabharwal, AR, reider, MJ, et al (1992). "The outcome of pregnancy following renal transplantation- the experience of a single center." Transplantation proceeding(54): 429.

Murray, J., Reid, DE, Harrison, JH, et al (1963). "Successful pregnancies after human renal transplantation." N Engl J Med: 269:346.

Nevins, T. E. and D. L. Dunn (1992). "Use of ganciclovir for cytomegalovirus infection." J Am Soc Nephrol 2(12 Suppl): S270-3.

Olshan, A., Mattison, DR, Zwanenburg, TS, (1994). "International Commission for Protection against Environmental Mutagens and Carcinogens. Cyclosporine A: review of genotoxicity and potential for adverse human reproductive and developmental effects. Report of a working group on the genotoxicity of cyclosporine A,." Mutat Res 317: 163-173.

Palmer, B. (1999). "Sexual dysfunction in uremia." J Am Soc Nephrol (10): 1381.

Pece, S., et al , (1979). "Prolactin in chronic renal failure, hemodialysis and transplant patients " Proc Eur Dial Transplant Assoc (16): 700.

Phe, V., M. Roupret, et al. (2009). "[Erectile dysfunction and renal chronic insufficiency: etiology and management]." Prog Urol 19(1): 1-7.

Price, D., Gingell, JC, Gepi-Attee, S,Wareham, K, (1998). "Sildenafil: Study of a novel oral treatment for erectile dysfunction in diabetic men." Diabet Med 15: 821-5.

Procci, W., Goldstein, DA, Adelstein, J, (1981). "Sexual dysfunction in the male patient with uremia; a reappraisal." Kidney Int 19: 317.

Pryde, P., Sedman, AB, Nugent, CE, Barr, M Jr. (1993). "Angiotensin converting enzyme inhibitor fetopathy." J Am Soc Nephrol (3): 1575.

Ramirez, G., O`Neil, W, Jubiz, W, et al (1976). "Thyroid dysfunction in uremia: evidence for thyroid and hypophyseal abnormalities." Am Intern Med 84: 627.

Redrow, M., Cherem, L, Elliott, J, Mangalat, J, (1988). "Dialysis in the management of pregnant patients with renal insufficiency." Medicine 67(4): 199-208.

Rizzoni, G., J. H. Ehrich, et al. (1992). "Successful pregnancies in women on renal replacement therapy: report from the EDTA Registry." Nephrol Dial Transplant 7(4): 279-87.

Safwenberg, J., U. Backman-Bave, et al. (1977). "The effect of blood transfusions on cadaver kidney transplants--an analysis of patients transplanted in Uppsala." Scand J Urol Nephrol Suppl(42): 59-61.

Salmela, K. T., L. E. Kyllonen, et al. (1993). "Impaired renal function after pregnancy in renal transplant recipients." Transplantation 56(6): 1372-5.

Sarikoski, S., Seppala, M. (1973). " Immunosupression during pregnancy: transmission of azathioprine and its metabolites from the mother to the fetus." Am J Obstet Gynecol(115): 1100.

Schaefer, F., R. Stanhope, et al. (1989). "Pulsatile gonadotropin secretion in pubertal children with chronic renal failure." Acta Endocrinol (Copenh) 120(1): 14-9.

Schen, F., Stallone, G, Schena, A, Manfredi, G, Derosa, C, Procino, A, Di Paolo, S. (2002). "Pregnancy in renal transplantation: immunologic evaluation of neonates from mothers with transplanted kidney." Transpl Immunol 9(2-4): 161-4.

Schrier RW (2001). Diseases of the kidney and urinary tract, Lippincott Williams&Wilkins.

Sciarra J (2001). Gynecology &Obststrics, Lippincot Williams & Wilkins.

Seethalakshmi, L., Diamond, DA, Malhotra, RK, Mazanitis, SG, Kumar, S, Menon, M, (1988). "Cyclosporine induced testicular dysfunction: a separation of the nephrotoxic component and an assessment of a 60-day recovery period. ." Transplant Proc 20 (Suppl 3): 1005-1010.

Seethalakshmi, L., Flores, C, Carboni, AA, Bala, R, Diamond, DA, Menon, M, (1990). "Cyclosporine: its effect on testicular function and fertility in the prepubertal rat. ." J Androl 11: 17-24.

Seethalakshmi, L., Flores, C, Diamond, DA, Menon, M, (1990). "Reversal of the toxic effects of cyclosporineA (CsA) on male reproduction and kidney function of rats by simultaneous administration of hCG and FSH." J Urol 144: 1489-149.

Seibel, I., Poli De, Figueiredo CE, Teloken, C, Moraes, JF. (2002). "Efficacy of oral sildenafil in hemodialysis patients with erectile dysfunction." J Am Soc Nephrol (13): 2770.

Sgro, M. D., T. Barozzino, et al. (2002). "Pregnancy outcome post renal transplantation." Teratology 65(1): 5-9.

Shotan, A., Widerhorn, J, Hurst, A, Elkayam, U, (1994). "Risks of angiotensin converting enzyme inhibition during pregnancy: experimental and clinical evidence, potential mechanisms and recommendations for use." Am J Med(96): 451.

Steele, T., Wuerth, D, Finkelstein, S, et al. (1996). "Sexual experience of the chronic peritoneal dialysis patient." J Am Soc Nephrol(7): 1165.

Stewart-Bentley, M., Gans, D, Horton, R. (1974). "Regulation of gonadal function in uremia." Metabolism (23): 1065.

Sturgiss, S. N. and J. M. Davison (1995). "Effect of pregnancy on the long-term function of renal allografts: an update." Am J Kidney Dis 26(1): 54-6.

Thurm JA (1976). " Effect of chronic renal disease on sexual functioning." Med Asp Human Sex 10: 81.

Toorians, A. W., E. Janssen, et al. (1997). "Chronic renal failure and sexual functioning: clinical status versus objectively assessed sexual response." Nephrol Dial Transplant 12(12): 2654-63.

Treloar, A., Boynton, RE, Behn, BG, Brown, BW, Brown BW, (1967). "Variation of the human menstrual cycle through reproductive life." Int J Fertil 12: 77.

Wang, H. Y. and Y. F. Huang (2009). "Vardenafil for refractory erectile dysfunction: the latest advances." Zhonghua Nan Ke Xue 15(11): 1035-8.

Yang, J., W. Ju, et al. (2008). "Efficacy and safety of vardenafil for kidney transplant recipients with erectile dysfunction." Zhonghua Nan Ke Xue 14(10): 911-3.

Zerner J, Doil KL, et al. (1981). "Intrauterine contraceptive device failures in renal transplant patients." J Reprod Med. 26(2): 99-102.

Zuber, J., D. Anglicheau, et al. (2008). "Sirolimus may reduce fertility in male renal transplant recipients." Am J Transplant 8(7): 1471-9.

12

Hypertension in the Kidney Transplant Recipient

Heather H. Jones and Daniel J. Salzberg
Division of Nephrology, University of Maryland Department of Medicine, School of Medicine, USA

1. Introduction

Despite normalization of renal function and improvement in volume control with kidney transplantation, the prevalence of post-transplant hypertension (HTN) is substantial. The prevalence of post-transplant HTN reported in the literature varies considerably depending on the study population and the criteria used to define HTN, although most studies report a prevalence of between 60-80% [1-3]. In one cross-sectional study of 409 adults with stable kidney allograft function, the prevalence of HTN, defined as BP > 150/90 mmHg, was 77.3% [4]. Most subjects (68.9%) required multiple antihypertensive medications. However, for patients with diabetes or estimated GFR below 60 mL/min, treatment guidelines recommend blood pressure (BP) goals below 130/80 mmHg. Applying these more stringent recommendations, the true prevalence of post-transplant HTN is likely in excess of 95%.

2. Pathogenesis and impact of immunosuppression

The exact pathogenesis of post-transplant HTN is poorly understood, as multiple factors impact its development. Important risk factors include preexisting recipient factors, donor specific factors, use of immunosuppressive agents, extra-allograft related issues, and both acute and chronic allograft dysfunction [1,2]. Ultimately, post-transplant HTN is characterized by sodium retention, enhanced sympathetic nervous system activity, renal vasoconstriction and relatively lower levels of plasma renin [5].

Post-transplant HTN demonstrates a distinctive characteristic regarding ambulatory BP monitoring, with patients having a high prevalence of nocturnal HTN [3]. In one prospective study, nearly 75% of subjects with post-transplant HTN demonstrated absence or reversal of the normal nocturnal fall in BP (i.e. non-dippers) [3]. In non-kidney transplant recipients, loss of nocturnal dip is associated with left ventricular hypertrophy, lacunar stroke and microalbuminuria [6].

3. Role of immunosuppression

Systemic steroid use contributes to the development of post-transplant HTN through various mechanisms, including sodium retention with resultant volume expansion, decreased prostaglandin biosynthesis, and increased smooth muscle pressor response [9]. In one systematic review comparing post-transplant recipients on immunosuppression regimens containing steroids versus those on steroid-sparing regimens, steroid-attributable incidence of HTN was reported to be between 2 and 17% [10]. A more recent meta-analysis of steroid avoidance or steroid withdrawal protocols examined impact on both graft and cardiovascular outcomes [11]. Steroid avoidance or withdrawal was found to be significantly related to increased risk of acute rejection and elevated creatinine at end of follow-up, with no difference in patient survival, graft loss, or death-censored graft loss. At the same time, steroid avoidance was associated with significant reduction in the risk of cardiovascular risk factors, including a 10% reduction in risk of post-transplant HTN.

However, some evidence indicates that chronic steroid use may not alter BP control. Vincenti and colleagues evaluated one-year outcomes and cardiovascular risk factors in kidney transplant recipients randomized to immunosuppressive regimens with complete steroid avoidance, early steroid withdrawal, and chronic steroid therapy. There was no difference in systolic or diastolic BP between any of the groups and no difference in the percent of patients requiring antihypertensive therapy [12].

Perhaps the most important factor in the pathogenesis of post-transplant HTN is the use of calcineurin inhibitors. Calcineurin inhibitors lead to the development of HTN through a myriad of mechanisms, including sodium retention with resultant volume expansion, enhanced sympathetic nerve activity, up-regulation of intrarenal renin biosynthesis, and vasoconstriction of the preglomerular vasculature via decreased production of vasodilatory factors and increased production of vasoconstrictive factors [5,13-14]. It has been shown that cyclosporine-induced renal vasoconstriction precedes the development of HTN [13]. Additionally, cyclosporine has been implicated as contributing to the loss of the normal nocturnal drop in BP [3].

In recent years, there has been a paradigm shift in the choice of calcineurin inhibitors from cyclosporine to tacrolimus, as short-term patient and graft survival appears to be equivalent between the two [15]. Likewise, the incidence of acute rejection is similar between the two groups when they are used in conjunction with mycophenolate mofetil. The advantage of tacrolimus over cyclosporine is a lower incidence of hyperlipidemia, hirsutism, and gingival hyperplasia. However, a difference between the two agents with regard to HTN is not as clear.

A large multi-center open label randomized controlled trial comparing cyclosporine-based versus tacrolimus-based immunosuppression regimens involving 412 kidney transplant recipients reported that at 3 years post-transplantation, the number of recipients requiring antihypertensive therapy was lower in the tacrolimus group, though this did not reach statistical significance (74.7% vs. 84.9%, $p = 0.06$) [16]. Another cross-sectional study evaluating predictors of post-transplant HTN, defined as documented diagnosis of HTN or use of antihypertensive medications, determined that significantly more patients on a cyclosporine-based regimen were prescribed 2 or more antihypertensive medications compared with those on a tacrolimus-based regimen [17].

There has been interest in the use of a mammalian-target of rapamycin (m-TOR) inhibitor-based immunosuppression regimen as an alternative to calcineurin inhibitor-based regimens, partially due to concerns over long-term effects of calcineurin-induced HTN and chronic preglomerular vasoconstriction. Thus far, the data regarding the relationship between m-TOR inhibitor use and HTN have been mixed. Comparison of a small cohort of patients on tacrolimus-based vs. sirolimus-based immunosuppression demonstrated that patients receiving sirolimus had significantly lower systolic BP on 24-hour ambulatory BP monitoring, though there was no significant difference in preserved nocturnal drop in BP [18].

However, two large randomized controlled trials evaluating the conversion of kidney transplant recipients from cyclosporine to sirolimus demonstrated no difference in BP [19-20]. The CONCEPT study, evaluating efficacy of conversion from cyclosporin to sirolimus 3-months post-transplantation in 237 kidney transplant recipients demonstrated no difference in systolic or diastolic BP one year post-transplantation [20]. There was, however, a tendency toward no need of antihypertensive medications in the sirolimus group compared to the cyclosporine group (51% vs. 38%), though this was not statistically significant. The CONVERT study, which followed a cohort of 830 subjects randomized to either sirolimus conversion or continuation of calcineurin inhibitor, found a statistically significant decrease in systolic BP at one month and in diastolic BP up to three months post-conversion [19]. However, by study endpoint two years, there was no significant difference in systolic or diastolic BP between the groups.

4. Renal artery stenosis

Transplant renal artery stenosis (tRAS) is a potentially important contributor to refractory HTN and unexplained graft dysfunction. The incidence of tRAS has been reported to range from 1 to 23%, with most of this variance attributed to differences in definition and diagnostic technique employed [21]. Most episodes of tRAS in the first three post-operative months are attributed to surgical complications, such as donor vessel trauma, intra-operative kidney malpositioning, or stenosis at the surgical anastamosis [22]. Transplant RAS occurring greater than 3 months post-transplantation is rarely related to surgical complications.

Several risk factors have been implicated in the development of late tRAS, including graft rejection, CMV infection, prolonged cold ischemia time, delayed graft function, and pediatric donor source [22-26]. A recent case-control study of 29 transplant recipients with tRAS found that CMV infection was associated with a five-fold increase in the risk for tRAS, while DGF increased tRAS risk four-fold [22].

Doppler ultrasonography may be an appropriate first-line screening test for tRAS, as it is non-invasive and avoids exposure to iodinated contrast media [21]. Sensitivity and specificity have been reported as high as 94% and 100%, respectively [27]. However, this diagnostic test is very operator-dependent, and such impressive results may not be obtained in centers without strong experience in kidney transplant imaging. Ultimately, the gold standard remains angiography.

Therapeutic options for tRAS include conservative management, angioplasty with or without stenting, and surgical repair. A recent case series compared the outcomes of these three strategies and determined that the highest success rate, defined as improvement in graft function, occurred in those who underwent primary angioplasty (36% conservative therapy, 82% angioplasty, 44% surgery) [28]. Graft survival at five years post-transplantation was also highest in the primary angioplasty group (63% conservative therapy, 86% angioplasty, 65% surgery). The primary angioplasty cohort was the only group in which a sustained improvement in BP was observed, with 63% of participants in this subgroup reaching target BP with a single agent post-procedure. However, angioplasty is not without risks. Four participants (6%) who underwent initial angioplasty had to undergo a transplant nephrectomy due to post-intervention complications, specifically uncontrolled bleeding and/or thrombosis. Furthermore, the presence of large or multiple stenoses may not be appropriate for primary angioplasty, leaving surgical intervention as the only viable option.

Another case-controlled series of patients evaluated the efficacy of angioplasty with or without stenting in participants with tRAS [22]. Both serum creatinine and BP control improved significantly post-procedure. Restenosis occurred in 27% of patients at a mean time of 26 months post-procedure, and 10% experienced immediate graft loss due to procedural complications.

Transplant RAS is an important entity to consider in subjects with new-onset or refractory HTN. It can be effectively treated in most cases with angioplasty, which appears to impact positively on graft function and potentially prolonging allograft life.

5. Outcomes

The precise role of HTN on allograft outcome has been difficult to define due to the complex interactions between HTN and worsening allograft function. Hypertension is both a cause and consequence of kidney disease. The presence of post-transplant HTN is associated with an increased risk for acute rejection, and allograft recipients who experience an episode of acute rejection have a significantly higher BP than those without rejection [29-30]. In a historical cohort study of adult allograft recipients, Mange and colleagues characterized the relationship between BP and subsequent allograft function [31]. For each 10-mm Hg increment increase in systolic, diastolic and mean BP, there was a 15%, 27% and 30% reduction, respectively, in the rate of allograft survival. Another cohort study by Opelz and colleagues demonstrated that systolic BP greater than 140 mmHg was associated with increased risk of graft failure, regardless of diastolic BP or history of acute rejection [32].

Post-transplant HTN is associated with increased mortality, chronic allograft nephropathy, acute rejection, and graft loss [7,30,32]. It is also an independent risk factor for the development of cardiovascular disease, the leading cause of death in kidney transplant recipients. The fact that more severe HTN has been associated with a higher rate of graft dysfunction, worse graft survival and a higher frequency of proteinuria is suggestive of a causative relationship [8].

6. Antihypertensive therapy

In patients with chronic kidney disease (CKD), therapy for HTN slows the progression of renal insufficiency [33]. This suggests that treatment of post-transplant HTN may likewise ameliorate the loss of allograft function. Current KDOQI guidelines recommend kidney transplant recipients maintain a target BP < 130/80, largely based on extrapolation from outcomes data in CKD patients [34]. Due to various contributing factors, post-transplantation HTN can be difficult to control. Multiple retrospective cohort analyses report a significant proportion of subjects fail to reach target BP, even with use of multiple anti-hypertensive agents. A review of the Collaborative Transplant Study, a database involving nearly 30,000 chronic transplant recipients at 400 international transplant centers, demonstrated that only 44.5% achieved systolic BP < 140 mmHg and that 24.5% achieved systolic BP < 130mmHg [32]. A smaller cohort study of 150 transplant recipients demonstrated that over 60% of patients required three or more anti-hypertensive medications and that only 40% reached the target BP of < 130/80 mmHg [35]. Although the risk of HTN is well documented, there are few published reports on the management of post-transplant HTN that clearly elucidate ideal target BP or choice of individual antihypertensive agents [22].

7. Calcium channel blockers

Calcium channel blockers (CCB) are effective medications to lower BP in kidney transplant recipients. In the general population, they have proven to be robust agents to lower BP regardless of age, gender, ethnicity, and salt intake, which may explain why they are also effective in the kidney transplant population (36). In addition, they also appear to reverse some of the intra-renal vasoconstriction caused by calcineurin inhibitors (*36-38*). One trial of 65 transplant recipients receiving cyclosporine-based immunosuppression randomized to the CCB or placebo at the time of transplantation demonstrated that those taking felodipine had a significantly higher renal plasma flow at 6 weeks [39]. Additionally, those randomized to the felodipine also group had lower systolic and diastolic BP, higher renal plasma flow, and higher GFR (49ml/min vs. 40ml/min, p = 0.05) at 12 weeks post-transplantation, despite a greater proportion of patients in the placebo group receiving other anti-hypertensive agents.

In a study of 123 immediate post-transplant recipients, subjects were randomized to nifedipine (CCB) or lisinopril as first line maintenance BP medication [40]. At three months post-transplantation 20% of all participants had achieved a goal diastolic BP of < 95 mmHg, with 38% in the CCB group reaching diastolic BP goal at one year. There was no difference in BP response between groups, but patients randomized to nifedipine had higher hemoglobin and lower creatinine levels compared to the lisinopril group at the study end. In an additional study comparing nifedipine and lisinopril, impact on left ventricular mass and function was assessed [41]. This study demonstrated that myocardial mass was significantly reduced in both groups one year post-transplantation, with a mean reduction of 15% in both groups. There was no statistically significant between-groups difference. The percentage of participants with persistent left ventricular hypertrophy (LVH) one year post-transplantation was similar between groups (45% nifedipine, 41% lisinopril p = NS). Another study of 99 kidney transplant recipients one year post-transplantation randomized subjects to 1 of 3 groups: (i) amlodipine (CCB) monotherapy, (ii) enalapril monotherapy, or (iii) combination amlodipine and enalapril [42]. At six months post-randomization, there was no difference amongst the three groups in terms of systolic BP or number of antihypertensive agents used. However, participants assigned to amlodipine monotherapy demonstrated improved creatinine clearance but no change in proteinuria, as compared with either angiotensin converting enzyme (ACE)-inhibitor monotherapy or combination. Results of this study should be interpreted with some caution, as they did not reach the target number of participants for adequate power.

A recent meta-analysis of randomized controlled trials involving antihypertensive agent use in renal transplant recipients was conducted [43]. This analysis concluded that use of a CCB versus placebo did not reduce the risk of death but did reduce the risk of graft lost by 25% at 12-months post-transplantation. Additionally, subjects receiving CCB had significantly higher estimated glomerular filtration rate (eGFR). When compared to ACE-inhibition. There was no difference detected in death, graft loss, or cardiovascular event risk.

8. Renin-angiotensin system blockade

Use of renin-angiotensin system (RAS) blockers in kidney transplant recipients was initially limited due to a number of concerns, including ineffectiveness in BP control, potential exacerbation of anemia, potential for inducing hyperkalemia, and the risk of precipitating acute kidney injury, [44-46]. The concern for ineffective BP control with renin-angiotensin blockade was related to the fact that post-transplant HTN, characterized by a low renin, volume expanded state, has been compared with the Goldblatt single-kidney, one-clip model of HTN, which potentially would not be very responsive to these agents [47]. However, this concern has not been borne out clinically, as multiple studies have demonstrated that RAS blockers have efficacy in reducing BP in post-transplant HTN [48].

Renin-angiotensin system blockade has now become commonplace in many transplant centers. Before 1990, approximately 9% of post-transplant subjects received treatment with an ACE inhibitor, which increased to roughly 47% in 2003 [49]. In the same retrospective review, only 38.5% (781 subjects) had never received an ACE inhibitor or an angiotensin receptor blocker (ARB). Six-hundred thirty eight subjects (31.4%) used ACE inhibitor or ARB therapy for the entirety of their follow-up, and 612 subjects (30.1%) received this therapy during various times of follow-up [49].

Furthermore, there are multiple theoretical benefits supporting the use of RAS blockers in the treatment of post-transplant HTN, such as (i) decreasing intraglomerular capillary pressure, (ii) decreasing the production and expression of the potentially damaging growth factors, (iii) decreasing proteinuria, (iv) for primary and secondary prevention of adverse cardiovascular outcomes, (v) decreasing cyclosporine nephrotoxicity, and (vi) blocking angiotensin type 1 (AT_1) receptor antibodies that may be associated with vascular rejection [50-51]. In the general population, RAS blockers have been shown to reduce both primary and secondary cardiovascular events [52]. Despite these theoretical benefits for their RAS blocker use, there are no prospective studies demonstrating the advantage of RAS blockers for the protection against allograft loss or for prolonging patient survival.

The largest study to date that has evaluated the efficacy of a RAS blocker is the SECRET trial, a multi-center double-blind randomized placebo-controlled trial involving 500 participants from several transplant centers in Europe [53] This trial was designed to evaluate the effects of Candesartan (ARB) therapy compared with placebo, on mortality, cardiovascular events, and graft failure. The study was discontinued prematurely due to a lower than expected event rate in both groups, which precluded conclusions regarding the primary endpoints. However, analysis of secondary endpoints revealed that reductions in BP and proteinuria were greater in the ARB group, but this was associated with a decrease in creatinine clearance and hemoglobin There was no significant difference in cardiovascular or graft outcomes between the two groups, though the overall event rate was quite low (5.1% with candesartan vs. 5.3% with placebo).

A much smaller study involving fifty recipients of living unrelated kidney transplants at least six months prior to enrollment were randomized to losartan (ARB) 50 mg daily or placebo for one year [54]. Of note, the subjects were not proteinuric at randomization. There was no difference in number of antihypertensives prescribed between the two groups and no difference in creatinine clearance at study end. However, systolic BP was significantly lower in the ARB group at 12 months (113mmHg vs. 126mmHg).

Although insufficient data exist to determine the impact of RAS blockade on overall cardiovascular outcomes, a small study has evaluated the impact of ACE inhibitor therapy on echocardiographic findings [55]. Evaluation of 74 transplant recipients randomized to lisinopril (ACE) or placebo and followed for 18 months demonstrated a significant decrease in left ventricular mass index in the ACE group while no difference was observed in the placebo group. There was no difference between the groups in terms of systolic BP, serum creatinine, urinary protein excretion, or number of antihypertensive agents used. The decrease in left ventricular mass index was observed exclusively in those concomitantly treated with ACE and cyclosporine, as opposed to tacrolimus. This small study is one more piece of evidence corroborating data from the general population, suggesting that drugs that block the RAS are capable of regressing left ventricular hypertrophy, both as part of their hemodynamic effect, but also through BP independent mechanisms. It is likely that regression of LVH may be a beneficial prognostic event that patients achieve with an appropriate BP control and an optimal class of antihypertensive therapy, with a potential for reducing adverse cardiovascular events. This study parallels efforts in older trials in the general population, illustrating the advantages of a RAS blocking drugs in the reduction of proteinuria and the risk for cardiovascular events and renal disease progression. Sadly, compelling data are still lacking in the kidney transplant population.

Although the number of randomized controlled trials regarding RAS blockade in transplant recipients has increased in recent years, much of the available data are from retrospective studies and systematic reviews. In one retrospective review of more than 2,000 recipients of kidney transplants at the University of Vienna, investigators noted that the ten-year patient survival rates were 74% in patients receiving either an ACE inhibitor or an ARB as part of their antihypertensive regimen and only 53% in patients not receiving these agents (49). Their results were even more remarkable when one considers that the group receiving the RAS blockers were older, required a higher number of antihypertensive medications, and were more likely to have type 2 diabetes and evident cardiovascular disease, when compared to the group not receiving these agents. Although selection bias limits the power of this study, the data are intriguing and suggest that there may be an important advantage to employ RAS blocking drugs as part of an antihypertensive regimen in an effort to reduce cardiovascular events.

Heinze and colleagues (49), studied 436 kidney transplant recipients who had delayed graft function. Approximately half of those patients (n=181) were given either an ACE inhibitor or ARB at the time of transplantation. Those patients who received RAS blocker had improved ten-year graft survival, when compared to those who were not treated with RAS blockers (44% vs. 32%, respectively). Hiremath and colleagues (56) performed a systematic review of 21 randomized trials of 1,549 patients to determine the effect of ACE inhibitor or ARBs on graft function and patient survival after kidney transplantation. In this analysis, drugs that block the RAS were associated with a significant decrease in GFR (-5.8 mL/min), proteinuria (-470 mg/day), and hematocrit (-3.5%)(51,57). However, there was insufficient data to determine their impact on patient or graft survival. Authors suggested that there may be a trade off between the beneficial effects of proteinuria reduction and potential cardiac protection with the development of possible anemia and lowered GFR.

9. Beta-blockade

Since kidney transplant patients are at much greater risk for cardiovascular events compared to the general population (58), due to both traditional and non-traditional Framingham Heart Study risk factors, beta-blocker use is often advisable. This may be important both during the peri-operative period to protect against myocardial ischemia, but also in the long-term management of HTN and cardiovascular disease. However, these agents have not been extensively studied. A recent meta-analysis of randomized controlled trials involving antihypertensive therapy in renal transplant recipients identified four studies involving beta-blockers [43]. Currently, there is insufficient data to determine relative benefits and harms of these agents. However, data from these studies indicate that beta-blockers are effective in BP reduction without appreciable impact on renal function, proteinuria, or left ventricular mass [59-61].

10. Alpha-blockers

In addition to their antihypertensive effects, alpha-blockers are often used to facilitate prostatic relaxation. This is particularly important in many older patients who may have occult prostatic hypertrophy, or some degree of bladder detrusor neuropathy due to diabetes. However, these agents, in general, tend to cause significant orthostatic symptoms, and have not been proven to reduce mortality (62). Both doxazosin and prazosin have been shown to decrease HTN in transplant recipients, although the literature remains sparse (63-64).

11. Conclusion

Taken together, the clinical trials of antihypertensive therapeutics in kidney transplant subjects illustrates that BP can be controlled. However, it usually requires multiple drugs. Although the data is not definitive, it appears that CCB and or RAS blockers should be included in an effective antihypertensive regimen. Subjects at risk for, or who have known coronary disease, may also derive benefit from beta-blockers. More studies are needed to define optimal levels of BP control and ideal combination of agents to facilitate better long-term patient and graft survival in kidney transplant recipients.

12. References

Raine AE. Does antihypertensive therapy modify chronic allograft failure? Kidney Int Suppl. 1995;52:S107-11.

Sanders CE Jr, Curtis JJ. Role of hypertension in chronic renal allograft dysfunction. Kidney Int Suppl. 1995;52:S43-7.

Oliveras A, Vazquez S, Hurtado S, et al. Ambulatory blood pressure monitoring in renal transplant patients: modifiable parameters after active antihypertensive treatment. Transplant Proc. 2004;36: 1352-4.

Budde K, Waiser J, Fritsche L, et al. Hypertension in patients after renal transplantation. Transplant Proc. 1997; 29: 209-11.

McNally PG, Feehally J. Pathophysiology of cyclosporin A nephrotoxicity: experimental and clinical observations. Nephrol Dial Transplant. 1992;7:791-804.

Lipkin GW, Tucker B, Giles M, Raine AE. Ambulatory blood pressure and left ventricular mass in cyclosporin- and non-cyclosporin-treated renal transplant recipients. J Hypertens. 1993; 11: 439-42.

Sorof JM, Sullivan EK, Tejani A, Portman RJ. Antihypertensive medication and renal allograft failure: a North American Pediatric Renal Transplant Cooperative Study report. J Am Soc Nephrol. 1999; 10: 1324-30.

Kasiske BL, Anjum S, Shah R, et al. Hypertension after kidney transplantation. Am J Kidney Dis. 2004; 43: 1071-81.

Whitworth J. Mechanisms of glucocorticoid-induced hypertension. Kidney Int. 1987; 31: 1213-1224.

Veenstra D, Best J, Hornberger J, Sullivan S, Hricik D. Incidence and long-term cost of steroid-related side effects after renal transplantation. Am J Kidney Dis. 1999; 33: 829-839.

Knight S, Morris P. Steroid avoidance or withdrawal after renal transplantation increases the risk of acute rejection but decreases cardiovascular risk. A meta-analysis. Transplantation. 2010; 89: 1-14.

Vincenti F, Schena F, Paraskevas S, et al. A randomized multicenter study of steroid avoidance, early steroid withdrawal, or standard steroid therapy in kidney transplant recipients. Am J Transplant. 2008; 8: 307-316.

Conte G, Dal Canton A, Sabbatini M, et al. Acute cyclosporine renal dysfunction reversed by dopamine infusion in healthy subjects. Kidney Int. 1989; 36: 1086-92.

Textor S, Taler S, Canzanello V, et al. Posttransplantation hypertension related to calcineurin inhibitors. Liver Transplantation. 2003; 6: 530.

Tanabe K. Calcineurin inhibitors in renal transplantation: What is the best option? Drugs. 2003; 63: 1535-1548.

Jensik S. and FK 506 Kidney Transplant Study Group. Tacrolimus (FK 506) in kidney transplantation: Three-year survival results of the US multicenter, randomized comparative trial. Transplant Proc. 1998; 30: 1216-1218.

Bohlke M. Barcellos F, Rocha M. et al. Predictors of hypertension following successful renal transplantation: A population-based study. Transplantation Proc. 2009; 41: 3743-3746.

Steigerwalt SP, Brar N, Dhungel A, et al. Improved 24-hour blood pressure control with sirolimus versus calcineurin inhibitor based immunosuppression in renal transplant recipients. Transplant Proc, 2009; 41: 4184-4187.

Schena F, Pascoe M, Alberu J, et al. Conversion from calcineurin inhibitors to sirolimus maintenance therapy in renal allograft recipients: 24-month efficacy and safety results from CONVERT trial. Transplantation 2009; 87: 233-242.

Lebranchu Y, Thierry A, Toupance O, et al. Efficacy on renal function of early conversion from cyclosporine to sirolimus 3 months after renal transplantation: Concept study. Am J of Transplant. 2009; 9: 1115-1123.

Bruno S, Remuzzi G, Ruggenenti P. Transplant renal artery stenosis.J Am Soc Nephrol. 2004 Jan;15(1):134-41.

Audard V. Matignon M. Hemery F, et al. Risk factors and long-term outcome of transplant renal artery stenosis in adult recipients after treatment by percutaneous transluminal angioplasty. Am J Transplant. 2006; 6: 95-99.

Wong W, Fynn SP, Higgings RM, et al. Transplant renal artery stenosis in 77 patients: Does it have an immunological cause? Transplantation. 1996; 61: 215-219.

Pouria S, State O, Wong W, Hendry B. CMV infection is associated with transplant renal artery stenosis. QJM. 1998; 91: 185-189.

Sankari B, Geisinger M, Zelch M, et al. Post-transplant renal artery stenosis: Impact of therapy on long-term kidney function and blood pressure control. J Urology. 1996; 155: 1860-1864.

Patel N, Jindal R, Wilkin T et al. Renal artery stenosis in renal allografts: Retrospective study of predisposing factors and outcome after percutaneous transluminal angioplasty. Radiology. 2001; 219: 663-667.

Loubeyre P, Cahen R, Grozel F, et al. Transplant renal artery stenosis. Evaluation of diagnosis with magnetic resonance angiography compared with color duplex sonography and arteriography. Transplantation. 1996; 62: 446-450.

Ghazanfar A, Tavakoli A, Augustine T, et al. Management of transplant renal artery stenosis and its impact on long term allograft survival: A single centre experience. Nephrol Dial Transplant. 2011; 26: 336-343.

Cosio FG, Pelletier RP, Pesavento TE, et al. Elevated blood pressure predicts the risk of acute rejection in renal allograft recipients. Kidney Int. 2001 Mar;59(3):1158-64.

Cosio FG, Pelletier RP, Sedmak DD, et al. Renal allograft survival following acute rejection correlates with blood pressure levels and histopathology. Kidney Int. 1999 Nov;56(5):1912-9.

Mange KC, Cizman B, Joffe M, Feldman HI. Arterial hypertension and renal allograft survival. JAMA. 2000 Feb 2;283(5):633-8.

Opelz G, Wujciak T, Ritz E. Association of chronic kidney graft failure with recipient blood pressure. Collaborative Transplant Study. Kidney Int. 1998 Jan;53(1):217-22.

Mimran A, Ribstein J. Angiotensin-converting enzyme inhibitors versus calcium antagonists in the progression of renal diseases. Am J Hypertens. 1994 Sep;7(9 Pt 2):73S-81S.

K/DOQI clinical practice guidelines on hypertension and antihypertensive agents in chronic kidney disease. AJKD. 2004; 43: S1-S290.

Malyszko J, Malyszko J, Bachorzewska-Gajewska H, et al. Inadequate blood pressure control in most kidney transplant recipients and patients with coronary artery disease with and without complications. Transplant Proc. 2009; 41: 3069-3072.

Sennesael JJ, Lamote JG, Violet I, Tasse S, Verbeelen DL. Divergent effects of calcium channel and angiotensin converting enzyme blockade on glomerulotubular function in cyclosporine-treated renal allograft recipients. Am J Kidney Dis 1996 May;27:701-8.

Curtis JJ, Laskow DA, Jones PA, et al. Captopril-induced fall in glomerular filtration rate in cyclosporine-treated hypertensive patients. J Am Soc Nephrol 1993:1570-4.

van der Schaaf MR, Hene RJ, Floor M, Blankestijn PJ, Koomans HA. Hypertension after renal transplantation. Calcium channel or converting enzyme blockade? Hypertension 1995; 25:77-81.

Madsen J, Sorensen S, Hansen H, Pedersen E. The effect of felodipine on renal function and blood pressure in cyclosporine-treated renal transplant recipients during the first three months after transplantation. Nephrol Dial Transplant. 1998; 13: 2327- 2334.

Midtvedt K, Hartmann A, Holdaas H, Fauchald P. Efficacy of nifedipine or lisinopril in the treatment of hypertension after renal transplantation: A double-blind randomized comparative trial. Clin Transplant. 2001; 15:426-431.

Midtvedt K, Hartmann A, Foss A, et al. Sustained improvement of renal graft function for two years in hypertensive renal transplant recipients treated with nifedipine as compared to lisinopril. Transplantation. 2001 Dec 15;72:1787-92.

Halimi JM, Giraudeau B, Buchler M, et al. Enalapril/amlodipine combination in cyclosporine-treated renal transplant recipients: A prospective randomized trial. Clin Transplant. 2007; 21:277-284, 2007.

Cross N, Webster A, Masson P, O'Connell P, Craig J. Antihypertensives for kidney transplant recipients: Systematic review and meta-analysis of randomized controlled trials. Transplantation. 2009; 88: 7-18, 2009.

Vlahakos DV, Canzanello VJ, Madaio MP, Madias NE. Enalapril-associated anemia in renal transplant recipients treated for hypertension. Am J Kidney Dis. 1991;17:199- 205.

Curtis JJ, Luke RG, Whelchel JD, et al. Inhibition of angiotensin-converting enzyme in renal-transplant recipients with hypertension. N Engl J Med. 1983 17;308:377-81.

Andres A, Morales E, Morales JM, et al. Efficacy and safety of valsartan, an angiotensin II receptor antagonist, in hypertension after renal transplantation: a randomized multi-center study. Transplant Proc. 2006; 38:2419-23.

Kornerup HJ, Pedersen EB, Fjeldborg O. Kidney transplant artery stenosis. Interrelationship between blood pressure, kidney function, renin-aldosterone system and body sodium content. Proc Eur Dial Transplant Assoc. 1977;14:377-85.

del Castillo D, Campistol JM, Guirado L, et al. Efficacy and safety of losartan in the treatment of hypertension in renal transplant recipients. Kidney Int Suppl. 1998;68:S135-9.

Heinze G, Mitterbauer C, Regele H, et al. Angiotensin-converting enzyme inhibitor or angiotensin II type 1 receptor antagonist therapy is associated with prolonged patient and graft survival after renal transplantation. J Am Soc Nephrol. 2006;17:889-99.

Traindl O, Falger S, Reading S, et al. The effects of lisinopril on renal function in proteinuric renal transplant recipients. Transplantation. 1993;55:1309-13.

el-Agroudy AE, Hassan NA, Foda MA, et al. Effect of angiotensin II receptor blocker on plasma levels of TGF-beta 1 and interstitial fibrosis in hypertensive kidney transplant patients. Am J Nephrol. 2003;23:300-6.

Weir MR. Providing end-organ protection with renin-angiotensin system inhibition: the evidence so far. J Clin Hypertens (Greenwich) 2006; 8: 99-105.

Philipp T, Martinez F, Geiger H, et al. Candesartan improves blood pressure control and reduces proteinuria in renal transplant recipients: Results from SECRET. Nephrol Dial Transplant. 2010; 25: 967-976.

Nouri-Majalan N, Ghafari A, Moghaddasi S. Effect of angiotensin II type-1 receptor blockers on stable allograft kidneys: Prospective randomized study. Transplant Proc. 2009; 41: 2832-2834.

Paoletti E, Cassottana P, Amidone M et al.: ACE inhibitors and persistent left ventricular hypertrophy after renal transplantation: a randomized clinical trial. Am J Kidney Dis 50:133-142, 2007.

Hiremath S, Fergusson D, Doucette S, Mulay AV, Knoll GA. Renin angiotensin system blockade in kidney transplantation: a systematic review of the evidence. Am J Transplant 2007; 7: 2350-60.

Cieciura T, Senatorski G, Rell K, Baczkowska T, Paczek L, Gradowska L, et al. Influence of angiotensin-converting enzyme inhibitor treatment of the carotid artery intima-media complex in renal allograft recipients. Transplant Proc 2000Sep; 32:1335-6.

Premasathian NC, Muehrer R, Brazy PC, Pirsch JD, Becker BN. Blood pressure control in kidney transplantation: therapeutic implications. J Hum Hypertens. 2004; 18: 871-7.

Tylicki L, Biedunkiewicz B, Chamienia A, et al. Randomized placebo-controlled study on the effects of losartan and carvedilol on albuminuria in renal transplant recipients. 2006; Transplantation. 81: 52-56.

Suwelack B, Gerhardt U, Hausberg M, Rahn K, Hohage H. Comparison of quinipril versus atenolol: Effects on blood pressure and cardiac mass after renal transplantation. American Journal Cardiology 2000; 86: 583-585.

Hausberg M, Barenbrock M, Hohage H, et al. ACE inhibitor versus beta-blocker for the treatment of hypertension in renal allograft recipients. Hypertension. 1999; 33: 862-8.

Ruggenenti P, Perico N, Mosconi L, et al. Calcium channel blockers protect transplant patients from cyclosporine-induced daily renal hypoperfusion. Kidney Int. 1993; 43: 706-11.

Curtis J, Bateman F. Use of prazosin in management of hypertension in patients with chronic renal failure and in renal transplant recipients. British Med J. 1975; 4: 432- 434.

Martinez-Castelao A, Hueso M, Sanz V, et al. Treatment of hypertension after renal transplantation: Long-term efficacy of verapamil, enalapril, and doxazosin. Kidney Int. 1998; 68: S-130-S-134.

13

Handling of Fungal Infections in Patients with Chronic Immunosuppression Post Renal Transplant

Ewa Swoboda-Kopec, Irina Netsvyetayeva, Magdalena Sikora, Mariusz Jasik and Piotr Fiedor
Warsaw Medical University
Poland

1. Introduction

Invasive fungal infections (IFI) are serious diagnostics-therapeutic problem in recipients of vascularised organs. The nature of the IFI is determined by the type of the transplanted organ. Invasive candidiasis mostly occurs in liver recipients and invasive aspergilosis - in lung recipients. The greatest risk of IFI is in recipients of simultaneous lung and heart and liver transplants. Morbidity for IFI in the first year after transplantation is estimated to be in recipients of heart and lungs 8.6%, liver 4.7%, pancreas and kidneys 4% and heart 3.4%.

Incidents of IFI among kidney recipients is estimated by differed sources to lay between 0.01 - 1.5%. Although, IFI occur rarely in kidney recipients in comparison to recipients of other organs, invasive fungal infections carries a high risk of graft loss and high mortality in this population of patients. Among recipients which have developed an IFI the risk of graft loss was determined in approx. 50% of patients, and mortality in this group was approx. 15%. Yearly survival of patients after an episode of invasive aspergilosis is 59%, for mycosis caused by mould fungi from species other then *Aspergillus sp.* 61%, invasive candidosis 66%, cryptococcosis 73%. There is definitely a greater risk for recipients of kidneys collected from cadavers, compared to living donors related to the recipient, respectively 16.5% and 7.3%. Additionally in cases of a deceased donor there is a high transfer risk for yeast-like fungi colonising in the urinary tract of a terminal state patient, in result of the breakdown of the defensive mechanism and contamination of preservative fluids, to the uninfected recipient.

Mortality is determined by the virulence of the microorganism, localisation of the infection, weakened inflammatory response of the macroorganism, frequent co-occurring of renal insufficiency and diabetes and other predisposing factors. Unspecific clinical symptoms, fast progression of the disease and, what appears to be particularly important, lack of a precisely set algorithms of diagnostic procedure, contribute to the fact that IFI in kidney recipients are a diagnostics challenge and has a questionable therapeutic result.

1.1 Factors for fungal infections

Factors for fungoid infections:

- impairment of cellular resistance
- congenital genetic defects in phagocythosis, complement system

- use of immunosuppressants, cytostatics, broad spectrum antibiotics, corticosteroids
- interruption of tissue continuity (insertion of a needle into a vessel, diagnostic puncture)
- inflammatory disorders and functional in the gastrointestinal tract (favourable factors for translocation of fungi from the intestinal lumen)
- catheterization of the urinary bladder
- parenteral feeding
- dialysis therapy
- surgical procedures, particularly in the abdominal cavity
- tracheotomy, intubation, endoscopy
- blood transfusion
- tuberculosis
- metabolic disorders
- endocrinological disorders
- pregnancy
- extreme age groups
- nutritional factors (intake of food containing moulds - strains used in food production or contaminants).

Patients with final renal insufficiency qualified for the transplant procedure, despite the main illness, often have also at least a few of the risk factors described above, are part of the population particularly predisposed to developed an IFI. There is a very high risk of IFI occurrence in recipients which had consecutive kidney transplant procedures, recipients of a simultaneous pancreas and kidney transplant and highly immunised recipients, requiring induction of the immunosuppression with anti-thymocyte globulin.

1.2 The remaining infection risk factors

The remaining infection risk factors differ depending on the period after the kidney transplant.

1.2.1 Early period

Early period - 1 month after kidney transplant. Mostly infections are caused by yeast-like fungi: *Candida sp., Trichosporon sp., Saccharomyces sp.* Risk factors in this period are related to the used surgical technique, transfer of the fungal infection form the infected organ or preservative fluid or fungal colonization form a period before the transplant. Infection with mould fungi of the *Aspergillus* genus are rare and are related to the prolonged operation time or organ transport.

1.2.2 Interim period

Interim period - from 2 to 6 months. Among etiological factors, yeast-like fungi responsible for infections in the early period are predominant, as well as mixed fungoid-bacterial infections. The basic risk factor in this time is a weakened immunological response due to:

- infections and/or reactivation of immunomodulation viruses: CMV, HIV, EBV, HBV, HCV and other
- site effects of transplanted kidney rejection therapy, with high doses of corticosteroids or other cytotoxic lymphocyte inhibitors.

1.2.3 Late period

Late period - over 6 months. Relatively often occurring infection in this period is the cryptococcosis, often in scattered form. Other etiological factors for IFI are yeast-like fungi, mould fungi of the *Aspergillus* genus and others. In this period the level of basic immunosuppression is remained on a low level, which means that in cases without complications the state of the recipients immunological system is close to the state of the general population's. IFI episodes are sporadic and caused by an individual course of the post-transplantation period or individual predispositions:

- complications in previous periods in graft function - treatment of acute rejection episodes
- exceeding of drug level limits of the basic immunosuppression protocol in systemic fluids
- reactivation of infections with immunomodulation viruses
- environmental factors.

1.3 Difficulties due to lack of an effective strategy for mycological diagnostics

Difficulties due to a lack of an effective strategy for mycological diagnostics and often sparse clinical symptoms are the reason that important data for diagnosis of invasive mycosis on kidney recipients are undervalued. Statistics on mortality due to disseminated mycosis do not contain, also for reasons outlined here, all cases. Lack of specific symptoms indicating an early period of an IFI, or transition of colonization into an active infection, lack of criteria allowing differentiation of infections and colonisations and in result lack of precisely described evidence for implementation of preventive - therapeutic treatment. Also important is to decide - does every positive mycological result, obtained by classic diagnostic methods, mean an infection and the necessity to implement antimycotic therapy, and does every colonising strain cause systemic infections, also which genotype and phenotype can benefit this process.

Additionally the treatment of a developed invasive fungal infection carries a high risk for patients due to frequent interactions between antimycotics and immunosuppressants. Taking this into account, it appears to be of outmost importance to develop a diagnostics algorithm minimising the risk of IFI in kidney recipients, based on an active surveillance of particularly predisposed recipients.

2. Invasive systemic mycosis: aspergilosis

Invasive aspergilosis (IA) is an acute infection with a mortality rate of almost 70%. Mostly it occurs in recipient of allogeneic bone marrow from an unrelated recipient - 10.3%. Among organ recipients lung recipients (Lung Transplant) are at highest risk, with morbidity at 8.4%. Among heart recipients (Heart Transplant) morbidity for IA is estimated to be 6.2%, liver (Liver Transplant) -1.7%, pancreas (Pancreas Transplant) -1.3%. Morbidity in kidney recipients (Kidney Transplant) applies for 0.7% of patient population.

An etiological factor in more then 90% of cases is *Aspergillus fumigatus*. Another species of clinical importance are: *Aspergillus niger*, *Aspergillus flavus* and *Aspergillus terreus*. Different species participation is to be observed in external and middle ear aspergilosis, in most cases *Aspergillus flavus* and *Aspergillus niger* are responsible.

Aspergillus spores are now generally present in the environment. Etiology of *Aspergillus* infections are usually results of *Aspergillus* inhalation. The invasive form is the most severe form of infection. In the initial stage, spores infect the lungs (pulmonary aspergilosis), next they get into cardiovascular vessels and to other locations eg.: sinuses (nasal sinus aspergilosis), eyes, skin, kidneys, bones, central nervous system (CNS aspergilosis).

The most common clinical manifestation is lung aspergilosis - 75% of all IA cases, *rhinosinusitis* (infection of the nasal mucosa and nasal sinuses) - 5 - 10%, disseminated multiorgan - 25%, IA with an affected central nervous system makes out 10 - 40% of all cases.

IA Diagnostic: an early diagnostic is critical for an effective therapy, also to avoid the unnecessary administration of a costly and toxic antimycotic therapy.

Traditional methods: as a „golden standard" in the diagnostic of invasive aspergilosis until now, remains the cultivation of a strain from the sample clinical material and identification fungi fimbriae by histopathology.

Appropriate test materials are bronchalalveolar washings in case of pulmonary aspergilosis and sinus washings in *rhinosinusitis* with *Aspergillus* etiology. The value of a mycological rest of sputum is restricted by its low sensitivity and specificity, difficulties in obtaining enough material (lack of a productive cough in the treated patient) or a frequent lack of morphologic elements of fungi and spore. In cases when it is not possible to sample material with invasive methods, morning sputum should be sampled a few times, on consecutive days, with securing of the material from contamination.

A difficult to diagnose form of aspergilosis is the disseminated multiorgan form. In this case the probability to cultivate an etiological factor from blood is infinitesimal compared to disseminated infections caused by other microorganisms (yeast-like fungi and bacteria). In case of invasive aspergilosis with the seizure of central nervous system, cerebrospinal fluid and serum become materials of questionable significance, the only valuable diagnostically material in this case is biopsy material sampled from the lesion. Diagnostic in this case should be based on precise analysis of all available tests: exact evaluation of the interview data, subject test results, biochemical tests results, assessment of the inflammation exponents, and results of imaging tests. As supportive tests can be used: detection of galactomannan antigen and genetic fungi material in cerebrospinal fluid and in serum.

Validity of the mycological test depends on the correct performance of every stage. Material sampling should be assisted by a microbiology specialist or a specially trained physician. It is necessary to take an appropriate number of samples and to sample material on the right microbiological medium for cultivation and direct microscopic preparation. Microscopic testing of clinical material and the correct evaluation are an immensely important stage of the diagnostic, which should be taken into account at sampling: sample material with a sterile smear dampened in a sterile 0.9% NaCl solution, transport medium should not be used for this purposes.

Histopathology diagnostic value is particularly important due to a relatively short time of waiting for results, high sensitivity and possibility to obtain positive results in an ongoing antimycotic therapy and is based on detection of fungal fimbriae. This method is restricted by lack of microorganism identification possibility and antimycotics sensitivity assessment, which can be preformed only on the basis of mycological cultivation.

Microscopic tests or cultivation are a limited possibility to retain testing material, only invasive methods and is connected to long results awaiting period.

Biopsy can be dangerous in case of weakened patients.

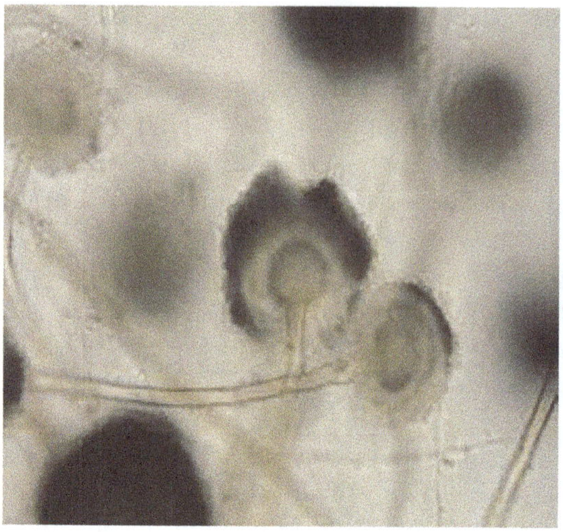

1

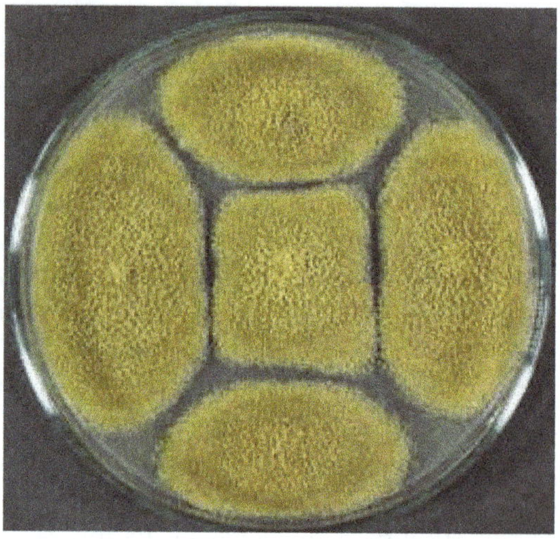

2

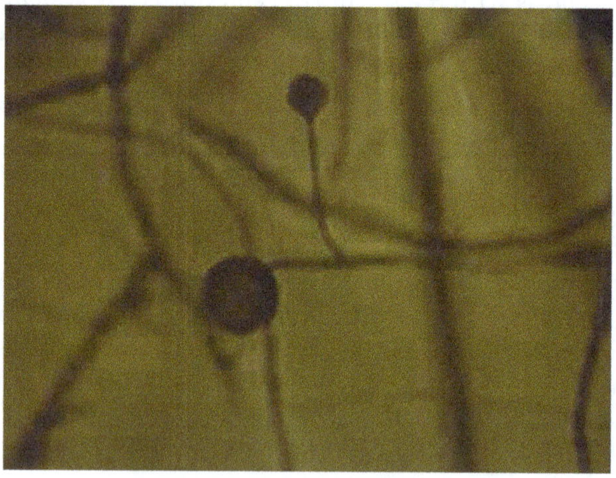

3

Fig. 1. *Aspergillus fumigatus:* **1** Microscopic slide (x400) Microscopic tests of expectoration or BAL, **2** Colonies on Sabouraud Agar. **3** *Mucor spp.* Microscopic sidle (x400).

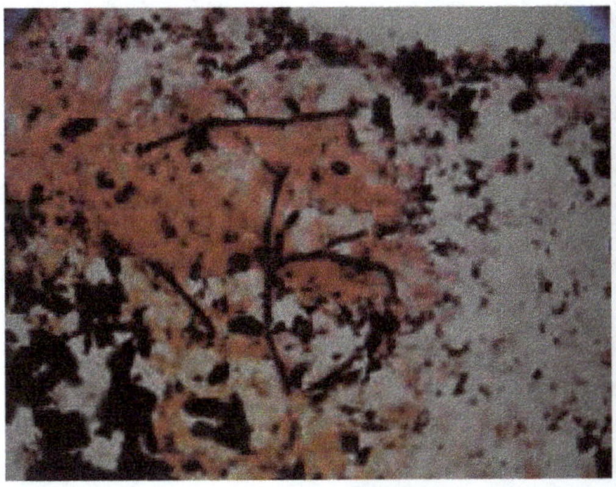

1

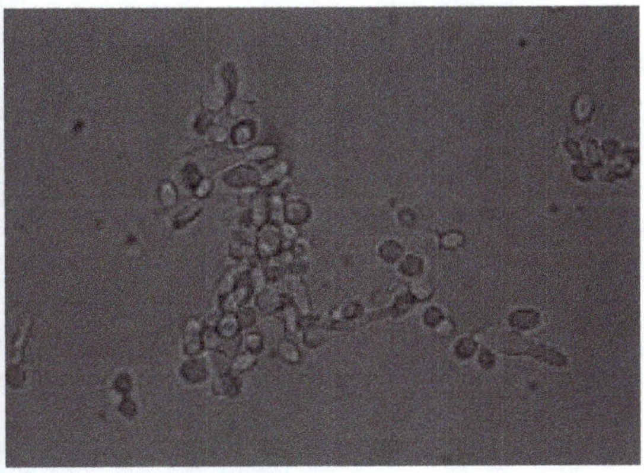

2

3

Fig. 2. **1** Invasive form of *Candida albicans* in blood (x1000), **2** *Trichosporon asahii*, microscopic slide (x400), **3** *Cryptococcus neoformans*. India Ink preparation (x400)

3. Infection with mould fungi other than Aspergillus supp. (non-Aspergillus mould infections): zygomycosis

Zygomycosis - is an invasive infection frequently with *Mucor spp., Rhizopus spp., Rhizomucor spp., Absidia spp.* fungi of the *Zygomycota* division. It has been noted in the past years that the number of zygomycosis in the general number of infections with mould fungi in a general population of recipients from 4% to 25% in the period between 2001 and 2003 has increased.
Mostly the infection will have a *sinusitis* form with a tendency to quickly spread to the central nervous system - *rhinocerebral* form. Additionally the following forms can be observed: pulmonary, cutaneous and subcutaneous tissue infection, renal, gastrointestinal tract and disseminated form, often diagnosed *post-mortem*.
Most important risk factors of this type of infection are: persisting acidosis caused by a badly monitored diabetes or renal insufficiency and immunosuppressive therapy, particularly in connection with chronic nasal sinus infection. In the organ recipients population as the most important risk factor was perceived a previous exposition to voriconazole therapy of a previous infection with yeast-like fungi or *Aspergillus spp*. Often

those are „infections with breaking-point" with strains belonging to species, which do not fall in the spectrum of this drug.
Cases of zygomycosis in kidney recipients population in industrialised countries are rarely documented, but in developing countries: India, Pakistan, and Iran - they are quite common. Also the trend of „transplant tourism" observed in the last years - travelling to „third world" countries for transplants due to economic reasons and greater availability of organs, while trivialising a great risk of complications.
Rejections of transplanted organs and infection complications are serious problems, which European doctors providing post-transplant care for patient in this group may have to face. Aspergilosis with mucormycosis are most common infection complications in patients who have practised this kind of „tourism".
The death rate in this group is estimated at 59%, and further 82% suffer from graft loss, or from a disseminated form of infection with an infection of the central nervous system. The diagnostic procedure for zygomycosis is norm for all mould fungi and has been described in the chapter in aspergilosis diagnostics.

4. Invasive yest-like fungi

4.1 Invasive candidiasis (IC)

The most important exponent of the invasive candidosis is candidemia - fourth in frequency etiological factor of in hospital blood infection (BSI): 6-10% of the total positive blood culture in hospitalised patients. In patients after vascularised organ transplantation, IC makes out 53% of all IFI.
Infections with yeast-like fungi occur in 5% of kidney recipients with a death rate between 30 - 70%. Most common forms of candidosis among kidney recipients are mucosa-cutaneous and oesophagus candidosis. Heavy complications endangering the survival of the transplant are urinary tract infections: *cystitis, pielonephritis* and *ureteral obstruction by Candida elements.*
In an early period it is often conditioned by a colonisation of yeast-like fungi in the insufficient kidney in a period before the transplant and presence of urinary catheters in a post operational period, the presence of which connected with a high level of immunosuppression makes the spreading of the colonisation to the membrane and an invasive infection easier. Also a very important mechanism of developing a urinary tract infection is the pathogen translocation form the intestinal lumen. In this case it is an endeogenic infection, but with the wrong medical care and hospital hygiene it can cause spreading of the yeast-like fungi from the exogenous source.
Urinary tract infections with occurrence of additional factors can lead to candidemia, spreading of the infection and vascular complications on the transplanted kidney. Invasion of yeast-like fungi to the vascular endothelium can lead to *arteritis* or aneurysms.
Complications can lead to graft loss or patients death. Other dangerous fungal infections are suprainfections of fluid vessels forming around the transplanted kidney, peritoneum infection and catheter fungemia.
The most important factor in invasive candidosis remains the species *Candida albicans but* there is an observed growing participation of non - albicans *Candida spp.* to which belong: *C. glabrata, C. tropicalis, C. parapsilosis.* This species are characterised by being more drug resistant compared to *C. albicans.* The species *C. glabrata* shows a natural lower sensitivity to Fluconazole, and *C. parapsilosis* - to echinocandin.

One of the reasons for a larger participation of species of non - albicans *Candida* spp. possibly can be related to the wide use of prophylactic antifungal drugs. *C. parapsilosis* is characterised by a larger adhesion ability and the ability to produce a biofilm on the surface of biopolymers, including vascular catheters, which often is related to spreading of microorganisms colonised in the catheter into the system.

Widely used fluconazole prophylactic can also be one of the reasons for a larger participation of the *Trichosporon* species as a etiological factor for IFI. *Trichosporon* spp. is not the most important etiological factor for fungal infections in immunocompetent patients.

It can be a reason for an invasive mycoses in patients after vascularised organ transplant, with a high death rate. *Trichosporon* spp. is a yeast-like fungi generally occurring in nature.

Trichosporon asahii mostly is connected with surface infections such as white piedra, skin and nails mycoses in immunocompetent patients. Among the species of *Trichosporon T. asahii* is the main reason for deep invasive infections in patients treated with immunosuppressants.

The most important factor predisposing for this kind of infections are renal insufficiency, phagocytolic disability and neutropenia. Mortality in result of infections with *Trichosporon* fungi is estimated to be 80-100%, which can be related to the late diagnosis of the etiologic factor, wrong treatment and lack of correlation between the efficacy of treatment and sensitivity of the strain *in vitro*.

Additionally one of the characteristics of this species, which makes the prognosis of the course of the infection pessimistic is the variable sensitivity to amphotericin B. It can enable the strain *Trichosporon asahii* to produce biofilm.

4.2 Diagnostics of yeast-like infections

Clinical symptoms of IFI in kidney recipients are sparse and lack specificity, which makes a quick diagnosis difficult and effects efficacy of treatment and the predictions.

Classic mycological diagnostic methods: microscopic tests, culture of clinical material, identification of biochemical strain of pathogen, testing of drug resistance remain standard diagnostics. Those methods are without doubt very important in most cases and allow to implement a target treatment including a minimal inhibitory concentration of specific antifungal drugs to the etiological factor IFI.

It has to be stressed that sensitivity and specificity of the classic mycological diagnostic method are insufficient to be used as a single element for the confirmation of IFI diagnostic.

An additional problem is the often occurring mucocutaneous colonization, which causes result interpretation difficulties - not every positive result for the mycological culture allows to implement an antifungal therapy and not every negative result of the culture excludes an invasive infection.

Sparse symptoms of a systemic infection and the difficulties in a quick mycological diagnosis are reasons for delays in implementing of an appropriate antifungal therapy, which can result in the loss of the graft and even the death of the patient.

The problem to identify the participation of the infection appears interesting, also in those caused by fungi in organ rejection.

The „golden standard" in diagnostic of invasive candidosis in patients in high risk groups remains blood cultivation, which has serious restrictions. The most important are:

- low sensitivity: approx. 50% of results in patients with a confirmed or possible IC can be a false negative
- long result waiting time: in most case the waiting time is longer then 2 up to 3 days, in patients receiving antifungal drugs even 14 days.

Developed are also other criteria allowing a rather quick identification, if the active monitoring strategy of the patients state has been adjusted to the mycological diagnostic. One of this criteria is determining if the yeast-like fungi in culture of clinical material is received from one or more parts of the body.

Diagnostic of the invasive candidosis leading to the implementation of the appropriate antifungal treatment consists of clinical, radiological and microbiological tests results.

4.3 Cryptococcosis

To the *Cryptococcus* belong 37 species. The most important pathogenic species for humans is *Cryptococcus neoformans* widely spread in nature globally.

Infection vectors are birds, mostly pigeons, infection sources are also soil particles containing bird faeces contaminated with the fungi, and the most common infection mechanism is inhalation.

A specific characteristic of the yeast-like fungi from the *Cryptococcus* species, used in diagnostic routine is a lack of a polysaccharide capsule with an antiphagocytic function.

Cryptococcosis is an opportunistic infection in patients with immunological defects, it is known as an indicative illness for AIDS. The primary infection localisation are the lower airway, from which it quickly spreads to the lungs and the CNS.

The most dangerous clinical form of cryptococcosis is menigoencephalitis, other clinical forms: chronic or acute pulmonary form or disseminated in relation to the CNS, skin and other tissue and organs. After the pulmonary stage and spreading to the CNS, in the blood serum and PMR rapidly appear dissolving capsule antigens, possible to detect with enzyme immunoassay methods.

The cryptococcosis diagnostic is based on:

- microscopic determination of yeast cells with a polysaccharide capsule in cerebrospinal fluid
- microbiological cultivation of *C. neoformans* from blood or cerebrospinal fluid. The waiting time for results of this test is longer then in case of diagnostic of fungal infections with *Candida* due to a longer incubation time and can take even up to 7 days.

Detection of capsule antigens *Cryptococcus spp.* in serum or cerebrospinal fluid. Sensitivity of the method increases the parallel marking of antigens in serum and PMR.

Diagnosis of cryptococcosis can be determined only based on joined results of clinical, radiological and microbiological tests, (microbiology, histology, serology), each of those elements should be carefully considered.

4.4 Serological diagnostic

The current use of serological diagnostic is based on the detection of specific fungi species – mannoproteins, which have the role pf antigen markers. In the period of sustained systemic fungal infection, those antigens occur in the blood stream temporarily, are easily eliminated by the formed immunological complexes and by way of endocytosis through the Kupffer cells in the liver. Regular monitoring of their presence in systemic fluids has a great practical value in high risk patients.

In diagnostics of invasive aspergilosis (IA) detection of the galactomannan (GM) antigen in the blood stream is valuable (GM). GM is a polysaccharide of the vascular wall of mould fungi belonging to the *Aspergillus* species *(A. fumigatus, A. flavus, A. niger, A.terreus* and other).

A positive test result for *Aspergillus* is one of the microbiological criteria recommended by the *European Organization for Research and Treatment of Cancer* and the *Mycosis Study Group (EORTC/MSG)* to determine IA, despite negative results in classic mycological tests in patients with haematological neoplasm.

Using of similar criteria seams to be justified for diagnosis of IA in vascularised organ recipients, including kidneys. For the purpose of maximising test sensitivity it should be performed at least once a week for patients in the high risk group.

For al patients with a positive result it is recommended to repeat the test with anew blood sample.

According to the *EORTC/MSG* criteria two consecutive positive results are necessary to classify the test as a real positive.

GM detection sensitivity depends on the infection localisation. In the localised invasive pulmonary aspergilosis the sensitivity of the method is significantly lower compared to the disseminated form. Monitoring of GM levels can be useful in infection course prognosis - a drop of the levels can be connected to good prognosis.

IC serodiagnostic (invasive candidosis) is based on the detection of mannan antigen circulating in serum, which is the main component of the cellular wall of a *Candida species fungi*. Mannan is a highly immunogenic polysaccharide antigen with immunomodular characteristics. It allows to use in IC diagnostics parallel monitoring of circulating mannan and titre of antimannan antibodies.

Parallel detection of both markers allowed to increase the sensitivity to 80% and to 93% the specificity of the method. Detection of circulating *Candida spp.* antigen in serum or plasma should enhance IC diagnostic in high risk patients regarding to sensitivity and detection time of infection development. Among *Candida* antigens, mannan which is the main component oft he cellular wall of yeast-like fungi from *Candida* species, appears to be one of the most important biomarkers in the diagnostic of invasive candidosis.

Regular testing of IC high risk patients, connecting the detection of mannan antigen is helpful in diagnostic of invasive candidosis.

The usefulness of testing levels of antibodies in patients treated with immunosuppressants is controversial, but in the period of graft stability in patients without additional problems can be helpful, as long as parallel marking of mannan antigen is performed.

It should be kept in mind that the highest sensitivity is proved in IC diagnostic for *C.albicans, C.glabrata, C.tropicalis* etiology. The lowest sensitivity of mannan detection and mannan antibodies, 40-50% applies for infections with *C.krusei, C.parapsilosis, C.quilliermondii* etiology.

Beta-glucan detection methods in serum (Fungitell-Associates of Cape Cod) proposed as marker in IC diagnostic has many gaps, a positive result does not allow to determine a fungal etiological factor, allows only to differentiate between a fungal and bacterial infection. Additionally the test has a low specificity and a high cost of marking and expensive equipment means that it is rarely used in routine diagnostic.

4.5 Molecular biology methods

Development of molecular techniques, which took place in past years allowed to introduce routine microbiological diagnostic to the tests based on detection of nucleic acids of microorganisms.

In mycological diagnostic genetic methods are used for microorganism detection in material sampled from patients, as well as identification of specific species in this material. It has to be underlines that they should be used as complimentary to the classic tests protocol or as a confirmation of its results.

Molecular methods should not be used instead of classic diagnostic techniques.

Their application with great success serve in diagnostic of infections difficult to detect with conventional cultivation methods.

Most tests are restricted to detecting of frequently occurring and consequently the most important clinically species, which are factors in general infection such as *Aspergillus fumigatus* or *Candida albicans*.

Although lately molecular identification tests are introduced for a wider group of fungal pathogens.

They have been developed for detection of some of the species *Aspergillus*: *A. flavus*, *A. niger*, *A. versicolor*, *A. terreus* and *A. nidulans* as well as etiological factors for zygomycosis isolated from clinical materials sampled from patients with a general infection.

In case of detection of ethological infections with yeast-like fungi, the newest application of molecular tests are for pathogens from the non-albicans group *Candida spp.*: *C. glabrata*, *C. tropicalis*, *C. parapsilosis*, *C. krusei*, species with an undeniable clinical expansion in recent years.

Detection methods in use are usually based on techniques which are modifications of the standard reaction PCR: real- time PCR, nested PCR, multiplex PCR to detect the ribosome gens RNA: 18s rRNA, 28s rRNA or regions ITS1 and ITS2.

Real-time reaction PCR is characterised by a fast analysis and does not require an electrophoretic test of products.

The reaction is based on the standard PCR method, allows a fast identification and quantitative assessment of the pathogen in a clinical sample. Nested PCR is a modified standard reaction in which two pairs of starters are being used: outer and inner , with different melting temperatures. The product received with outer starters becomes a live matrix for reaction with inner starters. The product received in the first stage - DNA fragment with a sequence specific for microorganisms in the second reaction stage is classified to the searched for species.

Multiplex PCR method differs from the classic method only slightly.

The reaction is performed in the same way, but with a use of more then one pair of starters with a similar melting temperature, which allows to detect more then one pathogen present in the clinical sample.

The choice of material for genetic testing is based on the localization of the infection.

In case of general infections, it is recommended to perform full blood tests on the patient, from which the DNA will be extracted in search of the pathogen.

Currently more often, particularly in mycosis diagnostics, applications are being used which do not allow for diagnostic in Rother clinical material:

- tissue biopsy,
- cerebrospinal fluid and Rother systemic fluids,
- bronchial washings (BAL),
- expectoration,
- tracheal aspiration.

Methods based on molecular techniques are characterised by higher sensitivity and specificity then classic cultivation.

It is estimated that real-time PCR sensitivity for *Candida* has 81-100% sensitivity and specificity from 97 to 86%.

While using the nested PCR method for *Candida* the reaction sensitivity can achieve 86-79%, and specificity 54%. Sensitivity in multiplex PCR is 98% with specificity of 88%.

Specificity and sensitivity in real-time PCR for *Aspergillus fumigatus* oscillates around 100% and depends on the amount of material sampled for testing.
Despite a sorter time needed for the performance of diagnostics, and in result of the waiting time for results, molecular methods hale some restrictions.
The first is the cost of testing, surely higher then in case of classic methods.
Another is a lack of possibility to determine sensitivity spectrum for antimycotics.
It is necessary to perform his test with the classic method.
It should be stressed that the possibilities of use for molecular testing is restricted to detection and identification of pathogens most frequently occurring in clinical material with the exception of the rare ones, which often cause serious infections.

5. Diagnostics algorithm for general fungal infection risk

5.1 Diagnostics algorithm for general fungal infection risk minimization in patients after kidney allotransplantation

In result of many years of observation of a 1301 kidney recipients from cadavers and/or a related donor (including 213 with diagnosed diabetes) a scheme of diagnostic procedure Has been developed, for timely diagnostic of fungal infection, differentiation from colonization with opportunistic fungi strains.
Influence of the fungal infections on an early and late function of the transplant has been analyzed and an algorithm has been developed for diagnostic procedure minimizing the risk general fungal infections in patients after a kidney allotransplantation.
For most patients a 3-drug immunosuppressive protocol has been used: Cyclosporine A (CsA) or tacrolimus (FK) with glucocorticosteroids (GS), with antiproliferative preparations: mycophenolate mofetil (MMF) or azathioprine (AZA), some of the patients received an immunosuppression induction with biological agents (ATG, OKT3).

5.2 An algorithm for an effective diagnostic procedure minimizing the risk of general fungal infections in kidney recipients

An algorithm for an effective diagnostic procedure minimizing the risk of general fungal infections in kidney recipients should include:

- strategy for a quick diagnostic of systemic mycosis in case of justified suspicion of such infection
- tactic of routine diagnostic minimizing the risk of developing a fungal infection in the general population of kidney recipients
- strict criteria for choosing of recipients from the high risk group for fungal
- programs for active monitoring of recipients from the high risk group.

5.3 Strategy for a quick diagnostic of systemic mycosis in case of justified suspicion

The diagnostic procedure should be based on all available testing methods: clinical, radiological, histological, classic microbiology diagnostic, serological methods, and molecular biology. It should be underlined that every diagnostic method has serious restrictions, the decision about the necessary implementation of a antifungal therapy should be based on the interpretation of a number of tests. The basic and crucial element of each of the schemes outlined above remains cultivation of etiological factor IFI from materials sampled from the patient: blood and other systemic fluids, biopsy materials, materials from lower airways, urine, smears from the oral cavity, throat, rectum and other parts, faeces and other materials sampled from the patient, regarding to the clinical situation at hand.

Microbiological criteria for diagnosis of general mycosis are:

- positive results for blood cultures and other physiologically sterile body cavities
- determination of fungi presence in the direct preparation from the tested material
- identification of antigens circulating by serological methods
- identification of genetic fungal material in clinical samples from usually sterile parts
- identification of specific antibodies
- determination of specific fungal enzymes in urine or other systemic fluids
- determination of morphological elements of the fungi in tissues sampled by biopsy.

Differentiation of colonization from infection:

- simultaneous cultivation of strains of the same species from different sampling locations (at least three)
- multiple cultivation of strains of the same species from one sampling location
- simultaneous occurrence of fungal antigens in serum or other naturally sterile systemic fluids
- significant (at least 4 times) of the antibodies titre in serum
- occurrence of hydrolytic enzymes specific for a species in systemic fluids.

The proposal of a procedure in cases of suspected invasive fungal infections scheme is presented in figure 3.

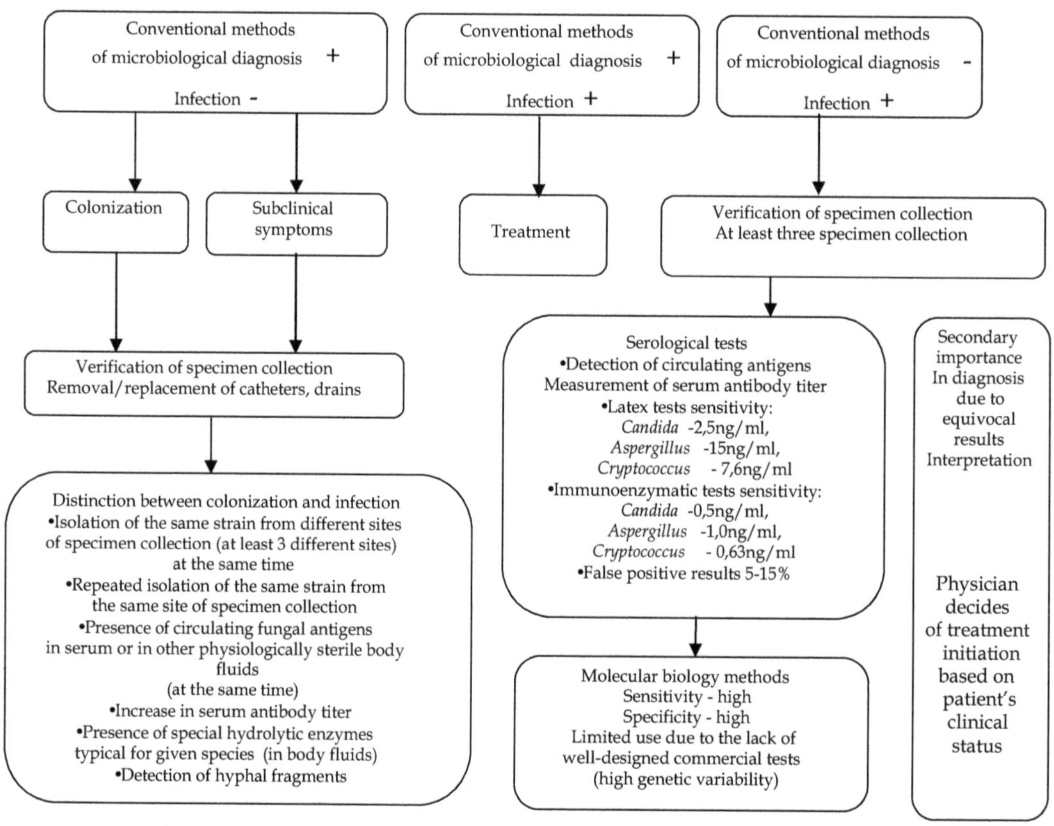

Fig. 3. Diagnostic algorithm for prevention of invasive fungal infection in solid organ transplant recipients.

5.4 Routine diagnostic tactic for minimizing risk of fungal infection in kidney recipients without risk factors disorders

Kidney recipients without additional risk factors should be monitored for a surviving skin, mucosa, urinogenital tract colonization with a classic microbiological method. Proposed is a regular cultivations for fungi in urine, oral cavity smears and qualitative diagnosis of yeast-like fungi present in the gastrointestinal tract.

Frequency of cultivations depends on the period after the Tx. In an early period it is justified to sample materials for microbiological testing not less then once every 5-7 days. In the second period once every 2-3 weeks. In the third - once every 1-2 months.

5.5 Strategy of diagnostics-prophylactic procedure minimizing the risk of a systemic fungal infection in kidney recipients with a specific predisposition

A more aggressive scheme should be applied in cases of additional risk factors for a general fungal infection.

In the early period after Tx, presence factors determined before Tx are very important:

- skin and mucosa colonization by yeast-like or mould fungi
- immunosuppression induction with biological agents in highly immunized patients
- therapy with broad-spectrum antibacterial agents
- blood transfusions
- a particularly important risk is a possibility of colonizing factor or causing a fungal infection in donor transmission from donor-recipient, especially in a diseased donor . To exclude such risk factors it is necessary to perform blood and urine cultivation for fungi
- contamination of preservative fluids with fungi
- risk factors occurring in the early period after Tx:
- skin and mucosa colonization with strains of yeast-like fungi
- bacterial infections
- another kidney transplantation
- acute insufficiency of the transplanted kidney
- repeated surgery due to early postoperative complications
- prolonged transplantation time
- treatment of acute transplant rejection with high doses of steroids or biological agents
- elevated levels of the basic immunosuppressive scheme

Risk factors in the second period after Tx:

- skin or mucosa colonization with yeast-like fungi strains
- treatment of acute transplant rejection with high doses of steroids or biological agents
- infection or reactivation of infections with immunomodulatory viruses: CMV, HHV, EBV
- leukopenia, hypogammaglobulinemia
- repeated bacterial infection
- long-term antibiotics therapy

Risk factors in the third period after Tx:

- skin or mucosa colonization with yeast-like fungi strains
- treatment of acute transplant rejection with high doses of steroids or biological agents
- infection or reactivation of infections with immunomodulatory viruses: CMV, HHV, EBV

- leukopenia, hypogammaglobulinemia
- repeated bacterial infection
- long-term antibiotics therapy
- chronic nephropathy of the transplanted kidney
- treatment of neoplastic diseases.

With the co-occurrence of two or more risk factors it a broader routine procedure, based on classic mycological diagnostic methods needs to be considered.

Together with performing cultivation of clinical samples for fungi on a regular basis, we recommend regular, weekly mannan, galactomannan and glucuronoxylomannan antigen marking, in serum with immunoenzyme method.

5.6 Therapeutic-prophylactic procedure - conclusions

Implementation of a therapeutic procedure, as far as it is possible, should each time be procedure by the identification of the etiological factor of the fungi infection species, taking into account natural resistance or a naturally lowered sensitivity to antimycotic substances.

In 7744 microbiological test of material sampled from kidney recipients, positive cultivation for fungi were received in 475 samples (6.13%). Fungi strains causing infections in his group of recipients belong mostly to the *non-albicans Candida spp.*, in which a large group are strains with a diversified sensitivity to antimycotics. *Candida albicans* was isolated only in 38.1%, where recently we domination of his species in vascularized organs recipients has been observed.

The participation of species which have replaced *C. albicans* is concerning, selected by an irrational treatment of prophylactic. Those are the strains with a restricted sensitivity to the available antimycotics, mostly from the azole group, resistant to flukonazole, namely: *C. glabrata, C. krusei, C. kefyr, C. inconspicua, Trichosporon asahi.* It has been proven that species with a natural resistance or natural sensitivity to flukonazole - *C. glabrata* and *C.krusei* make up for 40%. The acquired resistance to flukonazole has been observed in 5.27% of strains. Clinical material from which the fungi hale been cultivated, were sampled mostly from the urinary and respiratory tract, then from drainage and postoperative wounds and blood. Fungemia were caused only by strains belonging to the *non-albicans Candida spp.*

From literature and our own data appears that the popular use of flukonazole in antifungal prophylactic caused a negative selection of resistant strains. In this period it has also an increased rate of deaths due to general fungal infections with the genus *Aspergillus* has been observed.

Antifungal infection prophylactic can not be used commonly, but only in clinically justified cases, and prophylactic should be even given up, on behalf of active monitoring of recipients and progressive therapy. In this cases an implementation of drugs other then flukonazole or amphotericin B, Itrakonazole, Posaconazole should be considered. In prophylactic the toxicity of the preparations and resulting growing resistance should be considered.

Empirical therapy. In cases of suspected invasive fungal infection based on clinical evidence the appropriate drug would be amphotericin B or its liposomal forms and Itraconazole and new azoles - Voriconazole, Posaconazole as well as caspofungin. Flukonazole can be used only in large doses only in wards, where natural species resistant to flukonazole occur rarely and no prophylactic product has been used.

Treatment of diagnosed mycosis. In confirmed cases of systemic mycosis, the drug used should take into account the sensitivity to the drug of the isolated strain with a marked MIC (minimal inhibitory concentration). The dose should be calculated for each patient individually based on the MIC value. In severe cases it is possible to use a joined treatment. The length of the treatment depends on the clinical state of the patient, it usually takes a few weeks. Postoperative complications requiring a new operation bear a high risk of a fungal infection.

Due to this it appears justified to begin antimycotic treatment from the start of a repeated surgery and to perform an earlier decontamination of the gastrointestinal tract from fungal flora.

Relatively new group of antimycotic drugs are echinocandins. To this group belong: caspofungin, anidulafungin, micafungin. The mechanism of echinocandins is based on the inhibition of the polysaccharide glucan synthesis (1-3β-D-glucan), which is one of the main components of the fungi cellular wall.

Diminishing the concentration of the glucan in the cellular wall leads to changes in the permeability of the membrane and its osmotic instability, which eventually leads to cell lysis. Echinocandins can be only administered intravenously due to very low bioavailability in oral administration.

In adult patients the pharmacodynamic of those drugs is similar - all of them are used intravenously in one daily dose. They are eliminated from the organism by way of a non-enzymatic decomposition All echinocandins do not require dose modifications in case of renal insufficiency and renal replacement therapy.

Caspofungin and micafungin are metabolized in a small way in the liver, but without the cytochrome P450 superfamily enzymes. Caspofungin is the only echinocandins which requires a diminished dose in cases of moderate or severe liver insufficiency.

Echinocandins due to their mechanism are effective for fungi of the *Candida* and *Aspergillus* species similar to classic and lipid forms of amphotericin B. In a multiple site, randomised double blind a similar efficacy of caspofungin therapy with liposomal amphotericin B in treatment of fungal infection of the oesophagus in adults has been confirmed. Caspofungin has been better tolerated by the patients.

According to the IDSA 2009 guideline echinocandins are recommended as first choice drugs in fungemia treatment, particularly caused by *C. glabrata* strains in patients with neutropenia and previously treated with antimycotics from the azoles group. In the population of patients without neutropenia echinocandins are recommended as alternative therapy. Particularly justified is the use of echinocandins in case of fungemia due to their unique ability to penetrate the biofilm environment and to inhibit outer-cellular matrix composition production. This characteristics of echinocandins can have great significance in the inhibition of pathomechanisms in fungemia

Echinocandins also find use in therapy of infections with mould fungi treatment, mostly those belonging to the *Aspergillus* species, though it is restricted due to fungistatic effect of echinocandins on this type of microorganisms.

Caspofungin is recommended in treatment of invasive cadidosis and invasive aspergillosis in patients who hale previously not responded to therapy or intolerant to other antifungal drugs.

Anidulafungin approved by the FDA for treatment of esophagus candidosis, candidemia and other complications of infections with *Candida spp.* It Has been proved in clinical studies that anidulafungin has higher efficacy compared to flukonazole in patients with invasive candidosis and fungemia.

Micafungin is recommended in treatment of invasive cadidosis, for treatment of esophagus candidosis, prophylactic of infections caused by *Candida spp.* in patients with allogenic blood stem cells transplants. An important advantage of micafungin is its small potential for drug interactions. This applies for immunosuppressants: cyclosporine A, tacrolimus, mycophenolate mofetil. With a simultaneous treatment with sirolimus, Itraconazole or nifedipine with micafungin the patent should be monitored for toxic effects and if necessary the dose should be decreased. Lately reports of clinical efficacy of micafungin in treatment of infections caused by appear more frequently *non-albicans Candida species* and *Aspergillus spp.* In patients with immunological insufficiency or without.

6. Conflict of interest

The authors declare that there is no conflict of interest.

7. References

Albano, L.; Bretagne, S.; Mamzer-Bruneel, M.F.; Kacso, I.; Desnos-Ollivier, M.; Guerrini, P.; Le Luong, T.; Cassuto, E.; Dromer, F.; Lortholary, O.; French Mycosis Study Group. Evidence that graft-site candidiasis after kidney transplantation is acquired during organ recovery: a multicenter study in France. *Clin Infect Dis,* Vol.48, No.2, (January 2009), pp. 194-202, ISSN 1058-4838.

Arendrup, M.C.; Bergmann, O.J.; Larsson, L.; Nielsen, H.V.; Jarløv, J.O.; Christensson, B. (2009). Detection of candidaemia in patients with and without underlying haematological disease. *Clin Microbiol Infect,* Vol.16, No.7, (July 2010), pp. 855-862, ISSN 1198-743X.

Ascioglu, S.; Rex, J.H.; de Pauw, B.; Bennett, J.E.; Bille, J.; Crokaert, F.; Denning, D.W.; Donnelly, J.P.; Edwards, J.E.; Erjavec, Z.; Fiere, D.; Lortholary, O.; Maertens, J.; Meis, J.F.; Patterson, T.F.; Ritter, J.; Selleslag, D.; Shah, P.M.; Stevens, D.A.; Walsh, T.J. Invasive Fungal Infections Cooperative Group of the European Organization for Research and Treatment of Cancer; Mycoses Study Group of the National Institute of Allergy and Infectious Diseases. (2001). Defining opportunistic invasive fungal infections in immunocompromised patients with cancer and hematopoietic stem cell transplants: an international consensus. *Clin Infect Dis,* Vol.34, No.1, (January 2002), pp. 7-14, ISSN 1058-4838.

Badiee, P.; Kordbacheh, P.; Alborzi, A.; Zeini, F.; Mirhendy, H.; Mahmoody, M. Fungal infections in solid organ recipients. *Exp Clin Transplant,* Vol.3, No.2, (December 2005), pp. 385-389, ISSN 1304-0855.

Clancy, C.J.; Jaber, R.A.; Leather, H.L.; Wingard, J.R.; Staley, B.; Wheat, L.J.; Cline, C.L.; Rand, K.H.; Schain, D.; Baz, M.; Nguyen, M.H. (2007). Bronchoalveolar lavage galactomannan in diagnosis of invasive pulmonary aspergillosis among solid-organ transplant recipients. *J Clin Microbiol,* Vol.45, No.6, (June 2007), pp. 1759-1765, ISSN 0095-1137.

Denning, D.W, .; Kibbler, C.C.; Barnes, R.A; British Society for Medical Mycology. British Society for Medical Mycology proposed standards of care for patients with invasive fungal infections. *Lancet Infect Dis,* Vol.3, No.4, (April 2003), pp. 230-240, ISSN 1473-3099.

Erjavec, Z.; Verweij, P.E. Recent progress in the diagnosis of fungal infections in the immunocompromised host. *Drug Resist Updat,* Vol.5, No.1, (February 2002), pp. 3-10, ISSN 1368-7646.

Holzheimer, R.G.; Dralle, H. Management of mycoses in surgical patients - review of the literature. *Eur J Med Res,* Vol.7, No.5, (May 2002), pp. 200-226, ISSN 0949-2321.

Jiménez, C.; Lumbreras, C.; Aguado, J,M.; Loinaz, C.; Paseiro, G.; Andrés, A.; Morales, J.M.; Sánchez, G.; García, I.; del Palacio, A.; Moreno, E. Successful treatment of mucor infection after liver or pancreas-kidney transplantation. *Transplantation,* Vol. 73, No.3, (February 2002), pp. 476-480, ISSN 0041-1337.

Khlif, M.; Mary, C.; Sellami, H.; Sellami, A.; Dumon, H.; Ayadi, A.; Ranque, S. (2009). Evaluation of nested and real-time PCR assays in the diagnosis of candidaemia. *Clin Microbiol Infect,* Vol.15, No.7, (July 2009), pp. 656-661, ISSN 1469-0691.

Kingspor, L.; Jalal, S. Molecular detection and identification of *Candida* and *Aspergillus* spp. from clinical samples using real-time PCR. *Clin Microbiol Infect,* Vol.12, No.8, (August 2006), pp. 745-753, ISSN 1198-743X.

Magill, S.S.; Swoboda, S.M.; Shields, C.E.; Colantuoni, E.A.; Fothergill, A.W.; Merz, W.G.; Lipsett, P.A.; Hendrix, C.W. The epidemiology of Candida colonization and invasive candidiasis in a surgical intensive care unit where fluconazole prophylaxis is utilized: follow-up to a randomized clinical trial. *Ann Surg,* No.249, Vol.4, (April 2009), pp. 657-665, ISSN 0003-4932.

Matignon, M.; Botterel, F.; Audard, V.; Dunogue, B.; Dahan, K.; Lang, P.; Bretagne, S.; Grimbert, P. Outcome of renal transplantation in eight patients with Candida sp. contamination of preservation fluid. *Am J Transplant,* No.8, Vol.3, (March 2008), pp. 697-700, ISSN 1600-6135.

Netsvyetayeva, I.; Swoboda-Kopec, E.; Sikora, M.; Jaworska-Zaremba, M.; Blachnio, S.; Łuczak, M. (2008). *Trichosporon asahii* as a prospective pathogen in solid organ transplant recipients. *Mycoses,* Vol.52, No.3, (May 2009), pp. 263-265, ISSN 0933-7407.

Nucci, M.; Marr, K.A. (2005). Emerging fungal diseases. *Clin Infect Dis,* Vol.41, No.4, (August 2005), pp. 521-526, ISSN 1058-4838.

Nucci, M.; Anaissie, E. Fungal infections in hematopoietic stem cell transplantation and solid-organ transplantation--focus on aspergillosis. *Clin Chest Med,* Vol.30, No.2, (June 2009), pp. 295-306, ISSN 0272-5231.

Pappas, P.G.; Alexander, B.D.; Andes, D.R.; Hadley, S.; Kauffman, C.A.; Freifeld, A.; Anaissie, E.J.; Brumble, L.M, .; Herwaldt, L.; Ito, J.; Kontoyiannis, D.P.; Lyon, G.M.; Marr, K.A.; Morrison, V.A.; Park, B.J.; Patterson, T.F.; Perl, T.M.; Oster, R.A.; Schuster, M.G.; Walker, R.; Walsh, T.J.; Wannemuehler, K.A.; Chiller, T.M. Invasive fungal infections among organ transplant recipients: results of the Transplant-

Associated Infection Surveillance Network (TRANSNET). *Clin Infect Dis,* Vol.50, No.8, (April 2010), pp. 1101-1111, ISSN 1058-4838.

Rüping, M.J.; Vehreschild, J.J.; Cornely, O.A. Patients at high risk of invasive fungal infections: when and how to treat. *Drugs,* Vol.68, No.14, (October 2008), pp. 1941-1962, ISSN 0012-6667.

Schabereiter-Gurtner, C.; Selitsch, B.; Rotter, M.L. Hirschl, A.M.; Wilinger, B. (2007). Development of Novel Real-Time PCR Assay for Detection and Differentiation of Eleven Medically Important Aspergillus and Candida Species in Clinical Specimens *J. Clin. Microbiol,* Vol.45, No.3, (March 2007), pp. 906-914, ISSN 0095-1137.

Sendid, B.; Tabouret, M.; Poirot, J.L.; Mathieu, D.; Fruit, J.; Poulain, D. New enzyme immunoassays for sensitive detection of circulating Candida albicans mannan and antimannan antibodies: useful combined test for diagnosis of systemic candidiasis. *J Clin Microbiol,* Vol.37, No.5, (May 1999), pp. 1510-1517, ISSN 0095-1137.

Sendid, B.; Caillot, D.; Baccouch-Humbert, B.; Klingspor, L.; Grandjean, M.; Bonnin, A.; Poulain, D. (2008). Contribution of the Platelia Candida-specific antibody and antigen tests to early diagnosis of systemic Candida tropicalis infection in neutropenic adults. *J Clin Microbiol,* Vol.41, No.10, (October 2008), pp. 4551-4558, ISSN 0095-1137.

Suarez, F.; Lortholary, O.; Buland, S.; Rubio, M.T.; Ghez, D.; Mahe, V.; Quesne, G.; Poiree, S.; Buzyn, A.; Varet, B.; Berche, P.; Bougnoux, M.E. (2008). Detection of Circulating Aspergillus fumigatus DNA by Real-Time PCR Assay of Large Volumes Improves Early Diagnosis of Invasive Aspergillosis in High- Risk Adult Patients under Hematologic Surveillance. *J Cli. Microbiol,* Vol.46, No.11, (November 2008), pp. 3772-3777, ISSN 0095-1137.

Swoboda-Kopec, E.; Netsvyetayeva, I.; Paczek, L.; Dabkowska, M.; Kwiatkowski, A.; Jaworska-Zaremba, M.; Mierzwinska-Nastalska, E.; Sikora, M.; Blachnio, S.; Mlynarczyk, G.; Fiedor, P. Algorithm of clinical protocol lowering the risk of systemic mycosis infections in allografts recipients. *Transplant Proc,* Vol.41, No.8, (October 2009), pp. 3264-3266, ISSN 0041-1345.

Tortorano, A.M.; Peman, J.; Bernhardt, H.; Klingspor, L.; Kibbler, C.C.; Faure, O.; Biraghi, E.; Canton, E.; Zimmermann, K.; Seaton, S.; Grillot, R.; ECMM Working Group on Candidaemia. (2004). Epidemiology of candidaemia in Europe: results of 28-month European Confederation of Medical Mycology (ECMM) hospital-based surveillance study. *Eur J Clin Microbiol Infect Dis,* Vol.23, No.4, (April 2004), pp. 317-322, ISSN 0934-9723.

White, P.L.; Archer, A.E.; Barnes, RA. Comparison of non-culture-based methods for detection of systemic fungal infections, with an emphasis on invasive Candida infections. *J Clin Microbiol,* Vol.43, No.5, (May 2005), pp. 2181-2187. ISSN 0095-1137.

Verduyn Lunel, F.M.; Donnelly, J.P.; van der Lee, H.A.; Blijlevens, N.M.; Verweij, P.E. (2009). Circulating Candida-specific anti-mannan antibodies precede invasive candidiasis in patients undergoing myelo-ablative chemotherapy. *Clin Microbiol Infect.,* Vol.15, No.4, (April 2009), pp. 380-386, ISSN 1198-743X.

Yera, H.; Sendid, B.; Francois, N.; Camus, D.; Poulain, D. (2001). Contribution of serological tests and blood culture to the early diagnosis of systemic candidiasis. *Eur J Clin Microbiol Infect Dis.* Vol.20, No.12, (December 2001), pp. 864-870, ISSN 0934-9723.

Permissions

All chapters in this book were first published by InTech Open; hereby published with permission under the Creative Commons Attribution License or equivalent. Every chapter published in this book has been scrutinized by our experts. Their significance has been extensively debated. The topics covered herein carry significant findings which will fuel the growth of the discipline. They may even be implemented as practical applications or may be referred to as a beginning point for another development.

The contributors of this book come from diverse backgrounds, making this book a truly international effort. This book will bring forth new frontiers with its revolutionizing research information and detailed analysis of the nascent developments around the world.

We would like to thank all the contributing authors for lending their expertise to make the book truly unique. They have played a crucial role in the development of this book. Without their invaluable contributions this book wouldn't have been possible. They have made vital efforts to compile up to date information on the varied aspects of this subject to make this book a valuable addition to the collection of many professionals and students.

This book was conceptualized with the vision of imparting up-to-date information and advanced data in this field. To ensure the same, a matchless editorial board was set up. Every individual on the board went through rigorous rounds of assessment to prove their worth. After which they invested a large part of their time researching and compiling the most relevant data for our readers.

The editorial board has been involved in producing this book since its inception. They have spent rigorous hours researching and exploring the diverse topics which have resulted in the successful publishing of this book. They have passed on their knowledge of decades through this book. To expedite this challenging task, the publisher supported the team at every step. A small team of assistant editors was also appointed to further simplify the editing procedure and attain best results for the readers.

Apart from the editorial board, the designing team has also invested a significant amount of their time in understanding the subject and creating the most relevant covers. They scrutinized every image to scout for the most suitable representation of the subject and create an appropriate cover for the book.

The publishing team has been an ardent support to the editorial, designing and production team. Their endless efforts to recruit the best for this project, has resulted in the accomplishment of this book. They are a veteran in the field of academics and their pool of knowledge is as vast as their experience in printing. Their expertise and guidance has proved useful at every step. Their uncompromising quality standards have made this book an exceptional effort. Their encouragement from time to time has been an inspiration for everyone.

The publisher and the editorial board hope that this book will prove to be a valuable piece of knowledge for researchers, students, practitioners and scholars across the globe.

List of Contributors

Bhadran Bose and David Mudge
Princess Alexandra Hospital, Brisbane, Australia

Xu Haiyan and He Xiaozhou
Third Affiliated Hospital of Soochow University, Changzhou, China

Masahiko Okamoto
Department of Organ Interaction Research Medicine, Kyoto Prefectural University of Medicine, Japan

Elijah Ablorsu
Department of Nephrology and Transplant Services, University Hospital of Wales, Cardiff, United Kindgdom

Chengguo Ge, Gang Yuan, Qiansheng Li, Wenqian Huo, Keqin Zhang, Gang Wu, Fengshuo Jin, Xi Lin, Xiaojiang Jiang and Dong Gao
Department of Urology, Institute of Surgery Research, Daping Hospital, Third Military Medical University, Chongqing, China

Alexandros Giakoustidis, Nikolaos Antoniadis and Dimitrios Giakoustidis
Division of Transplantation, Department of Surgery, Medical School, Aristotle University of Thessaloniki and Hippokration General Hospital, Thessaloniki, Greece

Shirin Ghazizadeh
Obstetrics and Gynecology Department, Tehran University of Medical Sciences, Iran

Phuong-Mai T. Pham
Department of Medicine, Greater Los Angeles VA Medical Center and David Geffen School of Medicine at UCLA, United States of America

Son V. Pham
Department of Medicine, Cardiology Division, Bay Pines VA Medical Center, Bay Pines, Florida, United States of America

Phuong-Anh T. Pham
Department of Medicine, Division of Cardiovascular Diseases, VA Medical Center, University of Tennessee Health Science Center, Memphis, TN, United States of America

Phuong-Chi T. Pham
Department of Medicine, Nephrology Division, UCLA-Olive View Medical Center and David Geffen School of Medicine, United States of America

Hans W. Sollinger, Jon S. Odorico, Glen E. Leverson, Barbara J. Voss and Anthony M. D'Alessandro
Department of Surgery, Division of Transplantation, University of Wisconsin, U.S.A.

Jean Herman and Rita Van Damme-Lombaerts
Department of Pediatric Transplantation, University Hospitals Leuven, Belgium

Mahboob Lessan-Pezeshki
Nephrology Research Center, Imam Khomeini Hospital, Tehran University of Medical Sciences, Iran

Phuong-Thu T. Pham and Parikh S
Department of Medicine, Nephrology Division, Kidney Transplant Program, David Geffen School of Medicine at UCLA, United States of America

Heather H. Jones and Daniel J. Salzberg
Division of Nephrology, University of Maryland Department of Medicine, School of Medicine, USA

Ewa Swoboda-Kopec, Irina Netsvyetayeva, Magdalena Sikora, Mariusz Jasik and Piotr Fiedor
Warsaw Medical University, Poland

Index

www.ingramcontent.com/pod-product-compliance
Lightning Source LLC
LaVergne TN
LVHW062235200926
848484LV00006B/1546